Nursing the Older Patient

Nursing the Older Patient

Edited by

Stephen G. Wright RGN, DIP.N. (LONDON), RCNT,
DANS, RNT, M.Sc.
Consultant Nurse
Nursing Development Unit
Tameside General Hospital

Harper & Row Publishers London
Cambridge Mexico City New York
San Francisco São Paulo Singapore Sydney
Philadelphia

First published 1988
Reprinted 1989

Harper & Row Ltd
Middlesex House
34-42 Cleveland Street
London W1P 5FB

British Library Cataloguing in Publication Data
Nursing the older patient.
1. Old persons. Nursing
I. Wright, Stephen G.
610.73′65

ISBN 0–06–318390–0

Typeset by Burns & Smith, Derby
Printed and bound by Butler & Tanner Ltd, Frome and London

for Matthew and Ruth

Contents

List of contributors

June Andrews, RMN, RGN, MA (Glas.) MA (Nottin.), Ward Sister Northwick Park Hospital.

Jean Faugier, RMN, RCNT, Dip.N. (Lond.), DANS, RNT, MSc, Dip. Psych., Senior Lecturer, Nursing Department, Manchester Polytechnic.

Steve Goodwin, RMN, Divisional Manager for the elderly and physically handicapped, Lancashire Social Services and joint winner of the 1985 *Nursing Times*/3M National Nursing Award for Innovation in Nursing Education.

Anne P. Kennedy, B.Sc., SRN, Ph.D., Nurse Researcher, University of Manchester, Department of Geriatric Medicine.

Betty Kershaw, SRN, DANS, M.Sc., is currently Director of Nurse Education at Stockport School of Nursing.

Paul Mangan, SEN, Northwick Park Hospital and joint winner of the 1985 *Nursing Times*/3M National Nursing Award for Innovation in Nursing Education.

Lesley Surman, SRN, OND, RCNT, formerly Joint-Appointee Clinical Teacher/Ward Sister at Tameside General Hospital, Care of the Elderly Units.

Linda Thomas, formerly Professional Adviser to the Royal College of Nursing Society of Geriatric Nursing, currently journalist with *Nursing Standard* and editor of *Geriatric Nursing and Home Care.*

David R. Thompson, B.Sc., SRN, RMN, ONC, Senior Nurse, Coronary Care Unit, Leicester General Hospital.

Lesley Wade, SRN, RCNT, formerly Joint Appointee Clinical Teacher/Ward Sister, Department of Medicine for the Elderly, Tameside General Hospital, and currently Clinical Teacher.

Rosemary A. Webster, B.Sc., SRN, Ward Sister, Coronary Care Unit, Leicester General Hospital.

Brysson Whyte, Nurse, Fellow of the Royal College of Nursing and retired Director of Nurse Education. At the time of writing, she continues to work as a voluntary helper in a local hospital.

Steve Wright, RGN, Dip.N. (London), RCNT, DANS, RNT, M.Sc., Consultant Nurse, Nursing Development Unit, Department of Medicine for the Elderly, Tameside General Hospital.

David Wise, Documentary Photographer working in the north-east of England.

Foreword

Texts to help nurses and others understand the special needs of infants and children are numerous; comparable publications on the special needs of the adolescent, the young adult, mature and middle-aged men and women are rare, but fortunately, books and articles designed to prepare health workers, who are often young, to understand the special needs of those past middle age are increasingly available. This book, *Nursing the Older Patient*, is refreshing. It is written partially and edited throughout by Steve Wright, an experienced nurse in this field and expresses the creative, non-institutionalized concept he and his associates have of caring for the older person. As the life span lengthens in most countries, there are more of us in this category. And, since most care-givers have not experienced old age, they need all the help they can get in understanding what it is like to be old and how it affects the desires and needs of those who are.

In the author-editor's Preface, the nature and intent of this work is clearly stated and in Chapter 1 written by Brysson Whyte, an experienced retired nurse who calls herself an 'Ancient Briton', a personal and engaging view of ageing is given. Both speak more eloquently than I can to the interest and value of this book. The concluding chapter, written by Linda Thomas, a journalist, summarizes with great insight the content of the text — chapter by chapter. It is possible that reading her analysis first might enhance the unquestionable value of this work. It is easy to see how a study of *Nursing the Older Patient* can help to breakdown the stereotype view and stultifying practices only too common in many agencies and institutions serving this element of society. As a grateful reader, I recommend this text to all those involved which includes most if not all of us.

Virginia Henderson
Yale University
January 1988

Preface

It has always seemed a little unfair to me that, as we approach the later years of our lives, lives in which we have given so much, the time can be filled with new and unexpected fears. I have nursed so many older adults who, freed of work and family, were looking forward to doing in retirement so much that they had denied themselves in earlier years. Then a crisis of health strikes, and dreams can be shattered.

As Brysson Whyte says in her introductory chapter, a little money and health are all that is needed for a happy old age. Nurses, as one of the major health occupations, have so much to contribute to providing a happier old age. Nursing, when is is done well, is one of the few things in a harsh world that can bring real happiness, relief and joy into people's lives. There is no body of people more deserving of that help than those who have grown old - it is nothing more than their just reward for struggling against all the forces that life has ranged against them and for their contribution, however great or small, to the wider world around them.

I wanted to produce a book that would help nurses to nurse well, written by nurses, for nurses. Almost all the contributors were directly involved in clinical nursing at the time of making their contributions. What clinical nurses do is valuable - how much more so if they consign their ideas to paper so that they can be handed on to others.

The rise of nursing models in recent years gave me the key for an approach to the book. The story of how a nursing model was developed on one site has been documented elsewhere (Wright, 1987). Part of that model included the 'activities of healthy living' framework which was used in the problem-solving approach applied to care. It is these which I have used to provide the basis for the book. There is, therefore, less emphasis on the medical model and more on the nursing model. If, reader, you want to find out about 'fractured femur', 'Parkinson's disease' or 'congestive cardiac failure' then look elsewhere. The authors will refer to these and other medical diagnoses where they are relevant, it is true, but we have all tried to move to a different perspective that takes account of the whole person. How does that *person* with Parkinson's disease feel when they cannot eat, wash or move as they want to? How do they cope with the difficulties that failing health and increasing dependence on others have brought? How do they *live* their old age as the complex, unique and fascinating individuals that they are? Taking all this into account - what is the role of the nurse?

Each chapter seeks to address itself to these issues, combining practical advice on how to manage a variety of health issues with evidence from nursing literature and research, and suggestions for further readings. In each of the chapters a number of problem studies are included to illustrate how some of the points each writer makes are applied in practice. A problem-solving/care-planning approach is used. The reader needs to note that these care statements are not intended to be definitive, merely to identify some principal aspects of care. They are often taken in isolation as examples extracted from the total plan of the patient's care. Each author has stamped his/her own style on their text, and I have deliberately not tried to force them all into a uniform mould. However, I believe all of them made contributions which are authoritative, thought-provoking and of direct practical use. The principles the authors identify can be used in any setting where older people are encountered, be it hospital ward or nursing home, specialist unit or private residence.

We have all deliberately avoided the word 'geriatric'. Our feelings about the word are coloured by the images it conjures up and, most importantly, by the impression it gives to actual and potential patients and the wider community. We have tended to focus on the more benign words 'older patient' or 'elderly', an issue which is discussed in more detail in Linda Thomas's chapter. All of us are challenged by the difficulties of old age - that nebulous concept so difficult to define - and no nurse, provided he or she lives long enough, can ultimately avoid them. If we survive, it comes to all of us. Slowly, imperceptibly, it is creeping up on you even as you read this.

All nurses have their horror stories to tell about 'geriatric' nursing. There are many clues in this text to help you put things right. The goal is a simple but noble one, to contribute to making the nursing of older people better - and hence their lives. It is, after all, in your own best interests - God willing, you will be there yourself some day.

Steve Wright

REFERENCE

Wright, S. G. (1987) *Building and Using a Model of Nursing*, Edward Arnold, London.

1. On Growing Old: A Personal View of Ageing

Brysson Whyte

AN ANCIENT BRITON SPEAKS ...

Everyone knows something about ageing. We age all our lives, passing from childhood to adolescence and from adolescence to maturity. The physical changes which accompany ageing come gradually to remind us that time is passing; our arms become too short to hold the telephone book where we can read it and our hair turns white. Finally comes the moment of truth when we realize that from men and women we have become *old* men and women. This happened to me one day when I saw a poor old woman in the street. She was wearing a shabby anorak and an old tweed skirt, her shoes were definitely sensible, her hat round and woolly. I was so sorry for her that I smiled at her and, to my horror, as she smiled back, I realized that I was looking at myself in a shop window! This aroused my interest in discovering how old people are regarded in our society and learning of the problems of looking old whilst feeling young. Some of what I have learnt is set out below, written from the heart and not the head, just the point of view of an elderly person – no, elderly person is too smug, Ancient Briton (with its flavour of defiance) suits my mood better. There has been no research, no serious reading, just experience gained from a little voluntary work and much meeting and talking with other Ancient Britons and their carers.

ATTITUDES TO AGEING

Attitudes to ageing differ in all cultures and at all stages in their history. If only our forebears had possessed the foresight to promote ancestor worship the present plight of old people in this country might have been different! If present attitudes are examined it will be seen that though the rich and famous are rarely thought of as being old at all, old people who are neither rich nor famous may be seen as a problem. Except to their friends and relatives, they appear as a vague threat, like some gigantic iceberg waiting to sink the ship of state. In real life people who make up the 'iceberg' are ignored as completely as if they are indeed under water, but the small percentage who find themselves in need of help and support may become the focus of a wealth of feelings that do not always include love or pity. We tend to get impatient with the old man who holds up the bus queue as he climbs slowly aboard. An incontinent old person may provoke anger and disgust, and those with whom it is difficult to communicate, such as the deaf, may make us feel inadequate or embarrassed. Poor old people may find themselves despised, as if their plight was the result of improvidence and not lifelong poverty. Only the confused may be mercifully unaware of the feelings they arouse in others. For all the rest, unless they are known to us personally, it is fatally easy to forget that they are individuals and to perceive them as a nameless, faceless group.

RETIREMENT

All old people have an attitude to retirement, some looking forward to it eagerly, making plans to do all those things they have always wanted to, while others dread the future, wondering how to fill the long empty days ahead. Whatever our attitude, it is a time of greater stress than is sometimes realized, when people are as vulnerable as a hermit crab between shells. There has always been the discipline of work at the centre of our lives, so now a new pattern of behaviour must be learnt. Old workmates do not always remain friends so a new circle of friends must be built up; this is specially difficult if it is planned to move house on retirement. Unions or professional organizations are no longer there to fight for our interests and we have to learn how to fight our own battles, or at least find out where to turn for help. Living on a pension rather than a wage or salary often requires considerable adjustment of life-style, and it may take time to find out about all the concessions, such as cheaper fares, which are available. Retirement classes may give guidance on financial and other matters, but the central problem is the acceptance of the fact that we have indeed retired.

After Retirement

Now that old people are living longer, it is possible to look forward to twenty or thirty years of 'old age'. The key to happiness is independence. Some of us are lucky enough to remain independent all our lives, others can only manage if they accept some help and support and some inevitably become dependent on others. These three stages of ageing bear no relation to chronological age and those who have good luck and good health may remain independent all their lives.

INDEPENDENCE

Provided you have a little money and your health, there is no doubt that old age can be one of the happiest times of your life. There is no limit to the choice of occupations and pastimes. Although some have no problems in deciding what they want to do, and others may need encouragement to find ways to take part in the activities of their choice, the key to enjoyment is that it *is* our own choice, with freedom to do as little or as much as we want. There are, however, certain important needs which should be met if the stage of independence is to be prolonged as long as possible. The secret of a happy old age is good health and to this end resources should be concentrated on two things. Firstly, information and advice about how to promote health should be freely available to all; secondly, just as a car is given an MOT, so should old people have regular health checks in order that potential health problems may be recognized and treated early.

Independence with Support

Once started down the slippery slope from independence to dependence, life is not so easy. It is the time of bereavement. Although most associate the word bereavement with the loss of loved ones, it must be understood that the curtailment of a life-style which has been planned and enjoyed for many years is just as much a bereavement as any other loss.

Independence is fragile and is potentially at risk at any time from even a minor malfunction of the nervous system or the blockage of an artery. The effects may range from the loss of such simple pleasures as visiting picture galleries or walking in the woods, to such serious problems as loss of sight or hearing. It is true that if the physical changes are gradual it may be easier to adjust to them and learn to cut our pleasures according to the cloth of our abilities, by watching birds at a bird table rather than going bird-watching or tending a window box rather than an allotment, but it is a time when help is needed.

However, helping those who have suffered loss in any form makes many people very anxious and we may either avoid them altogether or else smother them with 'reassurance' as though we were a fire blanket and they a fire, whose flames of misery must be damped at all cost because they are too painful for us to cope with. It must never be forgotten that whatever the reason for the bereavement, all those who have suffered loss go through the same reactions of shock, denial, anger and depression before their final acceptance of the situation. What is most needed at this time is support and counselling to allow the grief and pain to be worked through. This requires real expertise for it is fatal simply to try and give advice (see Chapter 4). Perhaps, to help the busy professionals, there is a role here for groups of specially trained volunteers who have been taught something of the art of listening. They would have both the time and the patience to help the bereaved come to terms with their loss. Their motto could well be, 'Don't just do something, sit there'!

It is also important to foster independence for as long as possible and this means trying to keep old people at home. The loss of a home, however ramshackle, may destroy all the reality on which life is founded. When the world that was once our oyster has shrunk to become our living room, that room is the centre of our world, the last remaining part of the old framework of familiar faces, known routines and loved objects. The latter become more important as we grow older. Faces may change, death takes family and friends, even the cat and the budgie die, but the little blue jug, the rose-patterned cup and the old clock on the mantelpiece develop an importance akin to that of the tattered 'baby' we took to bed as a child. No wonder that when we finally have to leave home we find comfort in taking them with us.

DEPENDENCE

As we get older we must accept the fact that other people may have to care for us and support us. In the past those who could afford it bought care for their elderly relatives. Those who could not afford to pay were looked after by their families (there was no shortage of dutiful daughters and maiden aunts to help) and only a small proportion of people 'went to the workhouse or poorhouse' to be cared for by the state. However, social changes come faster than we are willing to accept them and we never seem able to plan for the consequences. The pattern is still basically the same: people who can afford it can buy care, ranging from employing domestic help or private nurses to using private nursing homes, while families try to look after their own and the rest are cared for by the state. It is those who would once have been cared for by their families who have been most affected by social changes. Families are smaller, children who are potential carers are scattered and the rising divorce rate brings its own problems. If family life was like a television commercial, kindly daughters and sturdy sons would be willing and able to care for their parents, but although nearly all families would indeed like to care and many do, under very difficult circumstances, many more people have to be cared for by the state, throwing an increasing strain on the health and social services.

There are other problems. For example, many single daughters do still care for their mothers, but, as people are living longer, it is not uncommon to find daughters of sixty and seventy caring for mothers of ninety or more. How can the priority between the needs of the mother and the needs of the daughter be assessed? Married sons and daughters have different problems, often running two homes and torn between their responsibility to their partners and children and that to their parents. The strains of caring for old people at home, particularly if they are confused, is considerable and all the nurses and social workers who provide help and support must consider the needs of the carers as carefully as they consider the needs of the old people. Some help may be provided by 'respite care' but sometimes the dependent old person has to be admitted to a long stay home or hospital.

HOSPITAL CARE

It is very important that those working in 'geriatric' units providing care for elderly people, realize that the happiness or misery of their patients depends on the quality of the care they receive. It is even more important to realize that this is not just dependent on the skills of the Sister, but on the integrity of every member of the caring team, not just the ward team alone but on the wider network of community staff and other disciplines as well. If the patient is to move from one group of carers to another, those working in different disciplines (for example the NHS and the social services) must learn to work in partnership. If they do not, the transition from home to hospital (or vice versa) may be mismanaged and the patient will suffer. So what do those coming into an institution need and expect from those who care for them? Firstly, it is important to remember that admission to a home or hospital is often an emergency precipitated by sudden illness or some tragedy at home, such as the sudden death or illness of a carer. Under these circumstances it is easy to understand how much help and support must be given on admission to an elderly person, often with impaired sight or hearing, suddenly meeting large numbers of strange people in a setting with which they are unfamiliar. If they are already confused then this only increases their confusion. The grief-stricken may weep silently and refuse to be comforted, the aggressive may reject all offers of help, but many sit trembling silently like wounded birds passively accepting what is done for them. It may take many days before they begin to relax and reveal their true personalities.

Those who care for old people know that nursing the elderly is among the most skilled branches of care; however, there are a few underlying principles which may serve as guidelines for those who are learning their skills.

The Patient Is a Person

Every patient is an individual and must be respected as such. In the old days a patient's care was fitted into the routine of the ward, but today we emphasize much more that care is planned individually and the skill of the nursing team is demonstrated by the way they fit the needs of each individual into the complex pattern of the ward day. This does not mean that each patient always gets what he or she wants but, with goodwill and some mutual agreement, patients can have the care which best meets their needs. It may not be possible, for example, to alter meal-times, but at least the patients should be able to control such things as the time they get up and go to bed. They should be able to choose their own clothes, and buy them with their own money. They should decide which of the ward activities and outings they wish to attend, and if these do not interest them, it is their right to say no. The last right of those who become dependent on others (provided they are able to make their wishes known) is the right of choice. Just because they are unable to do something, it does not mean that they should have no say in how it should be done. It is all too easy for carers, with the best of intentions, to offer others what they imagine they would enjoy, rather than finding out their real wishes. How many old people are trapped in their wheel-chairs in front of a television set without even the option of changing the channel, when they would far rather have been alone and silent? How many old ladies have their fingernails painted red whether they like it or not? Of course grooming is important, but if the patient is not consulted about the form it should take, it reduces her to the status of a doll to be dressed. We do not all appreciate having blue bows in our hair.

Preserving Independence

The aim of all care is to preserve independence for as long as possible and to this end nurses must learn the most basic skill of all, that of knowing when to do and when forbear. For example, it may have been agreed that patients should dress themselves, but, just as there are days when they are left to struggle to button their own cardigans, there are days when they are obviously too tired and need a helping hand. The skill lies in knowing which day is which. Of course there are times when what patients want and what the nurse thinks they should have are different. For example, patients may refuse to bath but in the interests of hygiene it is best if they maintain a reasonable degree of cleanliness. The nurse must deal with such situations with tact and patience until a reasonable compromise is reached - perhaps the patient may consent to have a shower! Similarly, sometimes the things which suit one patient affect another; the bedside lamp of one may keep another awake, for example, and the nurse must make arrangements which satisfy both. The most important thing is to focus on the needs of the patients and not see their care as a series of unconnected and repetitive tasks.

REWARDS

The rewards of caring for old people are not always financial but they are very real. Their courage and dignity never cease to make their carers feel humble. There is also the fascination of hearing about life as it was lived when they were young and listening whilst they recount the joys and sorrows of their lives. The satisfaction of helping such people live their lives to the full for as long as they are able and then to be with them as they accept death makes their care a challenging and satisfying skill.

SUGGESTED FUTURE READING

Blythe, R. (1979) *The View in Winter. Reflections on Old age*, Allen Lane, London.

Elder, G. (1977) *The Alienated – Growing Old Today*, Writers and Readers Publishing Co-operative, London.

Newton, E. (1980) *This Bed My Centre*, Virago, London.

Norton, D., McLaren, R. and Exton-Smith, A.N. (1962) *An Investigation of Geriatric Nursing Problems in Hospitals*, National Corporation for the Care of Old People, London (reprinted Churchill Livingstone, Edinburgh 1985).

Robb, B. (1967) *Sans Everything, a Case to Answer*, Nelson, London.

Wells, T. (1980) *Problems in Geriatric Nursing*, Churchill Livingstone, Edinburgh.

2. Images of Ageing

Linda Thomas

ATTITUDES TO AGEING

Nobody grows old overnight; the process of ageing is something in which we are involved from the moment of birth. This concept of ageing as a normal, continous process throughout life is difficult to reconcile with the widely held belief that old age begins abruptly with retirement. Gerontophobia, the fear of ageing, is something we all experience to a greater or lesser degree. Old age itself is often seen as a condition from which people suffer, or at least a time of life when disease and decrepitude are inevitable. Discrimination against people because of their chronological age has been dubbed 'ageism' (Butler, 1974). In a kind of collusion, the tendency for old people to act out the negative and declining role society has created for them, thus becoming a self-fulfilling prophecy, has also been described (Phillipson, 1982).

Once beyond the age of retirement, the tendency is to regard people as part of a homogeneous group – 'the elderly' – sharing exactly the same characteristics. The fact that their ages range across four decades patently makes nonsense of this generalized viewpoint; a generation separates the oldest from the youngest. However, population studies from the late 1970s (Figure 2.1) indicating a growth in the numbers of very elderly people in the next few decades have produced a negative method of subdivision into 'young old' and 'old old' categories. This has brought its own stereotyping, the former being slotted into a sentimental mould and the latter regarded as an incontinent, senile, rising tide of problems. The fact is, of course, that old people are neither problems to be solved nor challenges to be met. They are individuals whose needs are as complex and multifaceted as those of any other age group.

THEORIES OF AGEING

The search for immortality has been a continuing one for centuries; legend has it that Juan Ponce de Leon was searching for the Fountain of Youth when he stumbled across Florida instead on Easter Day in 1513 – ironic given Florida's modern attraction to those who have retired. Rejuvenation – ironing out the evidence of ageing – continues to be promised, as it always has been, by a multifarious selection of pills, potions and lotions. 'Corrective' surgery is one modern-day addition to the Peter Pan ethic, with anything from a face-lift to a bottom-lift on offer to smooth out wrinkles and boost sagging morale.

The Biblical pronouncement in Psalm 90 that the days of our years are threescore years and ten, with passing reference to the fact that fourscore years might be achieved 'by reason of strength' has remained remarkably constant, although demographic studies now draw attention to the increasing number of over 75-year-olds in our society. Nevertheless, the maximum human lifespan (the length of time a human being can expect to live in optimum conditions with no interference from disease or accident) is unlikely to alter significantly. Reports of incredible longevity are rare in Western civilizations and difficult to substantiate in areas lacking accurate records.

What has changed, however, is our ability to deal with the factors that have prevented more people in the past from living to the end of their 'normal' lifespan. As Alex Comfort (1977) notes, while medicine has done nothing to alter the human lifespan, it has been strikingly successful in helping us live to the end of it.

Heredity does influence lifespan to a certain extent both positively and negatively; some families are well known for being long-lived, but on the other hand disorders such as haemophilia or Huntington's chorea are examples of genetically transmitted disorders which may curtail lifespan (Ferguson Anderson *et al.*, 1982).

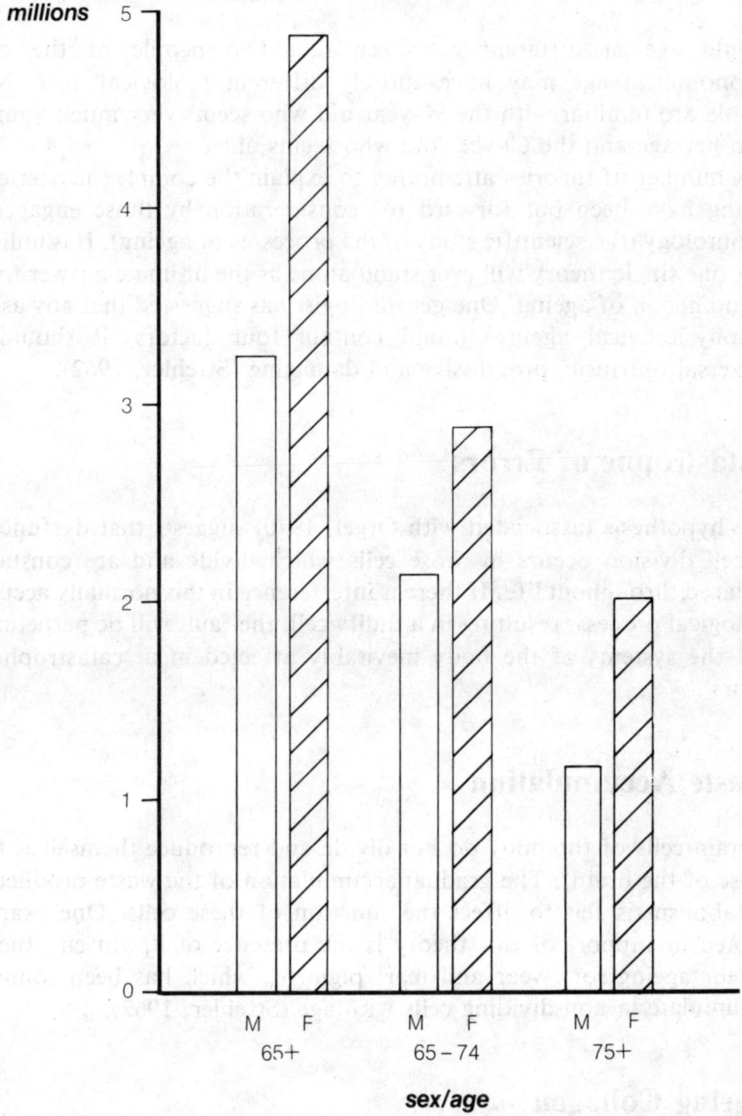

Source: Office of Population, Censuses and Surveys (1978).

Figure 2.1 Elderly population in Great Britain (1978) by age.

EXPLAINING AGEING

People age at different rates, so that two people of the same chronological age may have entirely different biological ages. Most people are familiar with the 90-year-old who seems very much younger than her age and the 60-year-old who seems older.

A number of theories attempting to explain the complex mysteries of ageing have been put forward for consideration by those engaged in gerontology (the scientific study of the processes of ageing). It is unlikely that one single theory will ever stand alone as the ultimate answer to the phenomenon of ageing. One gerontologist has suggested that any aspect of physiological ageing should contain four factors; it should be universal, intrinsic, progressive and damaging (Strehler, 1962).

Catastrophe of Errors

One hypothesis (associated with Orgel, 1970) suggests that dysfunction in cell division occurs in those cells which divide and are constantly replaced throughout life. If there is interference in this normally accurate biological process, resulting in a faulty cell, the fault will be perpetuated and the systems of the body inevitably affected in a 'catastrophe of errors'.

Waste Accumulation

Certain cells of the body do not divide and reproduce themselves (e.g. those of the brain). The gradual accumulation of the waste products of metabolism is felt to affect the function of these cells. One example quoted in support of this theory is the presence of lipofuscin, the so-called 'ageing' or 'wear and tear' pigment, which has been found to accumulate in non-dividing cells with age (Strehler, 1962).

Ageing Collagen

Collagen is the protein material which makes up the white fibres of connective tissue and which becomes cross-linked and rigid with age, a change that has been compared with similar age changes in such substances as rubber and old glue. As the number of cross-linkages increases, the effects obviously accumulate. Comfort (1977) points out that antioxidants might be used to slow ageing as they are used to slow perishing in tyres.

Programmed Ageing

Hayflick (1965) demonstrated that certain human cells, when cultured outside the body, had a finite capacity for reproduction; the older the donor, the less the reproductive capacity of the cells, suggestive of a kind of 'biological clock'.

Immunological Ageing

The performance of the auto-immune system becomes less efficient with age, leading to a corresponding increase in susceptibility to infection and disease. Auto-immune reactions also become more common, where the system fails to recognize the body's 'normal' cells and sets about destroying them; myxoedema is one example of an auto-immune disease, the thyroid gland having been attacked (Coni, Davison and Webster, 1980).

Evolutionary Ageing

Mortality is an essential component of life; the implications of immortality are obvious if procreation continues. One theory suggests that ageing and death are the deliberate inbuilt 'control' mechanisms which ensure mortality, thus allowing for evolutionary adaptation with birth.

Gerontology is a relatively new area of research. As Coni, Davison and Webster (1980) comment, none of these hypotheses is mutually exclusive; ageing may even have a combination of causes.

RECOGNIZING NORMAL AGEING

The physical changes of ageing are common to us all, although we may experience them at different rates. It is important to distinguish between the normal process of ageing and any disease or trauma which may be superimposed on the ageing process.

Physical Changes of Ageing

Appearance

The visible characteristics of ageing are easy to identify, although Mary Stott is quick to point out that although the wrapping may have got somewhat discoloured and tatty with long use, the content is not greatly changed (Stott, 1981)! Hair becomes grey or white due to loss of pigment cells, and both body and scalp hair thins with age, although women may find an increase in facial hair.

The epidermis changes with age, leading to loss of elasticity, increased fragility, dryness and wrinkles, all graphically described by Barbara Macdonald, an American septuagenarian, who speaks of 'the skin hanging loosely' from the forearm (Macdonald and Rich, 1983). Comfort (1977) points out that the best way to get wrinkled all over is to be a fanatical nudist in a sunny country, since wrinkles are accelerated by sunlight.

There is a loss of subcutaneous periorbital fat; the distribution of body fat generally changes, more being concentrated on the trunk than the arms and legs. Bones become more porous; there is a decrease in body size and height. Nails become more brittle and longitudinal ridges can often be seen on them.

Sensory Changes

Presbyopia is the term used to describe the normal changes in the eye due to age, the most striking of which is loss of elasticity of the lens. The effects tend to be felt for the first time during the fourth decade, when difficulty is experienced in focusing the eye for near vision and reading material has to be held at arm's length to be seen properly.

Presbyacusis, the natural failure of hearing caused by degenerative changes in the internal ear, tends to occur at around the same time. Difficulty is increasingly experienced in hearing high frequency sounds.

Cardiovascular System

There is no significant change in the 'at rest' heart rate with age. The systolic blood pressure rises by 20–30 per cent between the ages of 30 and 70 but there is only a slight rise in the diastolic pressure (Coni, Davison and Webster, 1980). The heart loses its elasticity and therefore responds less well to increased demands, for example as a result of exercise.

Respiratory System

Kyphosis (curvature of the spine in which the concavity of the curve is directed forwards) and increased anterior-posterior diameter of the chest both occur in old age. There is decreased blood flow to the pulmonary circulation and decreased diffusion, together with a lessening of lung elasticity. In order to maintain normal blood oxygen level, it is necessary to breathe harder.

Nervous System

Bennett (1986) points out that comparatively little is known of the function of the brain of the normal adult and even less of the changes with age. It is known, however, that brain volume and weight decrease. There is impaired temperature regulation, so that older people are particularly susceptible to extremes of temperature. Sleep patterns alter and the sense of balance is less efficient.

Alimentary System

The sense of smell becomes less sensitive and taste buds atrophy, 'sweet and sour' being the first to go. There is a lessening of salivary secretions and reduced gastro-intestinal motility (leading to increased likelihood of constipation).

Genito-urinary System

The size and weight of the kidneys decrease with age with a reduction in renal efficiency; the ability to conserve water is lessened and the filtration capacity of the kidney is reduced dramatically (an important consideration in drug administration). Bladder capacity and muscle tone diminish.

Reproductive System

The production of oestrogen decreases in women following the menopause while the uterus decreases in size and mucous secretions cease. There is diminished breast tissue. Vulval skin shrinks and the epithelial lining of the vagina atrophies. Vaginal secretions become more alkaline.

In men, production of testosterone decreases. There is no change in the volume of the testes and spermatogenesis continues. Erectile tissues of external genitalia may respond more slowly to arousal in both men and women due to less efficient vasocongestion.

PSYCHOSOCIAL THEORIES OF AGEING

Several psychosocial theories of ageing appeared in the 1960s, each suggesting that old people adapt their life-styles in a clearly defined, specific way in order to cope with the ageing process. The most widely quoted are the disengagement theory, the activity theory and the developmental (or continuity) theory. They should all, perhaps, be treated with a degree of caution in the light of Gladys Elder's comment, written when she was in her 70s, that old people can never do the right thing, nor make themselves acceptable. If they are too active, they are labelled dissatisfied and discontented. If they are too resigned, they are accused of disengagement (Elder, 1977).

Disengagement Theory

The theory of disengagement (Cumming and Henry, 1961) suggests that both society and old people benefit if there is a gradual mutual withdrawal. As the responsibilities of middle age are removed, old people become increasingly self-centred; their life-styles alter to accommodate narrower interests and they no longer look out for new challenges. This is felt to be to their benefit as they can concentrate on reflective self-fulfilment. Society benefits in that its future is safeguarded by the devolution of power from one generation to the next as its elders die.

Mandatory retirement perhaps exemplifies disengagement; the idea that the time has arrived to put your feet up and enjoy yourself is certainly a popular one. However, the notion that older people no longer have any useful contribution to make to society, and that they will become frustrated and discontented unless they disengage and take a passive back seat is less easy to accept. Differentiating between successful disengagement and apathy or depression might prove difficult if this theory was universally applied; it is a controversial generalization.

Activity Theory

At the other end of the scale, the activity theory (Havighurst, 1963) supports the idea that in order to age successfully, the life-styles of middle age should be maintained and new interests pursued. Some modification may be necessary – for example, substituting intellectual activities for physical if mobility is impaired – but continued active involvement in society will ensure adjustment is successful in old age.

Developmental Theory

This theory (Neugarten, 1968) – also referred to as the continuity theory – suggests that ageing brings no dramatic change in a person's unique personality, character traits or patterns of behaviour. People who have been involved and active throughout youth and middle age will continue this tendency as they age. Similarly, those who have always been reserved by nature will remain so as they age.

While the theories of activity and disengagement tend to be stereotypical and prescriptive in their approach, the developmental theory seems to allow for more individualism.

CARING FOR OLDER PEOPLE – A HISTORICAL PERSPECTIVE

The provision of care for older people is inextricably linked with the history of poor law resources. The stigma of the workhouse lingers on, not only in the living memories of some old people today but in the forbidding former workhouse buildings where elderly people are still cared for. Prison-like exteriors give little indication of the progressive care carried out within, nor of the many imaginative and innovative upgrading schemes which have transformed former workhouse interiors.

The Poor Relief Act of 1601, passed initially for a limited period only but eventually made perpetual in 1641, allowed for the 'necessary relief of the lame, impotent, old, blind and such other among them being poor and not able to work'. In 1832 a commission was appointed which proposed considerable alterations in the law, most of which were incorporated in the Poor Law Amendment Act of 1834. One of the intentions of this Act was to ensure that the only relief available to able-bodied paupers and their families would be within workhouses, and that there would be no 'outdoor' relief for such people. Furthermore, to act as a deterrent the level of relief within the workhouse was not to exceed anything outside.

Under the Local Government Act of 1929, the boards of guardians elected by ratepayers to supervise the Poor Law Unions were abolished and their functions taken over by public assistance committees of counties and county boroughs. Workhouses would become known as public assistance institutions; there was provision under this Act for workhouse infirmaries to become the responsibility of public health committees in order to improve standards of care for the aged sick within them. However, Evers (1986) suggests that this led to the infirmaries becoming highly selective of the patients they admitted so that many elderly people could no longer gain access to them.

The Impact of the Second World War

In their detailed and fascinating account of the development of welfare services for elderly people, Means and Smith (1984) devote considerable discussion to the impact of the Second World War. They point out that prior to the outbreak of war, an Emergency Medical Service (EMS) was planned based on predictions of civilian casualities from air-raids. When war was declared, thousands of patients were discharged from hospitals in a matter of days. However, for the first year of the war there was little demand for these beds vacated for the EMS; while they stood empty, the resources of hospitals and institutions not involved in the EMS were stretched to the limit.

The advent of severe bombing raids highlighted the fact that while casualties were fewer than had been predicted, the problems of homelessness had been underestimated. Initially, to ease pressure on overcrowded air-raid shelters, frail elderly people were evacuated to EMS hospitals throughout the country, although this plan was later abandoned due to shortage of beds as the war progressed. Means and Smith (1984) go on to suggest that consideration for sick and frail elderly people was shown only when their plight was seen as a threat to the morale of the rest of the civilian population. Whether or not this is a fair comment – and another side to the argument is published in their account – it is true to say that the upheavals and confusion of life in wartime Britain served as a melting pot for many existing social policies.

Post-War Reform

Phillipson (1982) comments that both the 1946 National Health Act and the 1948 National Assistance Act were regarded as heralding major changes in the quality of life enjoyed by elderly people, sweeping away the workhouse and removing all trace of the poor law. Additionally, financial needs would be met by the 1946 National Insurance Act. The joy with which these legislative changes was greeted by the population at large is reflected in the reminiscences of older people today, some of which have been captured in writing (Schweitzer, 1985).

National Insurance Act 1946

The Act established the first compulsory contributory insurance system, guaranteeing payment of benefits during unemployment or sickness; for the first time, the Act made retirement a condition for receiving old age pensions.

National Health Service Act 1946

The Health Service Act became law in November 1946, effective from July 1948. Its aims were to provide diagnosis and treatment of illness, at home or in hospital, which would be paid for by general taxation rather than at the point of treatment. When the Act became law, three types of hospital existed: voluntary (charitable) and public health hospitals, both of which tended to concentrate on the 'acute' sick, and public assistance hospitals catering for the 'chronic' sick, most of whom were elderly (Means and Smith, 1984). The Act also empowered local authorities to provide home help and home nursing services.

National Assistance Act 1948

Much emphasis was placed on the provision of residential care in this Act; under Part III of the Act, it became a statutory obligation for every local authority to provide residential accommodation for persons 'who by reason of age or infirmity are in need of care and attention which is not otherwise available to them'. The Act, amended in 1951, also contains the contentious Section 47, which allows for the compulsory removal to hospital or a residential home of a person, who on account of grave disease, is in a serious state of self-neglect and whose health would be endangered by remaining at home. This issue is addressed in some detail in an Age Concern discussion document (Age Concern England, 1986).

Despite the evident air of reforming zeal in the immediate post-war period, the National Assistance Act in effect seemed to perpetuate the old poor law customs, emphasizing as it did a system of institutional care. This view is supported by Townsend's (1964) graphic and disturbing word portraits of the appalling conditions in residential care institutions in the 1950s.

DEVELOPMENT OF GERIATRIC MEDICINE AND NURSING

The term 'geriatrics' – the branch of medicine that is concerned with the clinical study and treatment of the disorders and diseases of old age – is said to have been coined by Nascher in 1909. The Greek derivation makes the reason for Nascher's choice obvious: *geron* = old man; *iatros* = physician. The adjective 'geriatric' has fallen into disrepute over the years, grammatically abused and used itself as a term of abuse.

The speciality of geriatric medicine was pioneered by Dr Marjory Warren of the West Middlesex Hospital in West London. In 1935, presumably as a result of the 1929 Local Government Act, Dr Warren assumed responsibility for elderly people in a public assistance institution – a former workhouse infirmary. By 1948, she had reduced the number of beds from 874 to 200 by introducing the concept of rehabilitation rather than custodial care.

Nursing was a little slow to catch on to this concept, although a booklet published by Dr Warren (1967) on the treatment and care of elderly patients seems to be directed specifically at nurses. For example, she states that 'upon the nursing care of the hemiplegic depends much of the ultimate success or failure', a sentiment to be reiterated decades later by a physiotherapist describing nurses as the key members of any rehabilitation unit in relation to handling new hemiplegic patients on admission to hospital and in the very early days (Johnstone, 1982).

One statement early on in Warren's pamphlet draws attention to the fact that 'at the present time there is pioneer work to be done by nurses in many places where as yet the elderly are treated under old-fashioned conditions and by out of date methods'. The stage was set for Doreen Norton, one nurse who picked up the challenge and began a career concentrating on the needs of elderly people and those caring for them.

Looking back at her early experiences in caring for elderly people, Norton paints a vivid picture of the nursing care they were receiving:

> As for the nursing, it was called 'custodial care' but here I can speak from experience as a student nurse. We cherished those old people like infants (albeit unknowingly robbing them of initiative to do anything for themselves) and indulged ourselves in the giving of tender, loving care, even to the point of bedecking the ladies with pretty bows in their hair – the ribbon purchased out of our meagre salary.
>
> (Norton, 1986)

Consternation beset nurses when the idea of rehabilitation found its way into these wards during the 1950s; patients who had been bedridden for years were no longer to be nursed in bed. Since no explanation had been forthcoming for this radical new approach to care, Norton describes her discovery of Dr Warren's booklet as a revelation; irremediable patients could be rehabilitated.

Among Norton's many publications in subsequent years, the best known is probably the collaborative work, 'An investigation of geriatric nursing problems in hospital' (Norton, McLaren and Exton-Smith, 1962/1975).

Her impressive achievements in the specialty were recognized when she became the world's first professor in gerontological nursing in Cleveland, Ohio, in the USA. Now retired, other nurses continue her pioneering work. Where once there was a dearth, there is now a plethora of textbooks and research studies available to nurses on the care of elderly people.

INTEGRATION OR SEGREGATION OF SERVICES FOR ELDERLY PEOPLE

Only a very small minority of elderly people is ever in institutional care at any time – probably between 5 and 6 per cent; the vast majority of them are to be found in the community. The fact remains, however, that elderly people occupy 45 per cent of all hospital beds with the obvious exclusion of paediatric and maternity (Wilcock, Gray and Pritchard, 1982). This begins to throw into question whether there is justification for a separate, segregated department in hospital offering specialized care to the select few. Defining what is, or is not a 'geriatric' patient is fraught with difficulty, even within the nursing profession, as recent research has highlighted (Fielding, 1986).

Arguments both for and against segregation are equally persuasive.

Horrocks (1982) suggests that there are three ways in which geriatric medicine can be envisaged in the future. The first option might be to concentrate on rehabilitation, long term and community care, and not acute illness. The second option suggests that two or three general physicians might work in conjunction with a geriatric physician in a system of ward sharing. The third option is that the physician in geriatric medicine should offer a comprehensive service to the old, accepting specialist clinical responsibility for the illnesses of an age-defined sector of the population. Horrocks concludes that the option for geriatric medicine to become age-related has significant advantages for old people who become ill and require treatment in hospital, giving them access to the specialist expertise they require.

Whether this ideal can be realistically met in nursing terms is difficult to say. In promoting geriatric nursing as a speciality, Walden (1986) poses the question as to whether a great disservice has been done to elderly people by allowing large numbers of the nursing profession to abrogate their responsibilities to such an important group.

One fact remains quite clear; against the demographic backcloth of increasing numbers of elderly people, who will continue to be the major users of health and social services, all nurses need to be skilled in their care.

REFERENCES

Age Concern England (1986) *The Law and Vulnerable Elderly People*, Age Concern England, Mitcham.

Bennett, G. C. J. (1986) The physiology of ageing, in S. Redfern (ed.) *Nursing Elderly People*, Churchill Livingstone, Edinburgh.

Butler, R. N. (1974) Successful ageing, *Mental Health*, Vol. 58, no. 3, p. 11.

Comfort, A. (1977) *A Good Age*, Mitchell Beazley, London.

Coni, N., Davison, W. and Webster, S. (1980) *Ageing: The Facts*, Oxford University Press.

Cumming, E. and Henry, W. (1961) *Growing Old: The Process of Disengagement*, Basic Books, New York.

Elder, G. (1977) *The Alienated: Growing Old Today*, Writers and Readers Publishing Co-operative, London.

Evers, H. K. (1986) Care of the elderly sick in the UK, in S. Redfern (ed.) *Nursing Elderly People*, Churchill Livingstone, Edinburgh.

Fielding, P. (1986) *Attitudes Revisited: An Examination of Student Nurses' Attitudes towards Old People in Hospital*, Royal College of Nursing, London.

Ferguson Anderson, W., Caird, F., Kennedy R. and Schwartz D. (1982) *Gerontology and Geriatric Nursing*, Hodder & Stoughton, Sevenoaks.

Havighurst, R. J. (1963) Personality and patterns of ageing, *Gerontologist*, Vol. 8, pp. 20–3.

Hayflick, L. (1965) The limited *in vitro* lifetime of human diploid cell strains, *Experimental Cell Research*, Vol. 37, pp. 614–36.

Horrocks, P. (1982) The case for geriatric medicine as an age-related specialty, in B. Isaacs (ed.) *Recent Advances in Geriatric Medicine No. 2,* Churchill Livingstone, Edinburgh.

Johnstone, M. (1982) *The Stroke Patient: Principles of Rehabilitation*, 2nd edn, Churchill Livingstone, Edinburgh.

Macdonald, B. and Rich, C. (1983) *Look Me in the Eye: Old Women, Ageing and Ageism,* Women's Press, London.

Means, R. and Smith, R. (1984) *The Development of Welfare Services for Elderly People*, Croom Helm, Beckenham.

Neugarten, B. L. (ed.) (1968) *Middle Age and Aging*, University of Chicago Press, Chicago.

Norton, D. (1986) The past is the key to the future. Unpublished paper given at the Royal College of Nursing Society of Geriatric Nursing Conference, Nottingham, 10 September.

Norton, D. McLaren, R. and Exton-Smith, A. (1962) *An Investigation of Geriatric Nursing Problems in Hospital*, National Corporation for the Care of Old People, London (reprinted 1975, Churchill Livingstone, Edinburgh).

Orgel, L. E. (1970) The maintenance of accuracy of protein synthesis and its relevance to ageing: a correction, *Proceedings, – National Academy of Science, Washington*, Vol. 67, p. 1476.

Phillipson, C. (1982) *Capitalism and the Construction of Old Age*, Macmillan Press, London.

Schweitzer, P. (ed.) (1985) *Can We Afford the Doctor? Memories of Health Care*, Age Exchange, London.

Stott, M. (1981) *Ageing for Beginners: Understanding Everyday Experience*, Basil Blackwell, Oxford.

Strehler, B. L. (1962) *Time, Cells and Aging*, Academic Press, New York.

Townsend, P. (1964) *The Last Refuge*, Routledge & Kegan Paul.

Walden, E. (1986) The future of elderly care, letter, *Nursing Times*, Vol. 82, no. 40, p. 13.

Warren, M. (1967) Treatment and care of elderly patients, reprinted from *Hospital and Social Service Journal*, Vol. 30, p. 1469.

Wilcock, G. K., Gray, J. A. M. and Pritchard, P. H. (1982) *Geriatric Problems in General Practice*, Oxford University Press.

3. Nursing the Elderly and the Goals of Care

Steve Wright

The status value given to nursing the older patient is intimately linked to the social value of this age group (see the previous chapter by Linda Thomas), so that the low status of nursing them agrees with the low status of the elderly (Phillipson, 1982). The attitude in nursing itself that geriatric nursing is 'just basic care' requiring little skill or intellect even influences its potential recruits (Fielding, 1986) and pervades the nursing profession both inside and outside the specialty.

Where nurses help the older patient, their models must take account of the high value of the client group. The values of the traditional, high technology, high status 'acute' areas of nursing are not always relevant to the needs of the older patient (Martin, 1984). Perhaps the best service that nursing can do to help the elderly is to start with the assumption that *older people and those who nurse them are valuable.*

A degree of job satisfaction has to be achievable and is necessary both to recruit and keep excellent nurses in nursing the elderly. There is a need to recognize that satisfaction from high turnover 'cure' rates is less applicable in non-acute situations with older patients. Instead, the skills of promoting independence, being a friend, helping the older person to feel loved and valued are needed, and to be equally valued to other 'acute' nursing skills (Norton, McLaren and Exton-Smith, 1962; Wells, 1980). Jones and Galliard (1983), for example, found very positive attitudes towards the elderly, attributed to a unified policy of caring for them, close liaison with community nurses, good working environment and to nurses feeling part of 'a dynamic family unit giving rise to a feeling of positive involvement'. Rudd (1967) urged nurses to see the patient 'in a new relationship', for 'in respecting herself, the nurse learns to respect her patients, to regard them as valued friends'. He goes on to suggest that when the elderly patient is 'respected as an individual, and given security, opportunity for privacy and some protection from complete dependency upon others' then the patient's whole life is altered for the better. This plea is echoed in Brysson White's words in the introductory chapter. Nurses first have to come to terms with their own attitudes about ageing before they can begin to help others, and unless they have themselves cast off any negative images they have about ageing, then the specialty is no place for them. The need for nurses to look at ageing positively is paramount. Unless they do they live in an unreal world. The over-65s form the bulk of most nurses' case-loads (except those who work in the exclusively youthful areas) and a sizeable proportion of the whole population. Nurses who continue to deny the elderly do their potential patients and ultimately themselves a disservice, because in contributing to the negative views of their profession they inhibit others from progress and a positive approach. The nurse who does not hold nursing the older patient to be valuable *now*, will have no excuse when her turn comes in old age and she finds that care for her needs is not all that it could be.

ORGANIZING CARE TO HELP THE OLDER PATIENT

Many nursing approaches stress the need to make care 'individualized', to tailor the plan of care to the specific needs and wishes of the patient, rather than the routine of the institution or the rules of the organization. The immense risks and challenges to nurses of this grand ideal must not be underestimated. The strength of organizations, bureaucracies or institutions is enormous, and the highly complex societies which both support them and make them up render them powerful agencies in the control of many human destinies.

Martin (1984) refers to over twenty-two major and minor government and health authority inquiries into the failure in particular of the hospital system. He asks 'How is it that institutions established to care for the sick and helpless can have allowed them to be neglected, treated with callousness and even deliberate cruelty?' While accepting that there may be some nurses whose individual psychopathology may play a part, it must not be forgotten 'that much turns on the attitudes of society to its weakest members, and the resources assigned to their care' and 'that what may occur is both a perversion of individual motives and social institutions'.

Thus the nurse may not only institutionalize patients, but may herself become institutionalized by 'perverting' the motives of care into something diametrically opposite. The classic texts by Goffman (1961) and Robb (1967) demonstrate the effects of this distortion of motives upon the recipients of 'care' and set the challenge to the professions to put their house in order.

A number of features appear to be crucial for this restructuring. Firstly, it is necessary to establish the beliefs and attitudes which underpin the subsequent nursing actions. The forging of a common philosophy which guides and directs nurses in what they do is the foundation stone for nursing models (Kershaw and Salvage, 1986; Pearson and Vaughan, 1986; Wright, 1986). Elder (1977) posits that 'A belief in the species, which is an integral part of the will to survive and therefore a belief in life, presupposes an acceptance of the doctrine that all individuals count and have a right to a full life.' The rights of patients need to be made explicit to them, perhaps in writing as they enter the home, clinic or hospital (Wright and Gartside, 1987) as well as to the staff themselves (Ely Hospital 1981). This theme of patients' rights has recently been taken up by the Royal College of Nursing (1987) as an important issue to which nursing must address itself.

Nurses, wherever they work, need to be constantly alert to the insidious danger of creeping institutionalization. It happens in nursing home, hospital and private residence, when the institutionalized nurse ignores patients' real needs at best or, at worst, treats them with cruelty. 'Perhaps the basic abuse', de Beauvoir (1977) argues, 'is the insult to the patient as a person. ... By stripping the patient of his will to live, by daily sniping snubs and slurs – a nursing home can kill a man.' She reinforces Elder's (1977) view that nurses first need to examine the basic philosophy from which they operate, and from there to develop ways of caring which accept patients' rights, their humanity and their personhood.

Many texts pay great attention to philosophies of nursing and a wide variety of them are available to nurses as a result. Many arise in the early works of nurse theorists in the USA (e.g. Henderson, 1966; Rogers, 1970; Orem, 1980; Roy, 1980; King 1981; Parse, 1981) and latterly in the UK (Roper, Logan and Tierney, 1983; Chapman, 1985; Pearson and Vaughan, 1986; Wright, 1986). While there are many variations within these ideas about nursing, they are variations on a theme. Humanistic, holistic concepts of patients' rights, patients as whole persons more than the sum of their physiological parts, and nurses as partners and advocates in care are important concepts common to almost all of them.

A diversity of ideas and philosophies must be seen as a strength in nursing. Reilly (1975) notes how every nurse carries 'in her head' an image of what nursing is. However, these ideas need to be made explicit and brought together in shared beliefs and goals so that neither patients nor nurses are confused by a multiplicity of directions. This point is aptly illustrated in Pearson and Vaughan's (1986) text, where it is suggested that nurses in the same setting using different models produce confusion for both patients and staff. For example, a patient may need two nurses on the same shift – one is of the rehabilitative school ('Come along, Mr Brown, you can try and wash yourself!') and one from the more institutionalized school ('There, there, I'll do all that for you!'). What do nurses feel like in such settings? What conflicts do they encounter with each other? More importantly, the consequences for both relatives and patients is uncertainty and mistrust over the direction the care is going.

Thus, whether being nursed at home or in hospital by a variety of nurses, a fragmented pattern of care can be set up where nurses do not share the same beliefs about nursing or accept common goals. However, as Johnson (1986) has pointed out, there is a great danger that philosophies of care can become 'paper exercises', little shared or practised by colleagues, especially when imposed from above. Leadership is needed, but as Towell and Dartington (1976) note 'it needs to be combined with a "bottom-up" approach which starts from how care staff define their situation, and helps them to discover for themselves their capacity to bring about change'. The 'bottom-up' approach is espoused by Ottoway (1976) and has been used in a number of settings (e.g. Wright, 1985; Pearson, 1985) to develop nursing philosophies and other aspects of nursing. What is clear from the current trend towards establishing nursing pholosophies (embodying notions of patients' rights) is that this must happen concurrently with the application of a change strategy, especially if applying personalized care in practice requires a move away from institutionalized pracitce. The nurse therefore needs also to be skilled and knowlegeable in change theory and the management of change in all levels of nursing.

These are summarized briefly by Lancaster and Lancaster (1982) as follows:

- The power-coercive (i.e. imposing change).

- The rational-empirical (drawing on peoples' self-interest to provide change).
- The normative-re-educative (helping nurses to identify areas for change for themselves).

The latter approach, embodying the ideas of Ottoway (1976) and Towell and Dartington (1976), appears to be the most appropriate to nursing, for lasting change requires numbers of nurses to commit and involve themselves in it personally. Otherwise, change influenced by the change enforcer (power-coercive) or the change seller (rational-empirical) runs the risk of reversal or burning out when these influences are lost or diminished. Real, permanent change requires the commitment of the energy and will of those at the grass roots. The process of changing nursing needs to be owned by nurses themselves.

The reader is urged to refer to some of the significant texts on change mentioned above. Being change agents is a vital role for nurses, but they need the knowledge and skill to do it. Knowledge is power, and power is needed to change things. If change is not to be random and chaotic, then nurses need just as much knowledge and skill in change agency (and all the social and economic factors which influence it) as in giving drugs correctly or helping an elderly woman to the toilet at home.

If knowledge is power, then nurses need to know how best to direct their energies. It is interesting that concurrent with the professionalization of nursing has come a closer definition of what nursing is and how it is done. This defining of nursing models is crucial to nursing. If nurses are weak in determining what nursing is and how to do it, then what they do is constantly open to being challenged and dominated by other models, not least the institutionalized one. On offer to nurses appear to be two extremes of a continuum which appear to have certain characteristics (Figure 3.1).

These kinds of approaches are found in all settings in home or hospital. The nurse brings it with her to the nurse–patient relationship wherever she works. Thus the institutionalized approach is not exclusive to the hospital or nursing home. It can infect the way the community nurse deals with the patient on a one-to-one basis at home. It can create, as Martin (1984) notes, a place where 'the degree of order necessary for running a ward would become soulless regimentation, and the need to protect patients from mishaps could lead to incarceration in bed or chair'. How many patients are still forced to eat, drink, dress, move or sleep according to the dictates of the ward routine or the community nurse's visit? Such effects persist and form a common basis of complaint

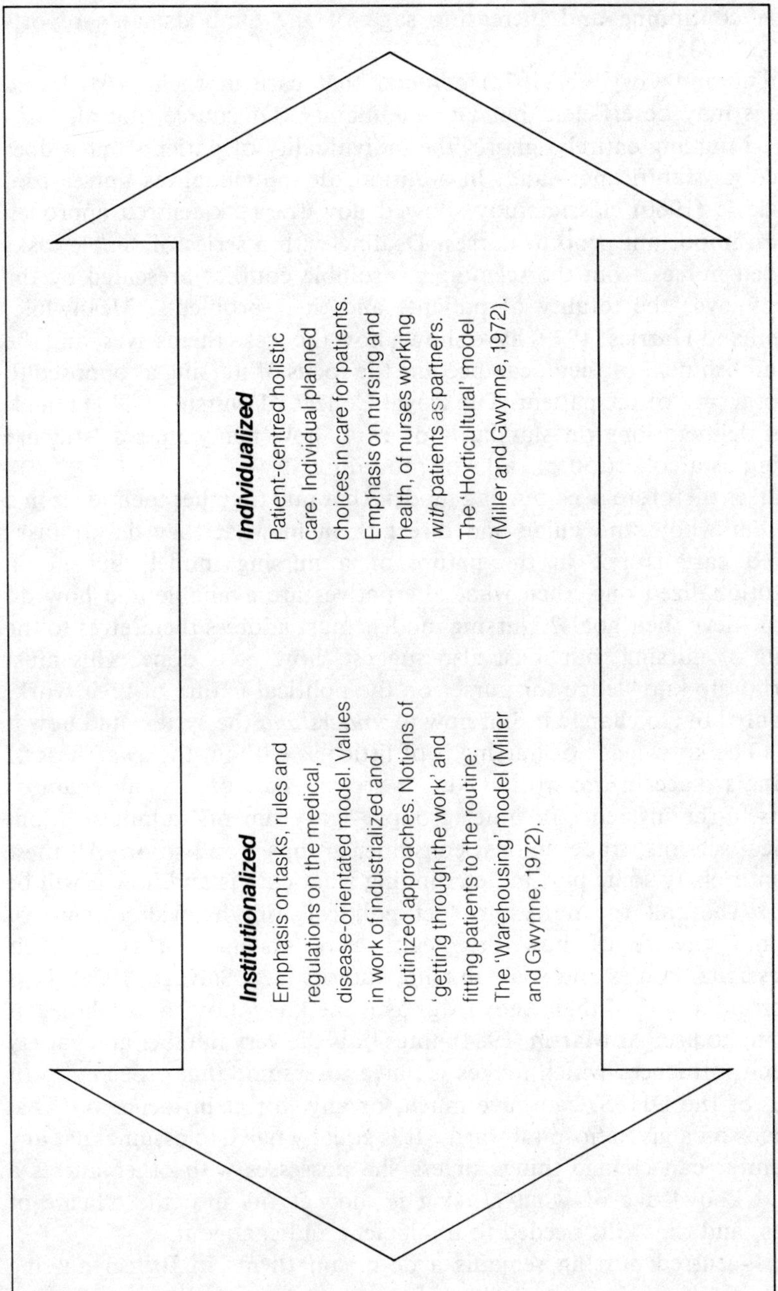

Figure 3.1 The nursing continuum.

in the continuing and increasing saga of the Ombudsman's reports (DHSS, 1985).

Miller and Gwynne (1972) contend that care in such task-centred settings may be efficient but lacks humanity. Of course, not all task-centred nursing entirely ignores the individuality of patients but it does reduce its significance, and, in addition, de-individualizes nurses too. Menzies's (1960) classic study showed how the task-centred approach was an important prop to nurses. Dealing with a series of simple tasks shielded nurses from the seemingly insoluble conflict presented by the anxiety over the totality of patients and their problems. Meanwhile, Towell and Harries (1979) have shown how the tasks themselves, and the accomplishment of them, can become the focus of nursing as opposed to the total care of the patient. The Royal College of Nursing (1981) noted, in its deliberations on standards of care, how many nurses 'still are nursing as a collection of tasks or procedures'.

Nurses therefore need nursing models that pull together their ideas in a coherent whole and guide and direct them in what they do. If task-centred care is not in the nature of a nursing model, but in an institutionalized one, then what alternatives are available and how do they achieve their goals? Nursing models must address themselves to the 'what' of nursing, but must also suggest 'how' it is done. This must incorporate knowledge for nurses on the political nature of their work, not only how to change it, but how to *understand* the system and how it ticks. The knowledge of nursing is of little use without the awareness of nursing's place in the world. Nurses are but part of a small chain of events in the influence of other groups – governments, administration, medical schools, trade unions, consumer groups – and so on. All these and more play some part in determining what care is and how it will be given. The call for nurses to 'get political' (in the widest sense of becoming aware of how the health care system works) by their professional bodies and some nursing authors (e.g. Salvage, 1985), is as important a part of their knowledge as is the know-how in the choice of dressing to use. As Martin (1984) notes 'it is the very number and variety of such influences which makes it naive to assume that a Secretary of State, or the DHSS, can have much, or any, direct influence on what happens on a given hospital ward'. It is equally naive to assume that any one nurse can change things unless she possesses with other nurses a shared knowledge of what nursing is, how it fits into the scheme of things, and the skills needed to implement and change it.

Task-centred nursing remains a dominant theme in British nursing

(Merchant, 1985). Yet it is ultimately dissatisfying to both patients (the elderly no less than other groups) and nurses. However, what are the alternatives? Universal in nursing models is the appeal to individualized, personalized or patient-centred nursing.

Beyers and Phillips (1971) draw interesting parallels between changes and developments in ways of organizing nursing and the historical events of the last century. Up to the 1920s and 1930s, the primary effort of nursing was seen in the 'case method' – exercising environment controls, often in the community working with families and individuals, with many of the ideas based on the writings of Florence Nightingale.

The massive expansion of hospital care systems was not seen as important until the early twentieth century when, by 1930, insurance facilities and rising living standards meant that more people could avail themselves of hospital care. The increase in hospital work and in the technology and complexity of nursing meant a review of the approach to nursing was necessary. After all, the 'case method' was 'expensive in terms of professional nursing salaries and impractical for most nursing units' (Beyers and Phillips, 1971). Thus the basis of change came not from nurses but from economic pressures to enable 'better utilization of large numbers of personnel', and this led to the growth of the 'functional method' where tasks could be doled out according to ability. Professional nurses were scarce and aides took on jobs 'in situations where there is a lack of professional staff on a limited budget for staffing'.

In the post-war period, the faults in the functional method of nursing were mainly as the result of nurses perceiving care as tasks to be done and not perceiving the total needs of the patient. The answer to these problems, it was felt, could be found in team nursing, where each contributes nursing care to the best of her ability under the supervision of the team leader.

A fourth era of nursing is seen to have developed in recent years with the demand for nurses with specialist skills, and along with this has been a regeneration of the idea of individualized nursing more far-reaching than previously envisaged.

Recent nursing literature has concentrated on the nursing process as a tool to make care individualized. Personal, tailor-made care of this nature requires a nurse with a deep understanding of the patient and his/her problems and arguments have been put forward in favour of patient allocation, team or primary nursing to achieve it (Marks-Maran, 1978; Kratz, 1979; Castledine, 1980).

TEAM NURSING

Waters (1985) describes team nursing as 'the allocation of a small group of nurses (team) to a group of patients, for whose care they are responsible and may be accountable'. The term can be applied to a wide variety of nursing situations varying from task assignment to almost primary nursing. The general aim is to make use of different levels of skill within the team to meet the needs of the patient. Thus small groups of nurses look after small groups of patients. Team leaders (whom Kron [1981] says must be registered nurses) co-ordinate the team's activities and plan the care, the team members following the leader's guidelines (Figure 3.2).

Waters (1985) further suggests that team nursing has been very widely interpreted, but believes it can promote satisfaction for both patients and nurses where there is continuity of allocation of nurses to patients and clear nursing care plans. However, misuse of team nursing can lead to working according to status of tasks and fragmentation of care.

Patient allocation requires not so much the allocation of patients to teams, but to specific nurses (Marks-Maran, 1978) with some degree of continuity, for example over several working shifts or perhaps longer.

Primary nursing as described by Manthey (1980) is seen as the return of the 'my nurse' concept in nursing. The Nightingale era saw the rise of this 'case method' which to some extent was lost with the rise of task-centred nursing, but is seen as still important to community-based nursing practice (Cumberledge, 1986). In the case method, the nurse performing

> all the nursing care for an individual was allowed autonomy and was able to form a close therapeutic relationship with the patient. A return to this is not economically viable at the present time and so primary nursing, with one nurse assuming 24-hour responsibility for a group of patients, is a feasible alternative.
>
> (Sparrow, 1986)

In primary nursing there is

- allocation and acceptance of individual responsibility for decision-making to one individual;
- assignments of daily care, that is individual receiving total care from one nurse;
- direct person-to-person communication; and

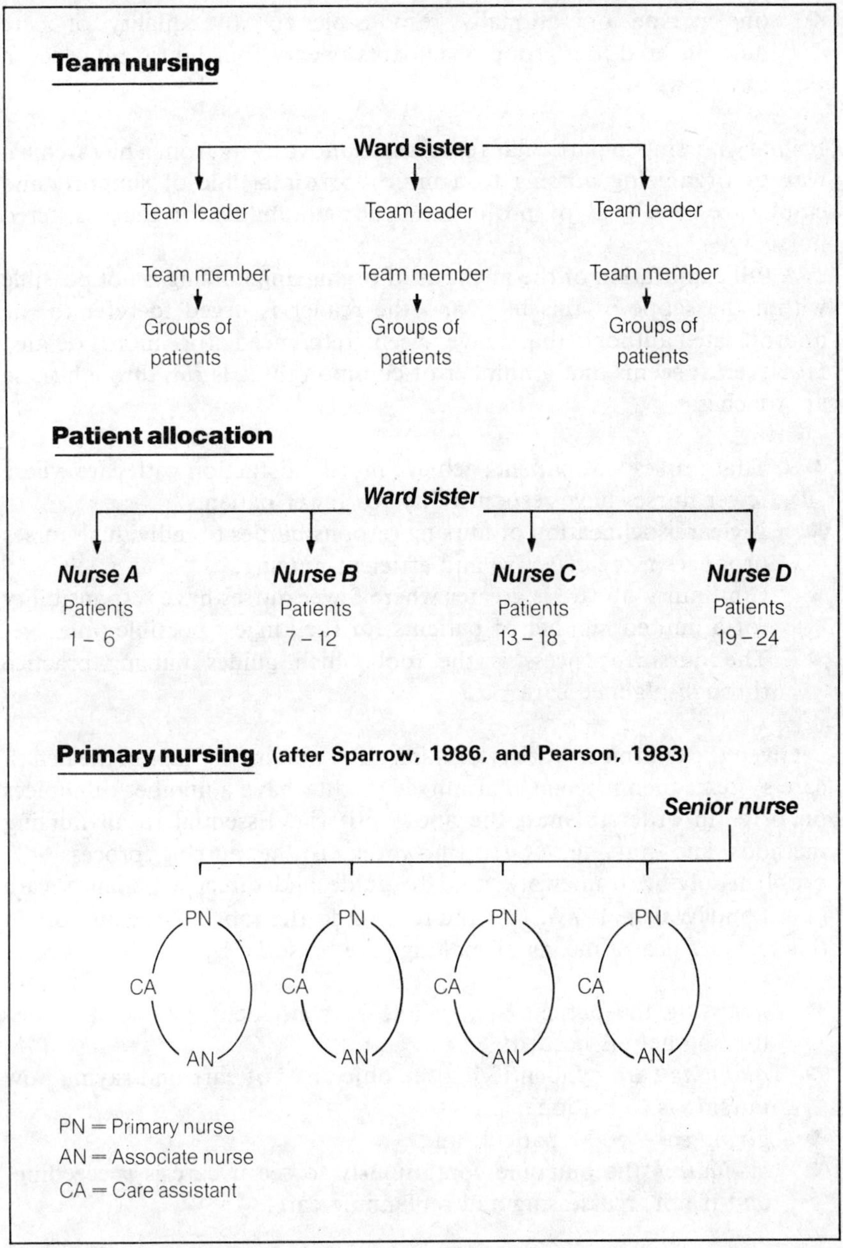

Figure 3.2 Examples of organizational charts.

- one person operationally responsible for the quality of care administered to a group of patients twenty-four hours a day seven days a week.

Primary nursing in particular represents a move away from a hierarchical way of organizing nursing to a more horizontal line of support, and emphasizes the goal of professional accountability for the registered nurse.

A full exploration of the methods of organizing nursing is not possible within the scope of this text, and the reader is urged to refer to the appropriate authors that have been referenced for more details. However, it seems that a number of common threads run through these approaches.

- That nurses and patients achieve more satisfaction with care where fewer nurses have responsibility for fewer patients.
- A clearer delineation of nursing responsibilities to individual nurses produces more effective and efficient nursing.
- Continuity of care is greater where fewer nurses have responsibility for a limited number of patients for the longest possible time.
- The nursing process is the tool which guides nursing practice through planned care.

Given the enormous variety of nurses and nursing settings in the health care system, then it seems that nurses need to have a number of choices on offer in order to meet the above criteria. Essential to all nursing methods and nursing models, however, is the nursing process - a problem-solving framework used to guide and direct a patient's care (Yura and Walsh, 1973). It is the tool to do the job. All the authors in this text use it as a means of making care personal by

- *assessing* the patient as a whole person, identifying areas where nursing help is needed;
- *planning* care by identifying the objectives of care and saying how nursing is to be done;
- *giving care* to the patient; and
- *evaluating* the outcome continuously to see if care is succeeding, and if not, reassessing and replanning care.

Arguments still rage in British nursing on the pros and cons of the nursing process. Problem-solving and care-planning, however, are seen as one of the hallmarks of skilled, professional nursing and they lie at the heart of the work of subsequent authors in this text. It is a crucial tool to helping nurses themselves to guard against the instrumental model of care.

THE NURSE AS PART OF A TEAM

Repeatedly throughout this text, the authors will refer to their work as being 'part of a team'. The work in nursing is not done in isolation, and in dealing with the multiplicity of health problems the older patient encounters, it takes more than the skills of one person to achieve solutions.

While nurses must work with a variety of disciplines – social workers, dieticians, physiotherapists, doctors, and so on – there has been relatively little work undertaken on evaluating multidisciplinary teams. Does the ideal of a team of equals, with each contributing to the patients' needs according to skills (rather than one discipline ruling overall on the basis of authority), work in reality?

To participate as equals in the team nurses must possess the necessary skill, information and training to meet the expectations of their role with others in the team (Harries, 1976). The concept of the multidisciplinary team means the bringing together of groups of colleagues involved in the care and treatment of an individual patient (Royal Commission, 1979). McFarlane (1980) claims that the narrow disease orientation of the NHS, coupled with undue emphasis on medical function, have served to concentrate attention on the role of the doctor and minimize the contribution and potential of other health workers. The level to which doctors will relinquish their traditionally dominant role in the team is debatable. Kyes and Hoffling (1977) see the development of a healthy climate where there is a minimum of negative competition, hostility and resentment as being the primary move to the development of positive clinical relationships. The success of the team depends upon the freedom of each member to use his/her professional skills independently in an atmosphere of mutual respect.

INDIVIDUALIZED CARE AND PATIENT INVOLVEMENT, ANOTHER SAFEGUARD

A further aid to guaranteeing the quality of care is for nurses to develop the assessment of it. This can happen at the initial level through the use of the evaluation phase of the nursing process. This alone is no guarantee of quality, that the patients' rights are being upheld or that planned care is being given. Filling in nursing care plans is no assurance that the care has been implemented. Other efforts need to be included.

Assessing the quality of care has become a new trend in nursing. Many efforts concentrate on questionnaires or assessments using staff, nursing records, and so on. While these may yield valuable information, it is argued here that patients too must be included. However, this area is fraught with many pitfalls. Some sources (Thompson, 1986; Wright, 1987) have shown how responses can be elicited from patients, but also demonstrated the difficulties of collecting the data. Will the patients in the home find fault with their community nurse when they may depend on her for regular visits? Can 'captive audience' patients in the hospital or nursing home give an honest view of the care if they depent on those carers to meet all their needs?

Patients, meanwhile, will have a very different perspective. Does the nurse (as the major health worker with 24-hour patient contact) take the blame because the ambulance is late, the X-ray delayed, the food unappealing? When patients' subjective feelings on good or bad care are added (for example, the patient who loves white bread and beef and the vegetarian who loathes it) the picture becomes even more complex. Some authors are therefore wary of including patient evaluation of quality of care (Hall, 1966; Pearson, 1983).

Much of the work on quality assessment has tended to focus on the views of nurses and others by questionnaire, interview or observation and assessment techniques. These perspectives may be too limited, however – a broad view of quality needs to take into account the perspectives of both carers and cared-for. The balancing of these ideas will then enable the nurse manager to make a realistic assessment. An amalgam of different approaches needs to be considered; each one yields some benefit, though alone its use is limited.

To promote quality of care for the elderly, four main themes may be evident from the foregoing discussion which may be represented as in Figure 3.3.

Whatever nursing approach is used, it needs to be open and dynamic –

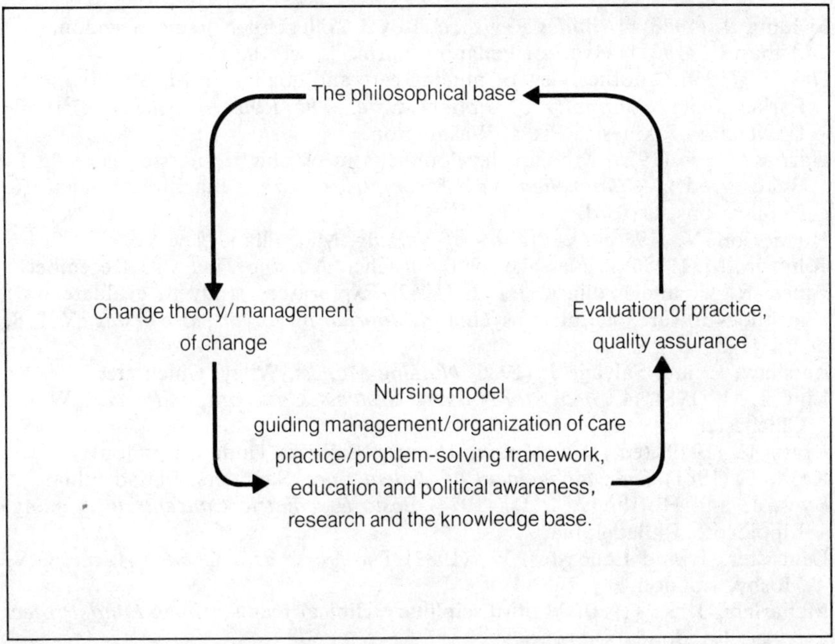

Figure 3.3 Promoting high quality care: key elements.

responsive to the changing needs of patients and their carers. A closed system becomes a narrow institutional box, confining nurses and patients to an inhuman and unresponsive mould.

REFERENCES

Beyers, M. Phillips, C. (1971) *Nursing Management for Patient Care*, Little, Brown, Boston.

Castledine, G. (1980) 'My nurse' and 'my patient', *Nursing Mirror*, Vol. 151, no. 6, p. 14.

Chapman, C. (1985) *Theory of Nursing: A Practical Application*, Harper and Row, London.

Cumberledge Review Team (1986) *Neighbourhood Nursing: A Focus for Care*, HMSO, London.

de Beauvoir, S. (1977) *Old Age*, Penguin, Harmondsworth.

DHSS (1985) *et seq*., Ombudsman's Reports, DHSS, London.

Elder, G. (1977) *The Alienated: Growing Old Today*, Writers and Readers Publishing Co-operative, London.

Ely Hospital (1981) The rights of residents, in J. P. Martin (1984) *Hospitals in Trouble*, Blackwell, Oxford.

Fielding P. (1986) *Attitudes Revisited*, Royal College of Nursing, London.
Goffman E. (1961) *Asylums*, Penguin, Harmondsworth.
Hall, L. (1966) Another view of nursing care and quality, in M. Straub and K. Parker (eds) *Continuity of Patient Care: The Role of Nurses,* Catholic University of America Press, Washington.
Harries, C. J. (1976) Modern developments in psychiatric nursing care, in E. Baker (ed.) *Comprehensive Psychiatric Care*, Blackwell Scientific Publications, Oxford.
Henderson, V. (1966) *The Nature of Nursing,* Macmillan, New York.
Johnson, M. (1986) A message for the teacher, *Nursing Times*, 31 December.
Jones, R. G. and Galliard, P. G. (1983) Exploratory study to evaluate staff attitudes towards geriatric psychiatry, *Journal of Advanced Nursing*, Vol. 8, pp. 47–57.
Kershaw, E. and Salvage J. (1986) *Nursing Models*, Wiley, Chichester.
King, I. M. (1981) *A Theory for Nursing: Systems, Concepts and Process*, Wiley, Chichester.
Kratz, C. (1979) (ed.) *The Nursing Process,* Baillière Tindall, London.
Kron, T. (1981) *The Management of Patient Care*, Saunders, Philadelphia.
Kyes, J. and Hoffling, M. D. (1977) *Basic Psychiatric Concepts in Nursing*, Lippincott, Philadelphia.
Lancaster, J. and Lancaster, W. (1982) *The Nurse as a Change Agent*, C.V. Mosby, London.
McFarlane J. K. (1980) Multi-disciplinary clinical teams, *Kings Fund Project paper*, London.
Manthey, M. (1980) *Primary Nursing*, Blackwell, Oxford.
Marks-Maran, D. (1978) Patient allocation *v.* task allocation in relation to the nursing process, *Nursing Times*, Vol. 74, no. 10, pp. 413–16.
Martin, J. P. (1984) *Hospitals in Trouble*, Blackwell, Oxford.
Menzies, I. (1960) A case study in the functioning of social systems as a defence against anxiety, *Journal of Human Relations*, Vol. 13, no. 2, pp. 95–121.
Merchant, J. (1985) Why task allocation? *Nursing Practice*, Vol. 1, no. 2, pp. 67–71.
Miller, E. J. and Gwynne, G. V. (1972) *A Life Apart*, Tavistock, London.
Norton, D., McLaren, R. and Exton-Smith, A. N. (1962) *An Investigation of Geriatric Nursing Problems in Hospital*, National Corporation for the Care of Old People, London.
Orem, E. E. (1980) *Nursing: Concepts of Practice*, McGraw-Hill, New York.
Ottoway, R. N. (1976) A change strategy to implement new norms, new style and new environment in the work organisation, *Personnel Review*, Vol. 5, no. 1, pp. 13–18.
Parse, R. R. (1981) *Man - Living - Health*, Wiley, New York.
Pearson, A. (1983) *The Clinical Nursing Unit*, Heinemann, London.
Pearson, A. (1984) The Burford experience, *Nursing Mirror*, 12 December, pp. 32–35.
Pearson, A. (1985) Nurses as change agents and a strategy for change, *Nursing Practice*, Vol. 1, no. 1, pp. 80–4.
Pearson, A. and Vaughan, B. (1986) *Models for Practice*, Heinemann, London.
Phillipson, C. (1982) *Capitalism and the Construction of Old Age*, Macmillan, London.

Reilly, D. (1975) Why a conceptual framework? *Nursing Outlook*, Vol. 23, no. 9, pp. 12–20.
Robb, B. (ed.) (1967) *Sans Everything: a Case to Answer,* Nelson, Edinburgh.
Rogers, M. E. (1970) *An Introduction to the Theoretical Basis of Nursing,* Davis, Philadelphia.
Roper, N., Logan, W. and Tierney, A. (1983) *Using a Model for Nursing*, Churchill Livingstone, Edinburgh.
Roy, C. (1980) The Roy adaptation model, in J. P. Riehl and C. Roy (eds) *Conceptual Models for Nursing Practice*, Appleton-Century-Crofts, New York.
Royal College of Nursing (1987) Standards of care, *Senior Nurse*, Vol. 6, no. 4, p. 13.
Royal College of Nursing (1981) *Towards Standards: A Discussion Document*, London.
Royal Commission on the National Health Service (1979) HMSO, London.
Rudd, T. N. (1967) Hospital geriatrics – the mechanism of success, *British Hospital Journal and Social Science Review*, 21 July, pp. 8–11.
Salvage, J. (1985) *The Politics of Nursing*, Heinemann, London.
Sparrow, S. (1986) Primary nursing, *Nursing Practice*, Vol. 1, no. 3, pp. 142–8.
Thompson, A. (1986) Patients' eye view, *Nursing Times*, 5 March, pp. 30–2.
Towell, D. and Dartington, T. (1976) Encouraging innovation on hospital care, *Journal of Advanced Nursing*, no. 1, pp. 391–8.
Towell, D. and Harries, C. (eds) (1979) *Innovation in Patient Care,* Croom Helm, Beckenham.
Waters, K. (1985) Team nursing, *Nursing Practice*, Vol. 1, no. 1, pp. 7–15.
Wells, T. (1980) *Problems in Geriatric Nursing*, Churchill Livingstone, Edinburgh.
Wright, S. G. (1985) Change theory: the application of change theory to practice, *Nursing Practice*, Vol. 1, no. 1, pp. 85–91.
Wright, S. G. (1986) *Building and Using a Model of Nursing*, Arnold, London.
Wright, S. G. (1987) Consuming interests, *Senior Nurse*, Vol. 6, no. 2, pp. 24–6.
Wright, S. G. and Gartside, P. J. (1987) Patient's rights, *Nursing Standard*, 9 April, p. 5.
Yura, J. and Walsh, M. B. (1973) *The Nursing Process*, Appleton-Century-Crofts, New York.

4. Promoting Safety and Comfort

Lesley Wade and Steve Wright

A HOSTILE ENVIRONMENT

An old chinese proverb begins 'To understand the man you must firstly understand his memories'. Suppose you have been transported by time machine to a time between the wars. Your senses tell you things are not quite right. The landscape is barely recognizable, your nostrils are unaccustomed to the many smells, your eyes take in a chaotic confusion of animals and machines producing sounds. People wear strange attire and their speech is strange both in tone and manner. You are not exactly at home here; the vaguely familiar serves only to emphasize how you do not fit in. This environment feels rather alien; you begin to feel uneasy, uncomfortable, you sense this environment is hostile to you; that you are unsafe.

Through this fantasy we can glimpse another generation's world. This insight into how it may feel to live in an unaccustomed society and environment is central in promoting safety and comfort for the elderly. How are the elderly to find ways of coping with this strange world – and with the attitudes of 'ageism': 'The notion that people cease to be people, cease to be the same people, or become people of a distinct and inferior kind by virtue of having a specific number of years' (Comfort, 1977). Their feelings are no different from the younger generation's. Consider for example the comments made of a ward environment.

There is a hint of sun today in my small wedge of sky, but it does not touch

> my room. The sense of segregation is so palpable, you feel as if at any moment you will be tightly enclosed in a cocoon of isolation. You never hear young people singing, speeding recklessly home from late parties. Only spasmodic screeching a few doors away, that would send cold shivers down anyone's spine.
>
> (Newton, 1980)

A full sense of safety therefore comes from the familiarity and comfort in the environment, which poses no threat to mind or body. Older patients may experience relocation stress, institutionalization and the need to adapt their abilities to maintain their own safety and comfort within an unfamiliar environment. This includes the essential idea of personal space. Ebersole (1981) described this space as geographically and perceptually defined, subject to enlargement and construction. He suggests that personal geographical space may be limited to five or ten cubic feet. The notion of personal space is dealt with in more detail in Chapter 5.

The legacy of poor law institutes and cramped living conditions within organizational structures erode this territory. As Morris (1977), states, 'When people move inside this space we are threatened, yet if they keep too far away we feel rejected.' Roberts (1978) carefully analysed many aspects of care within a hospital that interfere with this personal space and its effect upon our sense of safety and comfort.

Many items of equipment, as well as 'tidying' nurses, may interfere with this sense of territory. Roberts (1978) notes 'The nurse by moving articles such as glasses, tissues or newspapers off the bed was observed as being a threat to personal security.' The aged person maintains a sense of personal space in three ways: by assembly of clutter, by environmental props such as personal items and also by possessiveness. This behaviour may be readily observed by those caring for the elderly. Sommer (1961) noted that the right to privacy and individual territory is one first forfeited and mostly ignored in institutions. This may well be because the institution, usually a hospital or nursing home, is perhaps viewed as the nurses' territory and space is arranged mainly for the convenience of staff rather than patients. In order to assess the individual's need for personal space certain oberservations could be made:

- A difference of culture has an influence on the amount of personal space an individual prefers.
- There are many differences among introverts and extroverts for personal space.

- The elderly individual reacts to spatial invasion in different ways. Some flee, others are verbally or non-verbally aggressive, some even withdraw into a private world, appearing confused or even apathetic.
- Spacing in small groups is not random, but rather follows from the personality and culture background of individuals.

Within this environment the nurse may be able to promote comfort and security by:

- Allocating the patient a single room.
- Avoiding transferring patients from ward to ward, room to room and area to area.
- Including objects of personal significance within the environment.
- Respecting the arrangements of the patient's space and not moving things without permission.
- Preparing for intrusive procedures, which is necessary even though they appear routine to the nurse. Personal items, e.g. for washing, need to be preserved and providing privacy to respect the individual's dignity when carrying out any procedure is essential.
- Asking patients whether they would like doors open or shut, curtains open or closed.
- Assessing each patient's needs as to his/her preferences for personal space and passing this information on to other colleagues.

In the community preservation of this territory and space can present many problems. Translocation, the removal of the individual from their home, can produce stressors which have been documented (Liberman, 1961).

Relocation of the elderly may have been for the best of motives, in order to maintain safety and comfort. There has been a tradition for local authorities and housing associations to provide rented accommodation for elderly people, and recently there has been a growth in private building firms producing houses and flats for those who wish to sell their home and buy into purpose-built schemes. For many elderly people this movement is seen as a crisis and many actually suffer from translocation shock (Muller, 1977). Recent recommendations in order to keep the elderly safe at home are laid down in *Staying Put* (Age Concern, 1984) which takes a pragmatic approach to the housing needs of the elderly. The aim of this report in 1980 was look at 'the practical difficulties that beset old people mainly owner-occupiers who wish or have no choice but to remain in their own house, which may be cold, lacking important repairs or amenities'. Other difficulties which emerge from this report showed how the problems of immobility inconvenienced the elderly at home (see Chapter 9).

A HOSTILE OR HAPPY ENVIRONMENT

> You are ill, you are over 65 years old, and as the ambulance arrives you know they are going to take you to the 'old workhouse'. It is the place designated for the 'undeserving poor'. Awaiting you the nurse is only too aware of the many problems of maintaining safety and comfort in that environment. As she gently lifts you onto the bed it is not only your personal space that comes under threat, the very territory appears hostile.

Fire is a constant threat, and despite obedience to regulations, fire-resistant coverlets, working fire doors and hoses, the risks from a lighted cigarette looms. Promotion of safety and comfort must ensure that all fire stairs are free from clutter, equipment is working and everyone on the ward knows and takes part in the drill. The nurse giving prescribed oxygen to the many elderly with breathing problems must develop a heightened sense of awareness to the risk of fire. Those identified as at risk should not be left smoking alone in day rooms or toilets. Another risk to environmental safety lies in the problems of infection control, particularly in narrow Nightingale wards. The control of infection officer, like the fire officer, should be sought for advice regarding bed spacing. In practical terms each member of the ward team must be made aware of the importance of hand washing and drying in stopping cross-infection. Bed spacing according to desirable areas is not always achievable. Wells (1980) recommends a minimum individual bed space of 5.57 square metres.

These are some of the more obvious problems that interfere with personal safety and comfort. Ergonomics is the study of the human being in the working environment, and it comprises psychology, biomechanics, engineering and instrumentation. By definition ergonomics aims to improve the work-place by producing greater efficiency and to improve the quality of the working life (Porter, 1986). However, nurses not only need to be able to take account of efficiency, they must also be able to take account of the aesthetics of equipment for the patients:

> Recently some colleagues were invited to preview a local engineer's mechanical skill. On display to the local hospitals were a new range of specifically designed chairs for the elderly. There they stood to be previewed, gleaming chrome, steel and clinically white, with the latest electronic wizardry included. The nurses stood speechless. Asked to sit in one of these 'it felt like awaiting for take-off at Cape Kennedy!' The nurses could not wait to jump off these starships and feel the earth beneath their feet!
>
> (Goodwin and Mangan, 1985)

Caring for the elderly and providing safety and comfort in a working environment calls for good problem-solving abilities and imagination most of all. Small things are important to improve the safety of the ward. The layout and bed formation can be altered. Is it always necessary to adhere to military straight lines? For example, to avoid isolation on traditional wards, perhaps the corner beds could be turned through 90 degrees to enhance space and privacy. To increase this it is desirable to have continuity of colour, and if possible some degree of matching bedspreads and curtains. Sitting arrangements are left to the individual's preference and small informal groups arrange themselves around bed areas or day rooms. As an extension of this, nurses and patients need to be involved in helping to plan the accommodation for the elderly and it is a good idea to get to know involved local committees, to make sure the nursing and consumer voice is heard.

Observations on the working environment made by nurses and others have led to a number of suggestions to help make the environment for the elderly both safer and more aesthetically pleasing (Kings Fund, 1979; Tinker, 1984):

- Excessive furniture causes clutter, resulting in restriction of movement for both staff and patients.
- Faulty equipment must be repaired promptly.
- The day room is everybody's lounge; it should not be used for storage or as a waiting room.
- The right type of bed, chair and bed table should be selected to meet individual requirements.

Perhaps a better understanding of ergonomics would help nurses to reduce the number of accidents that occur within the ward. Roberts (1985) states that nursing staff in particular feel guilty and fear recrimination about accidents that occur in hospital. The degree of control by nurses was seen to be one of the main causal factors in maintaining a safe environment. The staff had to be competent in using equipment and it was noted how staffing levels and organization of patient care contributed to safety. Above all, it was found that nurses need to collate information and evaluate why accidents occur. The dual accident form HN 55 66 for both staff and patients should be filled in promptly and accurately; in this way the nurse can keep an accurate history of accidents and evaluate them to discover factors for action, to avoid recurrences.

ACCEPTING RISK

The desire to promote the safety of the patient (and, to some degree, a fear of litigation) leads many nurses to become over-protective towards patients. The patient becomes an object, to which many things are done 'in his best interests' when the interest is really the staff's sense of security and degree of control over patients (Goffman, 1961). As Goodwin and Mangan (1985) point out:

> Once admitted to hospital or residential care, the biggest risk they face is that the cushion of care and concern for their physical well-being suffocates normal fuctioning. It can intrude upon their civil liberties so that even their moral and legal rights are abused to such an extent that legal buffs and courts would reel. However, only a murmur of disapproval is muttered against the howling pessimists who see no alternative to restraint and seclusion for wandering and confused elderly folk.

It is certainly true that elderly people are more at risk from falls and injury. Smith (1976) identifies the main predisposing factors:

- *Drop attacks* -usually due to arteriosclerotic problems or diseases such as myxoedema, vestibular disease, cervical spondylosis, epilepsy, etc.
- *Trips* – related to hazards in the environment as well as the tendency of the elderly to develop a shuffling gait.
- *Vertigo* – the sensation of instability or disorientation in space, for example as produced by visual disturbances, disturbed vestibular function (head injury, drugs, Ménières disease etc.) or lesions affecting the mid-brain and cerebellum, etc.

- *Postural hypotension* - especially when associated with a sudden rise from the chair or bed.
- *Leg and foot abnormalities* - 90 per cent of people reaching old age have some type of abnormality in the lower limb causing difficulty in walking, such as corns, overgrown toenails, arthritis or osteo-arthritis.
- *Contraction of the visual field* - from the fourth decade onwards there is a gradual reduction of the visual field increasing, for example, the risk of road accidents.
- *Environmental* - poor living conditions, lack of pedestrian crossings, badly designed furniture and so on.

While noting the danger, Smith goes on to suggest that the nurse has a major role to play in accident prevention, by taking action on dangers identified in the environment and selecting equipment that is safe for the elderly use. However, she urges nurses, in their enthusiasm to prevent accidents, not to indulge in excessive restraint of patients:

> However, to abandon the policy of activity in geriatric wards is unthinkable. The solutions are to be found in well designed wards, chairs and equipment; lower beds for patients not requiring full nursing care, and bed-rails to be fastened, especially at night.
>
> (Smith, 1976)

The use of bed rails, however, has remained a contentious issue in nursing. The Royal College of Nursing has produced its own guidelines for nurses on restraint in response to the pressure from the profession (RCN, 1988). Among their guidelines are the following:

- Restraint should only be used in exceptional circumstances, and should only be of a temporary nature.
- Restraint should only be used following a comprehensive assessment of the patient's condition at the time. This assessment should itemize the alternatives to restraint.
- The period of restraint should be specified before the restraint begins and the decision to continue should be constantly reviewed, for example, every fifteen minutes.
- The decision to restrain should only be made by a trained nurse following consultation with other qualified staff and with the explicit approval of the nurse in charge of the ward.
- The clinical nurse manager should monitor all instances where

restraint is used and produce monthly statistics, which should be publicly and freely available, that indicate the amount, type and reason for restraint (whilst ensuring that patient confidentiality is protected).

- No patient should ever be restrained by means of a harness.
- Sedative medication should be reviewed on a daily basis by medical staff.

Generally, prevention is better than cure, and many measures can be taken by nurses in advance. They can, for example, attend to the following:

- Identify why the patient is disorientated/falling and deal with the underlying problem.
- Promote good orientation.
- Remove hazards in the environment, e.g. rugs that slip.
- Ensure that the patient is in a place where he/she can be easily observed.
- Use beds/chairs at a height that are safe for the patient to use.
- See if the patient prefers sitting in a chair to lying on the bed.
- Lower the bed to a minimum height where possible, providing pillows or mattresses along the floor in case of a fall from bed does occur.
- Remain with the patient where possible; engage others (e.g. relatives) to assist in supervision.
- Keep lockers, personal items, etc. within easy reach.
- Provide a call system for the patient to summon help.
- Provide clothing that is well fitting - especially footwear.

Certainly any kind of restraint needs to be used with extreme caution, for it has serious implications for both nurse and patient. Cubbin (1970), Isaacs (1979) and Johnson (1980) suggest the following:

- 'Cot sides' in use makes practical nursing of the patient more difficult, risking injury to both nurse and patient.
- In an effort to escape restraint, the patient may actually suffer more serious injury.
- They are infringements of the personal rights of the individual.
- The motivation of the patient to become independent is reduced.
- They increase the risk of complications of immobility, pressure sores.

- They may promote anger, resentment and confusion in the patient.

As Isaacs (1979) notes, the risk of a fall is often more of a problem to the nurse than the patient:

> It isn't only coroners and accident forms that frighten us. We are anxious to avoid distress and alarm which a fall causes to a patient under our care. We also feel that to allow a patient under our charge to fall is a slur on our professionalism, that we, quite literally, have let the patient down.

Case study

Mr Hayward had been a patient on the 'long stay' ward for several weeks, and there had been several incidents of falling out of bed at night. He was disorientated for much of the time, and when the nature of his falls was assessed it was found that he rolled from the bed while restless. He was too weak to stand or climb back for himself. To keep him safe, the nurses, reluctant to use any kind of restraint discussed the issue with his wife and decided on the following rules for coping with the problem:

- Nurse him in a part of the ward where he could easily be observed, with bed close to the wall at night.
- Keep his bed lowered to a minimum height.
- Check with him if restless - does he want a drink, toilet etc?
- Use of safety rails if he cannot be continuously observed (protective pads must also be applied).
- Explain purpose of rails to him and his relatives.
- Promote orientation of time/place - explain where he is, what is happening, etc. (see Chapter 5 for further details).
- Review use of the rails every twenty-four hours.

Another patient also had similar problems at home. Joan, now 74, was sleeping in a single divan-type bed downstairs and was nursed, for the most part, by her husband. After her 'stroke', Joan sometimes rolled while asleep from her bed at night, causing much concern to her husband that she would be injured. In addition he could not lift her easily back into bed and sometimes disturbed the neighbour for help. To keep her safe, the district nurse helped and advised her husband on several alternatives:

- Place the bed against the wall at night and place the back of an armchair at the other side.

- Place pillows on the floor alongside the other side of the bed in case she should fall.
- Place the mattress on the floor for Joan to sleep on.
- Place extra pillows along the underside of one side of the mattress to reduce 'rolling', with the other side of the bed against the wall.

In the end, her husband found the first option most easy to use and Joan remained safely in bed thereafter.

The choice for nurses, restrain or not to restrain, is often a difficult one. The UKCCN (1984) gives advice in the professional code of conduct. The nurse must 'have regard to the environment of care and its physical, psychological and social effects on patients/clients' and 'act always in such a way as to promote and safeguard the well-being and interests of patients/clients'. The nurse must also ensure that 'no action or omission on his/her part or within his/her sphere of influence is detrimental to the condition or safety of patients/clients'. The nurse often has both a professional and personal dilemma when making judgements about the best action to take for the patients' safety.

THE ELDERLY PERSON'S USE OF MEDICINES

It is not surprising that drug therapy can cause confusion in the elderly patient, putting safety at risk. The amount and variations of drugs (polypharamacy) they have to cope with is staggering. Exact figures on the quantities of drugs used by the elderly in the UK are not readily available. What is certain is that both prescribed and non-prescribed medicines increase with age (Williamson, 1978). Due to the risk of multiple pathology with older people medicine regimes may become complex. A project paper on the elderly and their use of medicines reports that many of the drugs prescribed for elderly patients are given not for recognized syndromes, but for symptoms related to this multiple pathology, and diseases associated with the ageing process. Many of the risks and complications of drug treatment in the elderly are related not only to the biopharmaceutical parameters affecting age, but to deteriorating mental and physical faculties. Also, many social factors isolate the aged from medical advice (Anderson, 1980; Crome, 1982).

Therefore, the physiological alterations due to ageing and the ability of the patient to comply affects safety and comfort. The effect of any drug upon a tissue is dependent on its concentration, and on the sensitivity of the tissue to that drug. Variations on these factors are determined by the absorption, distribution, metabolism and excretion of the drug. There is little evidence to show that absorption from the gastro-intestinal tract changes in the elderly. Distribution of drugs may be delayed as a result of cardiovascular decline. There is a greater danger in older patients of toxic drug levels because of fewer binding sites. The elderly are more susceptible to drug competition when two or more drugs are given owing to changes in protein binding, so that one drug may interfere with the action of another, or displace it (Anderson, 1980).

Adverse reactions and side-effects take many forms, and the nurse must be able to recognize changes in state from nausea or a rash or be able to discern changes in toxicity from irritability, confusion or drowsiness. One of the worst problems of detecting toxicity is its likelihood to be misinterpreted as dementia. To ensure safety with the complex drug interaction involved with the elderly, the nurse must have knowledge of the adverse reaction drugs may have on her/his patient. Some of these drugs are in common use but require special care in prescription and administration. They include diuretics, hypotensive agents, digoxin, hypnotics, tranquillizers, antidepressants and anti-Parkinson drugs. Medical regimes must be as simple as possible, using the fewest possible drugs in the lowest possible dose. Complicated schedules with poor labelling and poor directions reduce the ability of the elderly to comply with therapy. Hall (1975) found that there were three main categories among the elderly in their ability to manage their own drugs. There were those who could manage their own drug therapy, those who were very meticulous and those who will always make errors. Again, it is the ability of the nurse to identify those in each area and act upon this information that increases safety (Barrowclough, 1982).

The pharmacist and nursing staff must work in close harmony in improving safety (Crome, 1982). Bottles must be labelled clearly and the patients taught to manage them themselves. This requires often prolonged teaching sessions, especially before discharge. Information on dosage and times should be clearly illustrated. The individual must be assessed as to the ease bottle tops may be removed. Child-proof containers present difficulties to many nurses let alone the elderly. Safety not only involves the right drug, right time, right patient maxim, but assessment and patient education (see also Chapter 10).

INFECTION AND THE ELDERLY PATIENT

There is some debate on how far the elderly patient is more at risk of acquiring infection than any other group of patients. It has been suggested that selected infections may attack the elderly in higher numbers (Yosikawa, 1985).

There is some evidence to show that the older person's defence mechanisms against infection, and the immune response are reduced (Bloom *et al.*, 1985). The older person entering hospital, for example, may well come into contact with highly virulent bacteria such as *Staphylococcus aureus*. The combination of less efficient auto-immune response and contact with more virulent organisms may therefore leave the older patient more at risk of succumbing to bacterial/viral infections. Assessment is made difficult as it appears advancing age may blunt the ability of an individual to mount a febrile response to an infection (Gleckman and Hibbert, 1982; see also Chapter 7). Gardner (1980) summarizes the main risk factors which contribute to the apparent propensity of the elderly for acquiring certain infections. These include:

- Environmental exposure, found in overcrowded wards or clinics.
- Physiological changes due to ageing.
- Diseases that increase susceptibility to infection.
- Reduced efficiency of the body's defense mechanisms.

Some of the main implications of these factors for nursing are:

- Recognition that a patient may be febrile, even though their temperature remains within the 'normal' range of the general population. Where possible baseline observation of temperature should be taken at an early stage. For example, the patient whose temperature is normally 35.5°C may have an infection if the temperature rises to 37°C (although this would be regarded as normal for other adults).
- Promotion of cleanliness, both personal and environmental, is essential, especially in situations where groups of patients are gathered together.
- All usual cross-infection methods must be sustained whether in home or hospital, and especially among those patients more 'at risk', for example, those already weakened through other illness or those living in communal settings.
- Patients' complaints of feeling unwell, aches and pains etc. should

be taken seriously and an assessment carried out, for example, through monitoring of temperature, collection of specimens, to obviate any underlying problems such as infections.

PAIN CONTROL AND THE OLDER PATIENT

There is no one accurate definition of pain. McCaffery (1968) may come nearest, when she states 'pain is whatever the experiencing person says it is, existing whenever he says it does!' If this is so the elderly may be at a disadvantage as many older patients do not verbalize their complaints as well as younger people (Dangott, Thornton and Page, 1978). Allied to this fact is the knowledge that the elderly have a loss of reserve capacity in many organs that makes them slower in reacting to physiological stresses. Hunt (1979) and Hayward (1979) both recognized the need to encourage the patient to state how he/she experienced pain. Hunt states that it is important to take into account the social environment and psychological factors that influence pain.

The nurse and patient may both benefit from a suitable assessment tool that enables pain control to be patient-centred. The Burford Nursing Development Unit in 1984 identified four benefits gained by using a pain assessment tool:

(1) Information obtained helped to establish what the pattern of the pain was.
(2) Recording when analgesia was given and relating the level of pain with the time and type of medication helped to evaluate the effectiveness of analgesia.
(3) Involving the patient in monitoring his feelings of pain helped him to think more objectively about pain.
(4) Using the assessment tool can help the nurse and patient to more specific goal setting.

The development unit at Burford adopted the painometer as the tool of choice. The painometer (Figure 4.1) shows a thermometer with graded scales corresponding to a range of statements about the pain. Patients are asked to point to the pain and indicate the level of pain they are feeling by use of this device. The information received from patients can then be used to control pain. Together, the nurse and patient may try

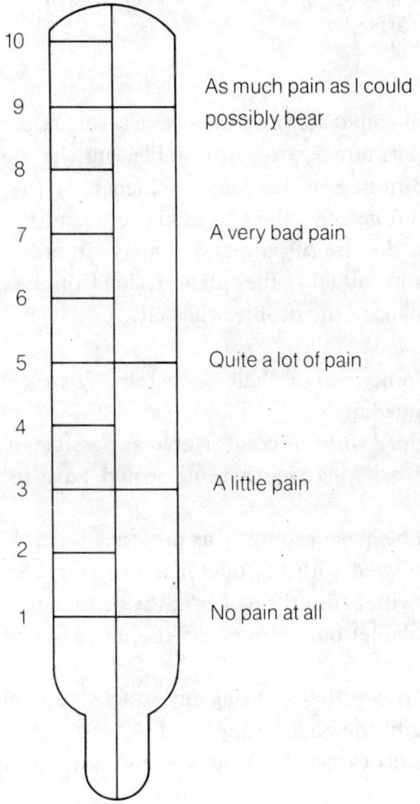

Figure 4.1 The pain thermometer or painometer.

alternative strategies before medication may be needed. These may include the use of music or rhythmical breathing to act as distractor to the pain, the use of ice packs or massage, but whatever the strategy adopted the choice will depend on the nature and intensity of the pain (O'Neill, 1985). Specific problems may be relieved by using specific treatments, e.g. lozenges to deal with painful mouth ulcers or consultation and expertly performed nerve block or radiotherapy to isolate bony metastasis.

Case study

Amelia Chisworth had come into hospital after a severe attack of chest pain. Her condition after the heart attack was fairly stable, but she was very distressed by the pain of her condition. She was very frightened by the mild sensations of 'tingling' and 'pins and needles' she had in her left arm. Each attack of angina resulted in a heightened sense of pain and anxiety. In order to relieve both her pain and prevent future attacks, the nurse decided on a plan which involved teaching Amelia to manage the problem herself.

- She was to rest in her bed or chair if she felt any attacks coming on and to tell her nurse immediately.
- She would be helped to be as comfortable as possible in bed/chair, with at least two nurses assisting, so that she would have to make little effort herself.
- Analgesia would be given promptly as prescribed and the effects monitored with her and reviewed with the doctor if necessary. She kept the glyceryl trinitrate tablets with her in the locker at the bedside (it reassured her if they were always available) but counted on the nurse to check how often they were needed.
- The nurse would stay with her during any attacks, teaching and explaining to relieve anxiety until the pain disappeared.
- Her general comfort (wash/drink etc.) as appropriate would be attended to at the same time.
- The nurse taught her self-medication and management of pain control, and involved her in the decisions about the planning of her care. She used question/answer techniques to ensure Amelia knew what to do in the event of a pain occurring either in hospital or at home and specifically in relation to the following:

    Taking her glyceryl trinitrate tablets.
    When to summon help and where from.
    Advising her family on how to help her if the pain recurred.

Devising a suitable exercise pattern at home to reduce the incidence of angina attacks.

The information booklet about her problem she was given to keep with her.

Ensuring that district nurse follow-up visits were arranged to continue care until Amelia was able to manage her problem confidently and independently.

When choosing analgesic drugs, Livesley (1986) states that 'it is important to become familiar with a few drugs and to use them well'. Aspirin and paracetamol are some of the most useful mild analgesics.

If given in adequate dosage the may often form the first line of treatment for bone pain. Analgesia may be introduced gradually, but if needed major analgesia should be given immediately. Livesley further recommends that patients with more severe pain of non-bone origin be helped by morphine sulphate twelve hourly in a time-released tablet. Diamorphine can also be used, having the advantage of being completely absorbed from the gastro-intestinal tract and thus reducing the effects of nausea. If administration of these type of medications produce nausea then prochlorperazine 5 mg or chlorpromazine 25 mg can be given.

Too much mixing of drugs in the elderly may cloud the consciousness and lead to coma. This alteration of mental function may cause confusion precipitated by peaks of pain. The nurse caring for the elderly in pain must aim to establish a balance between effective pain relief which does not over-sedate the patient.

Thus the major roles for the nurse in pain relief are the participation in assessing the nature of the pain, giving suitable relief measures, and in monitoring with the patient the effectiveness of pain control.

Case study

Rose Martin, who happened to live several streets away from Amelia Chisworth, had problems with pain too, but of a very different nature. With the intention of keeping her pain-free during the terminal stages of her illness (bronchial carcinoma with metastases in the vertebrae) the approach had to take account of a variety of other needs. Apart from her general comfort (she was now very weak and spending most of her day in bed) and attention to hygiene and toilet needs, the family too needed help and guidance in how to support her. The specific pain issue could not be easily separated from a number of others (the nurse was involved for example in teaching the family how to manage her and liaising with the priest who was important to her for her spiritual comfort). In relation to the pain, however, the following were found of particular help:

- Regular twice-daily visits from the nurse, not necessarily revising any treatments, but simply spending time with her, checking how comfortable she was, if the pain was well controlled, advising the family and acting as a link with the GP to identify other sources of help.
- Checking that the twice-daily doses of morphine sulphate tablets were enough to keep pain away. She appeared well controlled in this and was able to remain alert. She spent long periods in sleep, but awoke to enjoy meals and to watch her favourite TV 'soaps'. The nurse's role in keeping her pain-free was important, and as the disease progressed, she was able to be kept pain-free with a small increase in the drug dosage.

THE OLDER PATIENT UNDERGOING SURGERY

The main principles of nursing patients to promote safety before, during and after surgery are much the same for older patients as for younger ones. Garrett (1983) notes: 'Despite the multiple pathology from which they frequently suffer and their reduced tolerance of shock, many elderly patients respond remarkably well to planned surgical intervention with perceptive skill and planned surgical support.'

Older patients can achieve improvements in the quality of life after surgery equal to those of younger patients (e.g. after hip replacement). However, there is little doubt that prevailing attitudes to ageing, combined with economic limitations in health care, may leave the elderly at a disadvantage (Phillipson, 1982). While greater 'value' is placed on youth (see Chapter 2) in Western cultures, this influences decisions about who shall/shall not have resources when those resources (e.g. the opportunities for kidney transplants) are limited.

An otherwise fit elderly patient should not be disadvantaged if surgery can alleviate a health problem, even if it is of a relatively minor nature. For example, failure to repair a troublesome hernia may lead to more severe problems later if strangulation occurs.

The stress of surgery may be accentuated in the elderly person. Wattis (1984) suggests that 'partly because of poor eyesight and hearing, and partly, in some cases, because of a decline in mental agility, many old people find it difficult to cope with sudden change'. He further points out that 'an old person who develops a physical illness and is rushed off to hospital may become confused simply because of the changes to which he is subject'.

To minimize the risk of confusion brought on by stress, adequate preparation is necessary. This may be difficult to achieve in many hospitals where 'rapid turnover' is the order of the day and there is little time to reduce the risk of 'translocation stress' (Muller, 1977).

The patient requires time to become familiar with the environment, and at least several days beforehand, wherever possible, to become accustomed to the idea of admission to hospital. The nurse, in hospital or community, has a vital role to play here in teaching and explaining to the patient what is going to happen. Deciding what the older patient wishes and needs to know (see Chapter 10) needs to be combined with the communication skills outlined in Chapter 5 – not least taking account of the possible communicating difficulties of the older patient. 'Careful – and often repeated – explanation of all procedures is vital and apprehension must be recognized and allayed by discussion and appropriate intervention' (Garrett, 1983).

In preparing for the operation certain measures need to be considered. The risk of disorientation can be minimized if the patient can retain communication aids (spectacles and hearing aids) right up to the point of anaesthesia. If patients still have their own teeth, there is a risk that some of these may be loose and these need to be checked (Walker, 1985). Long periods of starvation are less well tolerated (Vowles, 1979) and the doctor may prescribe intravenous therapies before even routine operations are carried out. Comfort in relation to oral hygiene and mouthwashes is essential at this time.

To minimize confusion from too many carers, nursing care must be organized, with preferably one nurse allocated as the patient's 'own nurse' (see Chapter 3). In forming a relationship with one patient, and seeing him or her through the pre- and post-operative periods, this nurse is far more likely to be receptive to the patient's needs and aware of any anxieties and alert to any subtle changes in his/her condition.

Emergency surgery is more likely to produce problems for the elderly, such as confusion and a lower post-operative success rate. Cardiovascular problems – particularly in relation to deep vein thrombosis, pulmonary embolism and poor wound healing – are more likely to occur in view of the effects of the ageing process on the cardiovascular system (Vowles, 1979).

In the post-operative period, factors affecting limited mobility add to the dangers, particularly in relation to the risks of pressure sores, dehydration and chest infection (Garrett, 1983). An important role for nurses is to be aware of these added difficulties, for which the earliest possible mobilization and measures to promote good nutrition are essential (see Chapters 9 and 11 on mobility, eating and drinking, etc.)

Above all, careful assessment and selection of patients before surgery is essential. There is a need to balance the need for and type of surgery, with the potential effects on the patient's quality of life afterwards. Many 'heroic' operations have been done which have done little to enhance the patient's quality of life (Vowles, 1979). On the other hand, careful assessment, preparation and medical/nursing support can produce happier, more comfortable and fulfilling lives for the older patient after surgery. *Age alone should not be the criterion for deciding upon the patient's suitability for surgery.*

CRITERIA FOR SELECTION FOR SURGERY

The following criteria are based on Vowles (1979).

- What will be the patient's quality of life without surgery?
- What are the patient's chances of surviving surgery?
- Should the operation be elective, or should it be left until emergency surgery becomes necessary?
- How extensive does the surgery need to be (radical or palliative)?
- Which is longer without surgery, the course of the disease or the expectation of life?

While being highly subjective, being 'comfortable' and feeling 'safe' underpin much of the equality of the nurse–patient relationship. The skill the nurse brings into a variety of aspects of care are crucial, and a number of authors in this book have looked at their own themes in relation to comfort (e.g. with breathing, personal hygiene, and so on). Unless the older patient feels comfortable and safe with the nurse then all other aspects of care can be undermined.

REFERENCES

Age Concern (1984) *Staying Put*, London.

Anderson, R. (1980) The rise of repeatedly prescribed medicines. *Journal of the Royal College of Practitioners,* Vol. 30, pp. 609-13.

Barrowclough, F. (1982) Do they really need all those drugs?, *Nursing Mirror*, 10 November, pp. 22–7.

Bloom, E. T., Peterson, N. J., Tasking, T. and Makinodan, T. Immunity and ageing, in M. S. J. Pathy (ed.) (1985) *Principles and Practice of Geriatric Nursing,* Wiley, Chichester.

Burford Nursing Development Unit (1984) Nurses and pain, *Nursing Times*, Vol. 80, no. 19, p. 58.
Comfort, A. (1977) *A Good Age*, Mitchell Beazley, London.
Crome, P. (1982) *Psychopharmacology of Old Age*, Oxford University Press.
Cubbin, J. K. (1970) Mechanical restraints - to use or not to use?, *Nursing Times*, 11 June, pp. 24-6.
Dangott, L., Thornton, B. and Page, P. (1978) Communication and pain, *Journal of Communication*, Vol. 28, no. 1, pp. 30-5.
Ebersole, P. (1981) *Towards Healthy Ageing*, C.V. Mosby, London.
Gardner, I. D. (1980) The effects of ageing on susceptibility to infection, *Infectious Disease,* Vol. 1, no. 2, pp. 801-10.
Garrett, C. (1983) *Health Needs of the Elderly,* Macmillan, London.
Gleckman, J. H. and Hibbert, B. (1982) A febrile bacteraemia: a phenomenon in geriatric patients, *Journal of the American Medical Association,* Vol. 284, no. 3, pp. 1478-86.
Goffman, E. (1961) *Asylums*, Penguin, Harmondsworth.
Goodwin, S. and Mangan, P. (1985) Cosmic nursing - solitude and sanity, *Nursing Times*, 7 August, pp. 45-7.
Hall, M. R. P. (1975) Use of drugs in elderly patients, *New York Journal of Medicine*, Vol. 1, pp. 67-71.
Hayward, J. (1979) *Information - A Prescription Against Pain.* RCN, London.
Hunt, J. (1979) Protracted pain and nursing care, *Nursing*, Vol. 1, no. 2, pp. 56-64.
Isaacs, B. (1979) Don't get up - you'll fall!, *Nursing Mirror*, 18 October, pp. 40-1.
Johnson, J. (1980) Thoughts on cot sides, *Nursing Focus*, December 1980, pp. 120-1.
Kings Fund (1979) *Old People in Hospital*, King Edward Hospital Fund for London.
Liberman, M. (1961) Relationships of mortality rates in homes for the aged, *Geriatrics*, Vol. 16, October, p. 515.
Livesley, B. (1986) The management of the dying patient, in M. S. J. Pathy (ed.) (1985), *Principles and Practice of Geriatric Nursing*, Wiley, Chichester.
McCaffery, M. (1968) *Cognition of Bodily Pain and Man: Environment, Interactions, Student*, University of California, Los Angeles.
Morris, D. (1977) *Manwatching*, Triad/Panther, London.
Muller, E. (1977) Relocation of the elderly, implications for nursing, *Journal of Gerontology Nursing*, Vol. 3, July/August, p. 13.
Newton, E. (1980) *This Bed My Centre*, Virago Press, London.
O'Neill, J. (1985) Nursing assessment of the cancer patient who has protractive pain, *Nursing Practice*, Vol. 1, no. 1, pp. 20-4.
Phillipson, C. (1982) *Capitalism and the Construction of Old Age*, Macmillan, London.
Porter, L. (1986) The development of an observation schedule for measuring touch using an ergonomic approach, *International Journal of Nursing Studies*, Vol. 23, no. 1, pp. 11-21.
Roberts, F. (1985) Accidents in hospital - learning from past mishaps, *Nursing Times*, 6 March, pp. 24-7.
Roberts, M. (1978) *Behavioural Concepts and Nursing Throughout Life Span*, Prentice Hall Inc., New York.

Royal College of Nursing (1988) *'Focus' report - guidelines on restraint*, London.
Smith, C. (1976) Accidents and the elderly, *Nursing Times,* 2 December, pp. 1872–4.
Sommer, R. (1961) Symptoms of institutional care, *Journal of Social Psychology*, Vol. 8, p. 254.
Tinker, A. (1984) *Staying at Home*, HMSO, London.
United Kingdom Central Council for Nursing, Midwifery and Health Visiting (1984) *Code of Professional Conduct*, London.
Vowles, K. D. (1979) *Surgical Problems in the Aged*, Wright, Bristol.
Walker, D. M. (1985) *Oral Disease, Principles and Practice of Geriatric Nursing*, Wiley, Chichester.
Wattis, J (1984) *Psychiatric Disorders in the Elderly,* in P. Young (1984) *Nursing the Aged*, Woodhead Faulkner, London.
Wells, T. (1980) *Problems in Geriatric Nursing*, Churchill Livingstone, Edinburgh.
World Health Organisation Report (1982) *Health Policy Aspects of Ageing*, Vol. 82, United Nations, New York.
Williamson, J. (1978) Prescribing problems in the elderly, *Practitioner,* Vol. 220, no. 5, pp. 749–55.
Yosikawa, T. T. (1985) Geriatric infectious diseases; an emergency problem, *Journal of the American Geriatric Society*, Vol. 31, pp. 34–9.

5. Communicating

Steve Wright

This chapter deals with the theme of communicating in the broader sense. 'Communication establishes a sense of commonness with another and permits the sharing of information, signals, or messages in the form of ideas and feelings' (Murray and Zentner, 1975). Thus, there is information for nurses here not only on helping with the physiological effects of the older patients' ageing process (hearing, sight, speech, touch, smell) but also with their psychology (loneliness, unhappiness, anxiety, depression, nurse/patient/family relationships, and so on).

SOME ASPECTS OF COMMUNICATION

'You cannot *not* communicate.' This succinct comment by Satir (1967) holds many lessons for nurses. For, as Porritt (1984) notes, 'Whether intentional or not every behaviour carried out in the presence of another person will communicate something.' Even sitting doing absolutely nothing conveys something about us to another person. Attenborough (1985) has referred to human beings as the 'compulsive communicators' for communication in all it aspects is the basis of all human interaction and thus it is also a social process.

With such an immensely complex and fundamental activity going on between nurse, patient and others, it seems logical that the nurse's skills in this field should be highly developed. However, the focus of nursing has tended to emphasize the ability to complete tasks, often involving a high level of manual dexterity, to the neglect of the psychosocial skills. In Bridge and MacLeod Clark (1981) it is noted how 'everyone in the nursing profession pays lip service to the importance of communication. However, the fact that we are forced to give so much time and thought to the subject bears testimony both to its complexity and to the fact that there is still so much to be learned about it.' The Ombudsman's reports (DHSS, 1985 *et seq.*) attest to the continuing weakness of nurses in understanding patients' needs and in giving information. Menzies (1960) states that this weakness lay in nurses' inability to communicate about nursing to patients or to deal with the patients' feelings. Hence they protect themselves by hiding behind a shield of tasks – focusing on task-centred care enables the nurse to avoid the unhappiness at being unable to cope with the patient's needs as a whole. Melia (1982) suggests that nursing students often deliberately evade patients' questions because they do not know how to answer. Others have shown the enormous gulf which lies between the nurses' view of old age and the reality of the patients' view (Fielding, 1986). This leaves some authors to wonder whether nurses can ever really understand the elderly patients' world (Blondis and Jackson, 1977) when their life experiences and language may be separated by a gulf of many years. Can the 18-year-old student nurse really comprehend the needs of the disabled 70-year-old when what separates them is not only time and all the life events that go with it, but also the changes in language that occur over that time?

The gulf, however, need not necessarily be unbridgeable. Continued development in nursing education (UKCCN, 1986) lays much greater emphasis on nurses developing communication skills and much work is emerging (MacLeod Clark, 1981; Wilson-Barnett, 1981; Faulkner, 1984) to guide nurses in this field.

Nursing older patients may tax the nurse's communication skills to the full, for she may have to leap across the generations in order to understand them and meet their needs. Older patients may see the world differently from younger ones, and in turn the world treats them differently (Elder, 1977). The nurse has to understand the alienation that may come with old age – so vividly described by Brysson Whyte in Chapter 1 of this book. As Blondis and Jackson (1977) note, 'for most of us, old age is a time of loss. Just as the worst of our struggles with the job and the family raising are behind, old age begins.' Added to the physical limitations that may be imposed by the ageing process are the other losses due to retirement or professional obsolescence. There may be a loss of income, families grow up and may move away, friends and loved ones are lost to death. 'With loss comes the sense of not belonging, problems with self-esteem, identity, and these feelings often bring about the greatest loss of all – loss of desire to continue living' (Blondis and Jackson, 1977).

For the nurse to help the patient and overcome these immense difficulties requires more than the ability with the spoken word. It demands empathy – the ability to get inside the patient's head and see the world from his point of view. For the nurse to achieve this degree of understanding, she needs to have examined very carefully her own attitudes to ageing (Chapter 2) and gained knowledge of how the ageing process – as a physical, psychological and social phenomenon – affects the older patient.

COMMUNICATION – THE MAIN ELEMENTS

Human communication is usually considered to have two main components, verbal and non-verbal. However, the two frequently interact in a highly complex manner. The obvious nature of speech means that 'the non-verbal ways we communicate are often outside our awareness' (Porritt, 1984). The nurse needs to have knowledge and skill in both to be an effective helper.

Non-verbal Communication

Argyle (1978) says that 'non-verbal' communication can have five times as much effect on a person's understanding of a message compared with the words spoken at the time'. The nurse who says 'how are you?' to a patient and busies herself with some other task without waiting for (or listening to) a reply, is 'saying' far more to a patient than the simple words. She is saying don't keep me, I'm busy, I haven't got time, there are other things on my mind and so on. The main avenues of non-verbal communication can be summarized thus (after Hames and Joseph, 1980):

- Facial movement
- Gaze and eye contact
- Gesture and body movement
- Body positive and body contact
- The use of personal space
- The use of time

- Smell, appearance and clothes

A few general aspects of these elements need to be explained in more detail before proceeding further.

The face is one of the main expressors of emotion, which may be shown involuntarily, for example by blushing or sweating. 'Our face is a vehicle for many different types of information and is the most expressive physical aspect of our self' (Porritt, 1984). It can be used to express a whole range of feelings, either genuine or false, happiness, surprise, fear, anger, interest, disgust, or it may be mask-like to hide feelings. When not hiding emotion, then the whole face in involved in expression, expecially the mouth and eyebrows.

Eye contact occurs when two people look at each other and it may vary in length between men and women, and from culture to culture. What is acceptable to one may not be acceptable to another (Henley, 1977). Eye contact, however, underpins much conversation, allowing observation of non-verbal messages, sending out information through length of contact and couples with use of facial expression, and also helps in synchronizing the conversation – whose turn it is to speak (Kendon, 1967).

Gesture and body movement may often be used to replace speech or may be used to emphasize it. Again these are strongly influenced by the expectation of different sexes and cultures (Argyle, 1978).

Body posture may reflect the situation or feelings being experienced, and can help assumptions to be made by interpreting what the various postures mean. Leathers (1978) notes how, even having controlled facial expression, feelings can still be conveyed by the uncontrolled 'leakage' of signals given out by body posture.

Hall (1966) describes personal space as being like a bubble which surrounds the person and which others may or may not enter depending on the degree of intimacy they accept. The nature of the duties nurses perform means that they must often engage in invasion of another's personal space. Hall defines four particular layers of personal space:

(1) Intimate distance – less than 46 cm from the body surface.
(2) Personal distance – from 46 cm to 1.22 metres.
(3) Social distance – from 1.22 metres up to 3.66 metres.
(4) Public distance – more than 3.66 metres.

Invasion of the closest spaces by nurses leads patients inevitably to develop close relationships with them (Porritt, 1984). Hames and Joseph (1980) argue that an awareness of body space by the nurse needs to be 'combined with the therapeutic use of touch'. Touch is a crucial aspect of most human relationships. It plays a part 'in giving encouragement, expressing tenderness, showing emotional support and many other things' (Knapp, 1972). Touch may say non-verbally to a patient 'I care about you. Between people who care about one another, touch can communicate feelings where words would fail' (Murray and Zentner, 1975).

Time can be used as Henley (1977) suggests as a message about power and who holds it. 'The person who holds the power in a relationship is often the one who keeps the less powerful person waiting' (Porritt, 1984). The nurse who says 'I haven't enough time' may be using the mechanism to avoid other things, as a coping mechanism to avoid dealing with the anxiety of the patient and the complexity of the nurse–patient relationship (Menzies, 1960).

Appearance and clothes play an important role in assumptions being drawn about a person's social status, occupation, financial state, group affiliation and attractiveness. This further influences assumptions about the attitudes the person holds. However, 'in nursing, making quick assumptions about a person on the basis of her appearance is a trap to be avoided' (Porritt, 1984). Nurses also need to be aware of the, often subtle, influence conveyed by smell and, to some extent, taste. The days are not long gone when tasting urine was a common test for diabetes mellitus! The sense of smell is often ignored as an agent in communication (Hames and Joseph, 1980) largely because people become accustomed to the presence of odours and may fail to notice them, or because they often relate to negative observations ('bad breath', 'body odour', etc). It may lead the nurse to make assumptions about the patient's hygiene state and habits. On the other hand, uncontrolled expression of disgust or distaste (e.g. at the smell of a patient's sore, which he is helpless to suppress) may lead the patient to infer that 'I don't like you because you smell' (Lewis, 1973).

Verbal Communication

This 'represents only a small segment of total human communications' (Sundeen *et al.,* 1976). Hames and Joseph (1980) note how 'communication often fails because the sender and the receiver do not have a common understanding of the spoken words used during the interaction'. A few principles need to be established here:

- To provide understanding, repetition of information is often necessary. This should preferably be backed up with other non-verbal forms, for example writing or pictures (Johnson, 1972).
- Words need to be spoken clearly and concisely, particular attention being given to the clarification of words and ideas that are being transmitted to the receiver (Sundeen *et al.*, 1976)

Clarification techniques are needed to check understanding. What the nurse understands by a word may not be the same as the patient. The language gap that occurs between different sexes, cultures and generations can lead to misunderstanding. For example, a patient may be told he is going for a 'test' in the X-ray department. To the nurse this may be routine, but to the patient the word 'test' may imply a painful procedure, fears of radiation, anxieties about blood tests, needles and so on.

Porritt (1984) argues that nurses must beware of the 'jargon trap' which may confuse or obscure information which the patient is trying to understand. Patients (and nurses) carry the meaning of a word within their mental constructs, 'but the word itself is not the meaning'.

The above is a brief résumé of some important concepts in communications theory. The reader is urged to follow up some of the references in the text, as a full exploration of these complex issues could not be attained within the scope of this section.

THERAPEUTIC COMMUNICATION AND THE OLDER PATIENT

As suggested in the first part of this chapter, to help the older patient with a communication difficulty, the first prerequisite must be the nurse's knowledge of how communication takes place. The second prerequisite is the ability to use this knowledge to helping the patient. This is more than just the communication skills we use in an everyday conversation. 'The practice of relying on previously learned social skills used strictly for developing friendships has proven to be unsuccessful' (Hames and Joseph, 1980) when attempting to develop a relationship with a client and help with his problems.

Communication skills can be learned like any other skill, although they may be seen as a lifelong acquisition and application of knowledge. It is not a case of picking up a few ideas and trying them out on a patient.

Sundeen *et al.* (1976) suggest a few important principles to bear in mind:

- There may be no right or wrong method of helping someone. Styles of helping are individual and each nurse develops her own unique fashion.
- The outcome of communication does not necessarily make the patient feel better. The main purpose is to help patients express their thoughts and feelings and to find ways of solving their difficulties. Helping to solve the problem may therefore not be the first task. Indeed, decisions made by the nurse may later inhibit help being given later on.

Nurses who are really successful with patients need to know more than the proper communication techniques. They need to develop a way of demonstrating to patients that they care about them as people, otherwise 'any use of therapeutic communication skills are totally ineffectual' (Hames and Joseph, 1980).

Some of the main skills the nurse can deploy are identified as:

- *Broad opening statements.* This technique allows patients to start defining their own feelings. Statements such as 'let's talk', 'tell me more about what brought you here' are sufficiently generalized to let the patient take the initiative in introducing topics and to think through problems (Murray and Zentner, 1975).
- *Reflection.* This is a technique nurses use to repeat or rephrase what patients have said so that they can clarify their thoughts. Murray and Zentner (1975) suggest that the main purpose of reflection is to help the patient to 'see his own attitudes', confusions, ambivalences and perceptions accurately (hopefully expressed by another person)... but with a new quality stripped of the complications of caution'. For example:

Patient: Nurse, I'm really fed up, I thought I'd only be here a few days.
Nurse: You're fed up?
Patient: Yes, I thought the tablets would get my legs going again.

Reflection, with the nurse adding no new ideas or suggestions helps the patient to clarify or give more details about his feelings.

- *Speaking the implied.* A technique described by Hames and Joseph (1980) as adding to what the patient states, thus encouraging him 'to continue with the conversation and to focus on the problem'. For example:

Patient: I've always looked forward to going home before, but with all the extra responsibilities, this time...
Nurse: This time you're dreading it?
Patient: Yes, I just don't see how I can look after myself and my husband as well, especially now that he's incontinent.

This technique differs from reflection in that the nurse is adding to what the patient has said to help her identify clearly what is bothering her.

- *Clarification.* An attempt by the nurse to clearly understand the patient's problem by getting him to clarify ideas which the nurse has found vague or meaningless. The nurse may have to say, 'I'm sorry I don't quite understand that, can you explain it for me.' Doing this in an unobtrusive manner, allowing the patient to express something more clearly in different terms will allow the problem to be identified. This does not mean that the nurse appears unhelpful or 'slow', for 'it is not necessary to understand everything he says as long as you are honest about it and do not pretend to understand what you do not. Attempting to discover what the person is talking about can help him to become clearer to himself' (Murray and Zentner, 1975).
- *Silence.* This is a non-verbal method of communicating which allows the patient to collect and organize his/her thoughts. The technique however, requires considerable skill to be used positively. Silences or lulls in conversation can feel socially uncomfortable. The nurse herself may feel the need to break the silence because of her own self-conscious feelings (Collins, 1977). However, silence is 'a golden opportunity to contemplate thoughtfully what has been said and felt, to weigh alternatives, to formulate new ideas and to gain a new perspective of the matter under discussion'.
- *Placing the event in time or sequence.* This technique helps the patient 'to develop a clearer perspective regarding a given event' (Hames and Joseph, 1980). Questions such as 'what were you doing before you fell?' or 'when did you first notice you couldn't see properly?' not only help the nurse get an idea of the patient's problem but also help the patient see the issue more clearly himself.
- *Offering oneself.* This may involve setting specific periods of time when you will be with the patient to talk. It may be as structured as making a specific appointment, for example: 'I'll be back at 3

o'clock tomorrow and we can talk some more then', or may be less formal: 'let's get together with your husband sometime this afternoon and we'll discuss this'. What is more important is that patients feel the nurse is ready and available to talk with them when they need it. It might require the nurse to select the time and place carefully (considering privacy and avoiding interruptions) as well as showing that she is ready to listen without necessarily saying anything. For example, a non-verbal technique might involve finishing one task, but then sitting with the patient in a relaxed posture (as opposed to standing over him, looking impatient to be away).

- *Summarizing*. All therapeutic communication needs to end with a summary of what has taken place. The summary will 'bring together important points of discussion and give particular emphasis to progress made toward greater understanding' (Murray and Zentner, 1975). Summarizing therefore helps to close the conversation, ensure that both parties are closer to understanding what has been said and may simplify plans and arrangements that have been agreed. Thus the patient and nurse will each have a clearer idea of what course of action they each next take as a result of the conversation.

SOME BARRIERS TO EFFECTIVE COMMUNICATION

Many barriers may exist, often used habitually in conversation, which may inhibit a nurse's ability to help a patient. Joseph (1980) summarizes some of the main aspects of these barriers thus:

- *Trust*. Without trust between nurse and patient there is little opportunity for a therapeutic relationship to develop. Trust is not innate to the relationship. It evolves, based on the nurse's acceptance of the patient, the competence she demonstrates, her willingness to be open, honest and committed to the care of the patient.
- *False reassurance*. Well-meaning statements are used, but which often belittle the importance of the patient's real feelings. For example, 'Don't worry, everything will be all right' or 'Never mind about that, there are lots of people worse off than you.'

- *Giving advice.* The purpose of therapeutic communication is to help the patient solve his/her own problems. Giving advice, namely attempting to solve patients' problems for them by making decisions or telling them how to act, removes this purpose. It may help the patient through some initial difficulty, but ultimately it promotes dependence on the nurse and discourages patients from making their own decisions and acting independently.
- *Probing.* Although it is necessary to ask questions in the conversation, the use of too many may inhibit patients expressing their feelings or serve to distract or sidetrack them from the main issues. It may make patients feel defensive. Therapeutic communication therefore requires the nurse to be able to judge the fine line between appropriate and excessive questioning.
- *Changing the subject.* The nurse changes the topic during the course of the conversation. It may be that she has failed to pick up what the patient is trying to say and unwittingly moves on to another issue. On the other hand, it might be used by both nurse and patient to avoid a subject that is too embarrassing or difficult to explore at present.
- *Minimizing the patient's feelings.* Belittling or trivializing what patients say may make them feel that their feelings are unimportant. Patients need to know that their views are valued and 'special' to the nurse. Thus, attempting to console distressed patients with comments such as 'Lots of women get lumps in their breasts, you've really nothing to worry about' goes against the grain of therapeutic communication.
- *Trite expressions.* Glib remarks may block communication. Expressions such as 'Don't worry, you'll get over it', 'Plenty more fish in the sea' or 'No use crying over spilled milk' abound in everyday language but have little place in a helping relationship.
- *Jumping to conclusions.* Here, the nurse responds too quickly without listening to all that the patient has to say, and exploring the issue more fully. For example:

Patient: I can't decide about these nursing homes, there's a lot of variation in the price.

Nurse: But this one's cheap and it looks nice.

Patient (hesitantly): Oh, yes, I suppose you're right.

- *Inappropriate use of facts.* Here, the nurse may be more concerned with giving factual information than in responding to the patient's feelings. The patient may wish to explore an issue more deeply, but the nurse remains distant behind a barrier of facts. For example:

Patient: I feel so ill, these tablets...
Nurse: Yes, they're Distalgesics. Sometimes they can make you feel off colour.
Patient: Yes, but I'm so fed up, what's going on?
Nurse: They're painkillers. I can see about adjusting the times, sometimes we just have to get the timing right.

- *Interruption.* This, in effect, is 'cutting patients off', interrupting them before they have had the chance to explore their feelings. The habit of listening needs to be developed to prevent interruption.
- *Prolonged silence.* Silence can be used to allow patients to gather their thoughts and express feelings, but a prolonged silence extends beyond the point of usefulness if both patient and nurse become uncomfortable. Therefore there is a non-therapeutic as well as therapeutic component to silence.

The previous summary of therapeutic and non-therapeutic communication techniques suggest that communication skills are vitally important in the helping process. Each nurse needs to examine very carefully how she communicates with others and must begin to develop the skill of thinking about responses in advance and becoming a real helper to the patient.

Case study
Mrs Ziegler was afraid and anxious because of her recent attacks of chest pains. Her admission to hospital for tests left her fearful for the future. To relieve anxiety, promote acceptance of her care and relaxation and understanding, her nurse identified the following principal points.

- Spend time sitting and talking with her – listen and problem-solve.
- Give her time to express fears and feelings, listen in accepting manner.
- Give accurate, appropriate explanations on problems and management, explain all procedures, tests and care in advance, give time for questions and answers to clarify understanding.
- Involve her in decision-making process about care. Involve relatives/other carers also. Give her access to her care plans and encourage her to participate in her care plan.
- Deal with the other problems (pain, discomfort) as planned.

- Maintain nurse/patient allocation to promote trusting relationships.
- Clarify nature of any problems and help to identify solutions.
- Remain with and offer comfort through touch if she is distressed.
- Encourage her to join with other patients in afternoon relaxation therapy sessions.

HEARING DIFFICULTIES

Birren and Woods (1985), noting the arguments around the ageing process and hearing loss, suggest that 'it is sufficiently widespread however, to be a likely accompaniment of advancing age for many older persons'. While primarily affecting day-to-day communication, they note also that there can be a secondary involvement of hearing loss in its detrimental effects on intellectual functioning. In addition, it is asserted that a tendency towards paranoia in some older adults is exacerbated by hearing loss.

Murphy (1987) suggest that one of the most significant contributions the nurse can make is helping with a thorough assessment of the extent of the patient's difficulty. Mills (1985) notes that it is necessary to distinguish between true hearing difficulties, which may prevent the brain receiving the information, and other pathological states in the brain (e.g. the dementias), which may allow the information in, but prevent the patient interpreting it correctly.

Murphy (1987) has identified two main sources of loss of hearing. The first is *conductive* loss, a breakdown of the ability of the ear to transmit sounds. This may be caused by changes in the character of the cerumen (wax) combining with a tendency to produce more dry scaling skin to result in a plug of debris in the outer ear. Alternatively it may be due to diseases in the sensitive structures of the middle ear. To some extent surgical or medical intervention may be able to correct the latter or specific aids may be used to increase amplification.

The second main cause of hearing loss is *sensorineural* or *perceptive*. This occurs in about 85 per cent of the elderly affected by hearing impairment. Generally there is little that can be done in the way of medical or surgical intervention because the damage in this case affects the neural elements of the inner ear or auditory pathways. This form of hearing loss due to the ageing process is termed presbyacusis.

Recent reports (Davies, 1983) show that over 5½ million people in England and Wales, aged 60 and over have hearing loss severe enough to cause problems in hospital or other healthcare circumstances. High-tone loss produces difficulty in discriminating speech. Tinnitus is also often associated with hearing loss producing 'head noises' which Murphy (1987) suggests may even lead to severe depression or suicidal tendencies. Another phenomenon known as 'recruitment' may also affect the elderly, where minor background noises (such as a radio or television in a day-room) may be perceived as being painfully loud.

Detection, diagnosis and appropriate treatment are crucial to helping the elderly with hearing loss. Nurses need not only to be aware of the factors causing hearing difficulties, but also the features such as those mentioned above which aggravate the problem and the means, such as the correct use of hearing aids, to alleviate them.

Murphy (1987) and Mills (1985) identify a number of major steps nurses can adopt to help:

- Be close enough to the patient when speaking so that the face (to aid lip-reading, expression, etc.) can be seen.
- Reduce background noise during conversation (e.g. turn TV or radio off).
- Maintain as much eye contact as possible during conversation.
- Control noise levels generally in the environment.
- Choose other means of communication to back-up the spoken word, for example written notes, pictures, alarm lights, call bells, higher volume telephones, etc.
- Use close contact/touch to attract attention and maintain contact.
- Check that any hearing aid is working and suitable (making a referral to an audiologist if necessary). Aids should be checked and cleaned regularly (Fountain, 1987), especially for accumulating secretions, condensation or failed mechanism.
- Avoid shouting, instead speak slowly and clearly, with obvious lip movements and in a low voice.
- Check the ears regularly for accumulation of cerumen, and carry out cleaning and irrigation if necessary.
- Rephrase and repeat statements to ensure understanding.
- Cupping the hand over the least deficient ear may be helpful.
- Keep the patient informed of help available and give information to promote understanding of care.

The Royal National Institute for the Deaf (see useful addresses at the end of the book) can provide much help and guidance to the hard of hearing and those caring for them.

VISUAL DIFFICULTIES

Changes of sight are common phenomenon in the older patient. Degenerative changes particularly affect the lens and iris as well as certain common disease processes (e.g. cataract and glaucoma) (Graham, 1985). As long ago as 1948, Sheldon's survey suggested that fewer than 6 per cent of the elderly are able to read without the aid of spectacles (quoted in Exton-Smith and Overstall, 1979).

Gould (1987) believes that defects of this nature may severely reduce the leisure pursuits the patient can enjoy, while noting that 'these problems are of major concern to nurses working in hospital, where the effects of anxiety and unfamiliar surroundings may exacerbate existing sensory deficits. In the community, the district nurse or health visitor may be the first to hear the patient complain about failing eyesight.'

Brocklehurst *et al.* (1976) indicate that declining vision is closely associated with an increased incidence of fractured femur. Wilder-Smith and Thorpe (1981) link the problem closely to an increasing incidence of falls in general while Begbie (1967) notes its detrimental effects on balance.

Gould (1987) and Eliopoulos (1980) note a number of important measures nurses can take to assist the elderly person with a vision problem:

- Ensure spectacles are clean, well fitted, and checked regularly by an optician.
- Minimize risk of falls in the environment by removing obstacles, having smooth, well-fitted non-slip mats or carpets. Avoid patterned floor coverings which may give impression of steps or objects.
- Well-fitting footwear needs to be supplied for walking.
- Provide good illumination (older people see better in good light, and adaptation in poor light takes place more slowly). Several soft lights are preferable to a single direct one.
- Objects are seen most clearly when set in contrast. Thus, books, prescriptions, etc. are better seen in conventional black and white (possibly in larger print) than in different shades of the same colour.
- Choose other aids to assist the visually impaired, for example watches where the dials can be touched, radio as an alternative to newspapers, games and cards etc. where the number marks are raised, large print books, notepads, luminous telephone dials, 'talking books', etc.

- Face the patient when speaking to him/her, possibly exaggerating facial gestures and expressions.
- Spending time sitting and talking with the patient, explaining what is happening and encouraging others such as relatives and visitors to do the same.

SPEECH DIFFICULTIES

Hearing loss may also affect speech patterns. Speech training may be needed by older patients whose hearing loss limits their ability to hear their own speech (Yurick *et al.,* 1980). Speech training may help to conserve normal speech and to correct problems associated with loudness, clarity or quality of speech. The work of the speech therapist is vital here, and the nurse needs to liaise closely with her in following the guidelines set.

Apart from speech difficulties associated with hearing problems, other factors may affect speech requiring the intervention of an expert therapist (e.g. facio-maxillary surgery) with nursing support. However, one of the most common factors affecting speech in old age is cerebrovascular accident (stroke). Edwards and Davies (1985) estimate that 'probably 3 to 4 per cent of the elderly have verbal communication problems', and assert that 'the restoration of even minimal communication restores human dignity and worth of the patient to all carers, including the person and family'. According to them, some of the main terms encountered with speech problems are:

The aphasias/dysphasias (loss or difficulty with understanding and expression of language)

- *Expressive aphasia.* Intelligence is not affected, but the patient has difficulty finding words and a loss of fluency. Reading and writing skills may also be affected, sometimes to the point of failure to be able to read aloud.
- *Sensory or receptive aphasia.* There is difficulty in comprehending the written or spoken word, especially if the words are presented in isolation rather than in, say, the context of a sentence. The more severe the lack of comprehension, the more difficult the patient's speech is to understand – the words expressed may be fluent but appear to have no meaning.
- *Anomia.* Aphasia where the patient has a disproportionate difficulty in word finding.

- *Apraxia, dyspraxia.* Difficulty in producing the movements required (e.g. of tongue or mouth) to produce words. Chewing, sucking and swallowing remain intact, but the patient is often unable to protrude the tongue to command, purse the lips or imitate gesture or movement voluntarily.
- *Agnosia.* Loss of recognition, usually confined to one sense organ, either vision, hearing or touch. The ability, for example, to identify objects and understand their purpose results. The patient may stare at a cup of tea before him and be unable to understand what it is for.
- *Alexia/agraphia.* Alexia is the impairment of reading ability due to brain damage (as opposed to dyslexia, which is a developmental disorder of children who have problems in learning reading skills). Often accompanying alexia is agraphia, impairment of writing skills. This may be exacerbated if, for example, the patient has to change to the use of the non-preferred hand for writing or has accompanying visual defects.
- *Global aphasia.* The persistence, for example after the stroke, of loss of comprehension of spoken, written and non-verbal language.
- *Dysarthria.* This is another group of speech difficulties, but in contrast to the language problem of the aphasic patient, the dysarthric patient knows what he/she wishes to say, but cannot articulate words or co-ordinate breathing to produce intelligible speech. This may occur, for example, after a stroke or in Parkinson's disease. Dysarthria is a collective term for a number of related speech disorders, depending on the site of the lesion and the nature of the deficit (Darley, Aronson and Brown, 1975).

Helping the Patient with a Speech Difficulty

It is important that the nurse works closely with the speech therapist in co-ordinating the care of specific speech difficulties. The team approach is essential here. However, even if there is no speech therapist available, 'the patient will still need understanding and help from those who are caring for him' (Mort, 1985). Isted (1979) writes with some feeling, from personal experience, of the ways the stroke patient, for example, can best be helped: 'I found myself thinking clearly enough, but deprived of the abilities to speak and write. The frustration was intense and often overwhelming. Confusion, fear, anxiety: I experienced all of these as my speech became involved and deteriorated almost completely.'

The following points are drawn from the work of Isted (1979), Silverman (1980), Borsig and Steinacker (1982), Edwards and Davies (1985) and Mort (1985):

- Enhance communication by listening, observing, interpreting, empathizing (asking oneself, *what* one is communicating, i.e. by body language, tone, expression, etc.).
- Use clear simple speech with a raised voice (but not shouting) and the faces of nurse and patient in good light.
- Use adult speech and language at all times, but keep speech and language simple, aided by repetition.
- Ensure that dentures, glasses, hearing aid and other appliances are functioning correctly.
- Learn alternative methods to speech with the help of the therapist, for example signs, writing and mechanical aids, such as the 'canon communicator', 'blisstalk memowriter', 'possum communicator' or 'microwriter' (for further details on these see list of addresses at the end of the book). The choice of these items of equipment should only be with the advice of the speech therapist.
- Work with other relevant therapists to enhance other aspects of communication (e.g. hearing, vision).
- Minimize background noise.
- Help with simple screening procedures.
- Provide mental stimulation (orientation to time, place, weather, outside events, etc.) to encourage and preserve communication.
- Involve family, friends, other appropriate patients in care to promote conversation. Help them to understand the patient's difficulties and advise on ways they can participate.
- Provide a bell, buzzer or telephone to attract attention if unable to do so by voice.
- Sit with patients when talking with them, avoid appearing to be in a hurry to be away.
- Choose questions which are simple and direct and which can be answered with one word or a nod of the head.
- Watch for facial expression, ask questions in another way if the patients response is unclear (e.g. he/she may not be able to differentiate between 'yes' and 'no').
- Listen for key words to try and get the gist of a sentence – perhaps repeating this as a question to ensure understanding (e.g. the toilet? a drink?).

- Do not be afraid to tell patients that understanding them is difficult. Ask them to repeat and speak a little louder or more slowly if necessary.
- If the patients are speaking clearly, but the words do not make sense, try to imagine what the correct word is and put it to them as a question.

Patient: I want a road.
Nurse: Do you want your wheelchair? The toilet? A drink?

- If the patient becomes distressed then consider postponing the discussion rather than adding to his/her frustration. If possible, the nurse can alleviate the patient's despair by taking some of the responsibility on herself, for example 'I'm sorry, I'm just not with it today, I'll come back later with some ideas when I've had a think.'
- Avoid assuming that patients' requests can be solved by an offer of the toilet, or taking them there if they cannot be understood (everyone else may do the same!).
- Co-ordinate care with a limited number of nurses (e.g. through patient allocation) to reduce confusion and promote understanding of the patient's individual needs and means of expression.
- Practise the patients' speech exercises with them. Encourage them by praising achievements.
- Deal with the patient's other problems (e.g. attention to hygiene, dressing, sleep, promoting hobbies and interests) to boost morale.
- Provide a relaxed atmosphere, with privacy and peace and quiet, especially during specific speech therapy sessions.

Case study

Mrs Patel had lost her speech after her 'stroke'. An additional factor was that her command of English was poor. The nurse worked with her family, who were keen to be involved in helping her, to identify the following main points of her care; to help restore her speech and help her understand where she was and what is happening, and to help her make her needs and wishes known:

- Use of alternative means of communication:
  Pen and paper if she can write simple English words.
  A picture communication chart.
  Gestures, for example squeeze of the hand, nodding of the head, blinking, etc.
- Speak to Mrs Patel slowly, preferably in full view of her so that lip

movement and facial expression can be observed. Do not shout.

- Once she has developed some vocabulary, speak to her from the affected side which is impaired.
- Give her time to understand and respond. Repeat words if meaning appears to be lost, avoid anticipating what lines to say or 'putting words in her mouth'.
- Give her assurance that she is understood and make every effort to understand her. Show that you have time for her, appear unhurried by sitting with her.
- Give praise for attempts made to communicate either verbally or by gesture, no matter how small.
- Use the same simple words frequently in short sentences.
- Avoid frustration and unhappiness by indicating encouraging signs of progress.
- Involve her in other activities on the ward to promote communication, for example sitting at the table with the other patients at meal-times. Ensure they are aware of her difficulties.
- Give her an opportunity to read the newspapers or other magazines if she wishes.
- Find out her interests and take time to talk with her about them.
- Involve relatives/others in care and advise on methods of helping with speech. They will help with interpretation when possible.
- Refer to speech therapist and follow techniques/advice given on helping patient with speech problems.
- Refer to patient always by her preferred name (Mrs Patel etc.).
- Give honest accurate information to patient and family when desired and repeat as often as necessary if uncertain.
- Teach relevant aspects of the above care to her family.
- Ask relatives etc. to maintain visits and talk with her, about happenings at home.
- Help her family to understand her care and participate in it as they wish.
- Spend time talking with patient and give her time to express fears/anxieties. Listen and help identify her problems and help with solutions.

TOUCH

A general loss in sensitivity to touch often accompanies the ageing process (Yurick *et al.,* 1980). This may be caused by disease, injury or cirulatory insufficiency, or by degeneration of the Meissner corpuscles (responsible for sensitivity to light touch) in the skin (Kenshalo, 1977). Sensitivity to changes in temperature, to painful stimuli or to recognizing objects by touch declines. These features are exacerbated in certain disease process such as strokes. Older patients may thus be at greater risk from the dangers of extremes of temperature or damage to the skin, because of diminished awareness of the dangers present. While being aware of these difficulties, and perhaps modifying the environment to take account of them, it is also important that the nurse does not produce a sheltered institutionalized setting (Yurick *et al.*, 1980) in an excess of zeal to protect the patient.

Touch also has a significant social and psychological function. 'Touch is not only a means of sensory stimulation, but also an expression of warmth and caring' (Eliopoulos, 1980). Touch is a vital part of communication with the elderly person, and becomes increasingly important with greater degrees of changes in vision and hearing. A squeeze of a hand, a gentle pat on the shoulder or an affectionate cuddle not only serve to gain the patient's attention, they restore the sense of being valued, and minimize the touch-deprivation that may come with old age. The elderly person who lives alone, or has limited friends or family, may not experience the warmth and affection that comes from the daily social contact of loved ones (Elder, 1977; de Beauvoir, 1986).

The nurse can fill this gap herself, in the day-to-day interaction with patients. It needs to be done with sincerity and with an assessment that the patient wishes for and accepts such close contact (Yurick *et al.*, 1980). In addition, there are alternatives which nurses can explore, not least the use of pets, to provide touch and companionship to the older patient. There is much evidence to show that pets, especially cats and dogs which allow close contact, are sources of love and companionship to the elderly (Levinson, 1969; Corson *et al.*, 1975) and serve to restore morale and promote interest in life. Pets which can be touched and held are particularly helpful, but interest and enjoyment in caring for another living thing can also be derived from fish, plants or birds. The nurse's imagination in suggesting or providing suitable choices is of considerable help. Other elements of touch in relation to pets and companionship are also dealt with in Chapters 11 and 15.

NURSING THE OLDER PATIENT WHO IS MENTALLY HANDICAPPED

Recent government policies have sought to establish more mentally handicapped people in the community. There are implications for nurses involved with older adults, for many of their mentally handicapped are or will become elderly people and may need help from nurses who have little experience or contact with them. For example, a patient may be admitted from home to hospital for medical or surgical intervention.

Essentially, mentally handicapped people require little that is different in care from other adults. The principles discussed throughout this text apply equally to the mentally handicapped (Sines and Bicknell, 1985). Often, the greatest disadvantage for patients with these problems - and the levels of their difficulties are very variable - is the limitation in making others aware of their problems and getting appropriate help (Sines and Bicknell, 1985).

The general nurse, however, is not alone when uncertainties arise in dealing with mentally handicapped people. Each district has its own resettlement officer co-ordinating the return to the community and each patient has a nurse with the specialist skills in the community, who can be contacted to advise management. They can give information for the assessment and help with the planning of care. Their work with clients includes attending hospital and remaining with them to help if necessary. Those with severe difficulties will need this degree of support, and an open and co-operative relationship between various nurses and other professionals is in the best interest of the patient.

A CONFUSED STATE OF MIND

Jean Faugier's section later in this chapter deals in more detail with disorientation, and the ways to deal with it, that may come with advancing years. At this point it is worth noting that the essential role of the nurse is to participate in assessment (to identify the cause) and to help minimize the effects.

Brooking (1986) defines dementia as 'a progressive and usually irreversible decline in previously normal mental function, which is associated with detectable brain pathology'. Confusion, on the other hand, is an 'acute or subacute alteration in previously normal mental function, which is often temporary and reversible, associated with impaired brain function usually secondary to a pathological process outside the nervous system'.

Pre-senile dementia is considered as that which occurs before the age of 65 and is associated with disease processes such as Huntington's chorea or syphilis (Miller, 1977). Over half the cases of the senile dementias are caused by Alzheimer's disease, which also accounts for many of the instances of pre-senile dementia, and is associated with a degeneration of neurones and cerebral circulation (Kastenbaum, 1979).

With dementia, the process is essentialy irreversible, as the patient becomes progressively disorientated in time, place and sense of self. Reasoning and emotions are disrupted and the patient's whole life-style is affected in terms of both social changes (affects on the family and marriage and family) and physical changes of general accompanying deterioration. 'Confusion' may produce essentially similar problems, and is often of a relatively rapid onset, depending on the underlying cause. Where this is dealt with, then the patient stands a good chance of recovery. For example, dealing with the chest infection causing cerebral hypoxia, teaching and explaining to the patient to overcome 'translocation stress' (see Chapter 4) or restoring hydration. Brooking (1986) identifies nine main areas for assessment of the cause.

(1) Pharmacological, either as a side-effect or withdrawal effect of a wide range of drugs, e.g. steroids, sedatives or diuretics.
(2) Nutritional deficiencies, e.g. of vitamins.
(3) General medical conditions, e.g. anaemia, hypotension.
(4) Infections, e.g. pneumonia, septicaemia.
(5) Endocrine disorders – almost any hormonal imbalance may produce confusion.
(6) Neurological conditions, e.g. trauma, neoplasms.
(7) Surgical causes, especially after major surgery or prolonged anaesthesia.
(8) Environmental causes – sensory deprivation due to loss of spectacles, inefficient hearing aids, loss of familiar environment, background noise and lights.
(9) Psychological – the 'self-fulfilling prophecy' as the patient who is confused becomes even more so because he/she is treated as such by the staff.

Yurick *et al.* (1980), Brooking (1986) and Stokes (1986) identify the major principles for nursing consideration (see also details in Faugier's section in this chapter):

- Offering both physical and mental sustained stimulation, e.g. games, outings, exercise, visitors, parties, and so on.
- Providing a physical environment conducive to social interaction, e.g. dining tables with *small* groups of patients; arranging furniture to permit conversation.
- Nursing patients in small groups with familiar nurses. Providing stimulation yet avoiding stress (e.g. constant television, noise in the home or irregular visits which may exacerbate rather than diminish confusion).
- Maintaining patient participation and choice in care. Explaining and teaching about what is happening around them and what care is being given.
- Avoiding restraint and restriction of activity.
- Using diversionary, reality, orientation, and reminscence therapy techniques as well as behavioural modification techniques, such as rewards for good behaviour.
- Maintaining maximum independence of the patient in managing other personal needs (e.g. hygiene) by guiding, teaching, helping rather than adopting an interventionist and custodial approach.

Case study

Harry O'Dowd was being nursed at home by his wife, who had been coping well since the onset of his Alzheimer's disease. Her sudden admission to hospital for urgent surgery led to his urgent admission to hospital until she was well enough to return. He was often disorientated in time and place, 'mixed up' as to where he was and what was happening to him. He had difficulty expressing his needs and feelings. The nursing care of this patient and his particular problem was aimed at promoting orientation to time and place and helping him to express needs/feelings so that appropriate help could be given.

- Refer to patient always by preferred name (Harry).
- Introduce yourself when speaking to him.
- Maintain nurse/patient allocation to reduce confusion of too many carers.
- Keep bed in same area of ward. A neighbour was asked to provide familiar personal effects from home, especially his own clothing and a photograph of his wife.
- Speak to Harry slowly, meaningfully and preferably in full view so that lip movement and facial expression can be observed. Do not shout.
- Give him time to understand and respond. Repeat words if meaning appears to be lost, avoid anticipating what he tries to say or 'putting words in his mouth'.

- Give Harry assurance that he is understood and make every effort to understand him. Show that you have time and appear unhurried by sitting with him.
- Use the same words regularly, repeat information as often as necessary to reinforce understanding. Keep him up to date with Mrs O'Dowd's condition.
- Involve him in other activities on the ward to promote communication and orientation, such as sitting at the table with the other patients at meal-times. Ensure they are aware of his difficulties.
- Allow him to listen to the radio and watch television and observe reaction to it. (Prolonged viewing or listening may serve to confuse or distress him.)
- Give him an opportunity to read the newspaper or other magazines if he wants to.
- Find out Harry's interests and take time to talk with him about them. He is known to have been a cricket and football fan.
- Give honest accurate information to patient when desired and repeat it as often as necessary if uncertain.
- Ask neighbours and friends to maintain visit and talk with him about happenings at home, the progress of his wife.
- Spend time talking with him, give time to express fears/anxieties and listen and help identify his problems and help with solutions.
- Involve friends and neighbours in care and advise on methods of helping with orientation.
- Guide/direct about ward area, indicate calendar, clock, signs/mirror, etc. to promote awareness of time/place.
- Help with other activities as planned.
- Use question/answer/reminiscence techniques to promote awareness of himself, both past and present.
- Provide opportunities for him to visit his wife, and vice versa when she is well enough, perhaps to have meals together or contact over the inter-ward telephone.

STATES OF MIND

Jean Faugier

The term 'elderly mentally ill' denotes an actual and potential cut-off point in many discussions about the care of older people. Often the label seems to indicate an enormous difference between those 'normal' elderly and those viewed as mentally ill. To anyone experienced in psychiatry, or with a passing knowledge of medical sociology the increased stigma attached to the 'mentally ill' elderly will come as no surprise.

Stigma and discrimination are, after all, the lot of the 'normal' elderly and the young mentally ill. To be both old and suffering from mental illness simply serves to intensify the alienation and isolation from society.

In discussing communication with the elderly mentally ill it should be stated at the outset that it is the similarities between the general elderly population and those diagnosed with a mental illness that are important, more so than the differences. The elderly mentally ill have all of the problems faced by the so-called 'normal' population of elderly people and as such will require the same consideration in communication from nurses. In a similar way the excessive confusion and forgetfulness of dementia, or other mental illness, is mirrored in a less severe form among many elderly people.

However, a substantial number of elderly people do suffer from either mild or more severe types of mental illness in old age, the most common being depression. Although a very normal human emotion, a response to loss or disappointment, depression can also be of great intensity, especially in the elderly. Feelings of utter hopelessness and despair may influence the whole being of the patient to such an extent as to make normal, active, participative communication virtually impossible. According to Pitt (1982), 'the depression is a representation of that state which is characterized by feeling totally without hope and impotent to change the unpleasant situation he/she faces'. Many old people in institutional care are all too familiar with such feelings of despair and hopelessness, and as such depression can often be said to be a normal reaction to environmental influences. Social factors interact forcibly with the psyche to produce depression, and as Simmons and Brooker (1986) point out, the isolated old person is much more likely to suffer deep feelings of loneliness, uselessness, and frustration. Loss of a loved one or a decline in one's ability which are often normal accompaniments of ageing are also important influences in producing a depressive reaction. Brown and Harris (1978) clearly link life events associated with loss and lack of meaning in life as being influential in producing a more pathological picture.

Severe depression can produce enormous difficulties in communication for the nurse. The marked characteristic, diurnal variation often means that many depressed old people are at their worst in the mornings, when quite complicated motor tasks need to be performed. The psychomotor retardation, a sometimes almost total slowing down of motor function complicates this further causing great anxiety for the patient and thereby creating a vicious circle. Giving time to the patient and ensuring that only a little information is given at one encounter will aid concentration and the ability to recall. Most essential however is the attitude nursing staff have to the inner despair and pain of the elderly depressed patient. Simply by being available to be with the patient as an active listener or to provide a comforting touch at times of most distress will help the patient feel more able to articulate the extent of the problem. It is very common in depressive illness to encounter feelings of guilt, unworthiness, auditory hallucinations and paranoid beliefs. Therapeutic communication (see earlier part of this chapter) means giving the patient the 'space' to articulate these intense and disturbing feelings whilst not seeking to argue or reinforce them. It is important that the nurse listens very carefully and doesn't dismiss as 'crazy' the sometimes bizarre worries or concerns of the patient. Often these are unconscious or symbolic communications which can assist in giving a clearer picture of the patient's mental state. Depressed old people often refer to the feeling of 'rotting away inside' from some dreadful disease. They may present to the nurse grossly disturbed images of bodily function. To communicate effectively with the patient nurses should be looking beyond the manifest content of verbal communication to the latent content. For example, a patient who feels that his flesh is rotting away from the inside may be communicating in a symbolic way how he feels about the disintegration of his personality or psyche under the weight of depressive feelings.

Other patients who suffer depression may, rather than becoming withdrawn and isolated, become extremely agitated. These troubled souls may pace the ward or constantly bother families and nursing staff seeking reassurance about some imagined wrongdoing. Unfortunately the reassurance they seek can never be accepted and nurses who believe so will simply be the victims of frustration. In psychiatric care, as Malan (1979) points out, reassurance often has the effect of attempting to dismiss or to cover the real feelings and conflicts of the patient. Sometimes it is of more value to allow patients to explore by the use of reminiscence therapy the areas of the past that have become distorted and are now troubling them. Weber (1980) points to the beneficial effort of taking the patient back through memories of their life events to examine how they previously coped with similar feelings in the past. The effect of such an exercise with some agitated or anxious depressive patients can, according to Weber (1980), have the effect of increasing self-esteem.

For a minority of the elderly population (approximately 0.66 per cent of the over-65s and up to 22 per cent of the 80s) the ageing process brings with it the fairly radical impairment of higher mental abilities known as dementia. Simmons and Brooker (1986) put the figure for the 65s–80s at 10 per cent or higher. Whatever the figure it remains true that whilst not being the most common mental illness among the elderly, dementia is the most serious. Alzheimer's disease, which is the most serious form, predominates in women and is characterized by gross impairment of judgement, self-criticism and abstract thinking.

In reality orientation, either a formal or an informal approach can be adopted (Brooking, 1986). The more formal setting is that of involving the patient with other similar people in a group setting. By meeting daily with the same people the group teaches information related to reality and reinforces interpersonal communication. A more common approach to reality orientation is the total immersion, informal approach. The entire therapeutic encounter of nursing staff and patients is used during the day to reinforce and stimulate learning of reality. Basic facts about time, place and persons are reiterated time and again throughout the day. Patients learn and relearn and are encouraged to repeat the information. Uses of commonly encountered objects, names of food and clothing are repeated by nursing staff whilst dealing with the patient. The whole approach of Reality Orientation is founded firmly on the notion cited by Pitt (1982) that 'The neurone is sick but not beyond recovery.' Evaluative studies such as those undertaken by Holden and Woods (1982) would suggest that reality orientation is useful in improving the patient's sense of being in the world. It is also undoubtedly important in providing a structure for nurse/patient communication, without which it may become more difficult for the nurse to see the reason to make efforts to communicate.

Reminiscence therapy, on the other hand, is not aimed at reinforcing the 'here and now' but makes use of the normal tendency of old people to remember the remote past more vividly than the present. Pitt (1982) points out that the remote past for many old people may be more vivid and interesting than the present so making this tendency all the more understandable.

Butler (1963) claims that the use of reminiscence therapy is based on a normal, naturally occurring universal mental process, the need to review one's life in old age. 'Ideally the review should result in new wisdoms and insights so that the old person can retire from life with an acceptable image and dignity' (Brooking, 1986). Using memories evoked by old songs, old photographs, old sounds, films, even the use of old tastes and smells, the nurse is able to provide an atmosphere in which such a positive life review may take place. Such a journey however requires sensitive communication skills on the part of the nurse; active listening, acceptance and interest all combine to make the memories seem worthwhile and pleasant. It should never be forgotten however that we all have in our past bad memories and deep sadness and regrets as well as proud moments and happiness. Reminiscence therapy can often evoke these times just as effectively as the good times and the nurse must be prepared to encounter sadness as a part of life review in an empathetic and sensitive way. In the same way the pleasures of the past may simply throw into sharper focus the futility of the future, or the absence of any future. 'A limited future and a frozen past: such is the situation that the elderly have to face up to. In many instances it paralyses them. All their plans have either been carried out or abandoned and their life has closed in about itself.'

The use of reminiscence therapy may, if used with skill and sensitivity, 'defrost' the memories of the past enabling patients not simply to enjoy pleasant memories but to stimulate interaction between patients around particular themes, thereby helping the patient to feel less isolated and affirmed as a useful communicating human being.

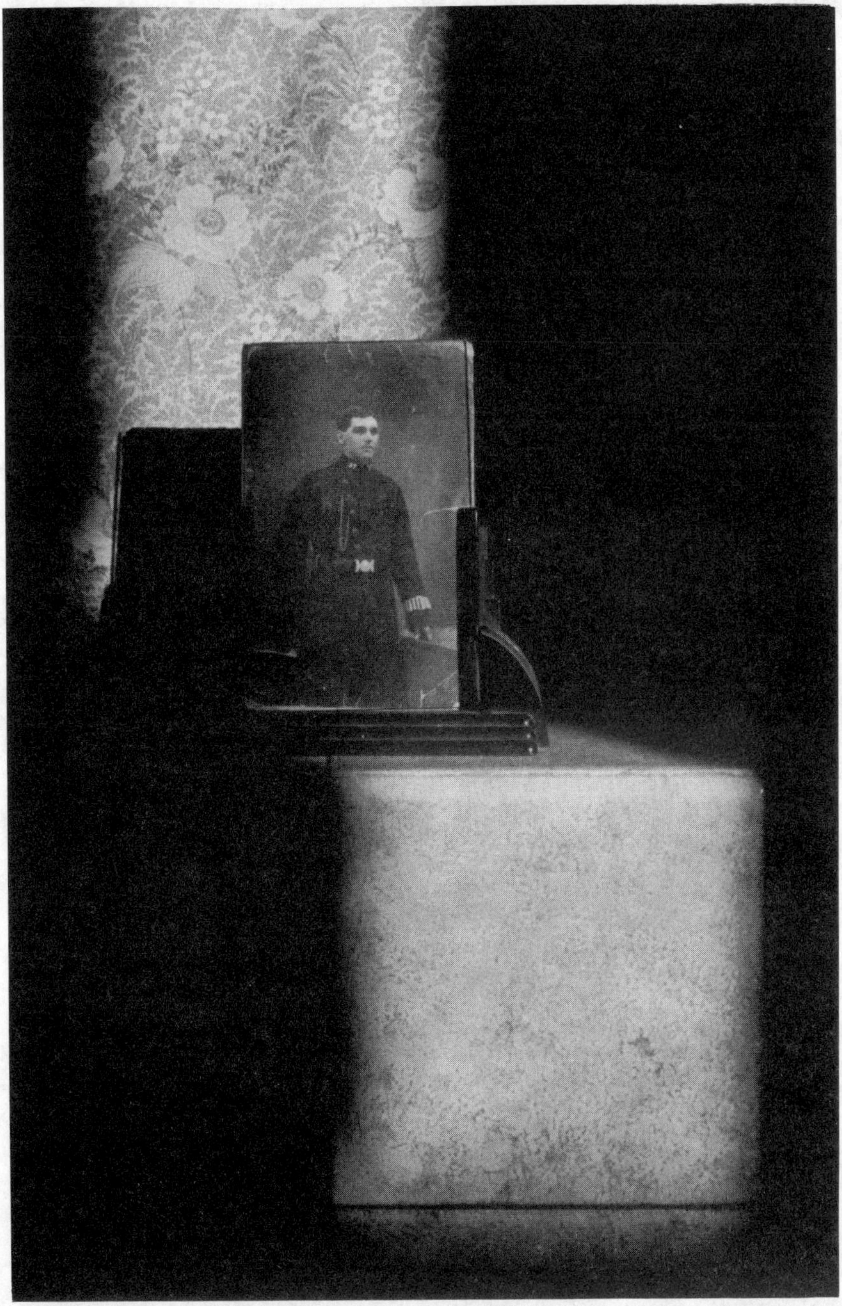

This chapter has suggested that the most crucial role for the nurse is that of effective communicator. Therapeutic communication is a skill requiring as much attention to detail as dealing with asepsis or giving medicines safely. For the nurse to be friend, partner and guide with patients, a trusting relationship built on shared understanding is a vital underpinning for a meaningful and productive nurse–patient relationship.

REFERENCES

Argyle, M. (1978) *The Psychology of Interpersonal Behaviour,* Penguin, Harmondsworth.

Attenborough, D. (1985) *Life on Earth,* Collins, London.

Begbie, G. H. (1967). Some problems of postural sway, in A.de Reuck and J. Knight (eds) *Myotactic, Kinesthetic and Vestibular Mechanisms. CIBA Foundation Symposium,* Churchill Livingstone, London.

Birren, J. E. and Woods, A. M (1985) *Psychology of Ageing,* in M. S. J. Pathy, *Principles and Practice of Geriatric Medicine,* Wiley, Chichester.

Blondis, M. N. and Jackson, N. E. (1977) *Nonverbal Communication with Patients,* Wiley, New York.

Borsig, A. and Steinacker, I. (1982) Communication with the patient in the intensive care unit, *Nursing Times,* (supplement) March 1982.

Bridge, W. and MacLeod Clark, J. (1981) *Communication in Nursing Care,* H. M. & M., London.

Brocklehurst, J. C., Exton-Smith, A. N., Lempert Barber, S. M., Hunt, L. and Palmer M. (1976) Fracture of the femur in old age: a two centre study of associated clinical factors and the cause of the fall, *Age Ageing,* Vol. 7, pp. 7–15.

Brooking, J. (1986) Depression and other mental disorders in the elderly, in S. Redfern (ed.) *Nursing Elderly People,* Churchill Livingstone, Edinburgh.

Brown, C. W. and Harris T. (1978) *Social Origins of Depression,* Tavistock, London.

Butler, R. N. (1963) The life review: an interpretation of reminiscence in the aged, *Psychiatry,* Vol. 26, pp. 65–76

Collins, M. (1977) *Communication in Health Care,* Mosby, St Louis.

Corson, S. A., O'Leary, J., Corson, E., Gwynne, P. H. and Arnold. L. E. (1975) Pet-facilitated psychotherapies in a hospital setting, in J. Masserma (ed.) *Current Psychiatric Therapies,* Grune & Stratton, New York.

Darley, F. L., Aronson, A. E. and Brown, J. R. (1975) *Motor Speech Disorders,* Saunders, Philadelphia.

Davies, A. C. (1983) Hearing disorders in the population, in M. E. Leitman and M. P. Haggard (eds) *Hearing Science and Hearing Disorders,* Academic Press, London.

De Beauvoir, S. (1977) *Old Age,* Penguin, Harmondsworth.

DHSS (1985) Ombudsman's Reports, London.

Edwards, J. and Davies, E. (1985) Disorders of communication, in M. S. J.

Pathy (1985) *Principles and Practice of Geriatric Medicine,* Wiley, Chichester.
Elder, G. (1977) *The Alienated: Growing Old Today,* Writers and Readers Publishing Co-operative, London.
Eliopoulos, C. (1980) *Geriatric Nursing,* Harper & Row, London.
Exton-Smith , A. N. and Overstall, P. (1979) *Geriatrics,* MTP Press, Lancaster.
Faulkner, A. (ed.) (1984) *Communication,* Churchill Livingstone, Edinburgh.
Fielding, P. (1986) *Attitudes Revisited,* RCN, London.
Fountain, D. (1987) Hearing aids and their care, *Geriatric Nursing and Home Care,* Vol. 2, pp. 10–11.
Gould, D. (1987) The biology of ageing: the special senses, *Geriatric Nursing and Home Care,* Vol. 7, no. 2, pp. 15–19.
Graham, P. (1985) The eye, in M. S. J. Pathy (1985) *Principles and Practice of Geriatric Medicine,* Wiley, Chichester.
Hall, E. J. (1966) *The Hidden Dimension,* Doubleday, New York.
Hames, C. C. and Joseph, D. H. (1980) *Basic Concepts of Helping: A Wholistic Approach,* Appleton-Century-Crofts, New York.
Henley, N. M. (1977) *Body Politics,* Prentice-Hall, Englewood Cliffs, NJ.
Holden, O. P. and Woods, R. T. (1982) *Reality Orientation: Psychological Approaches to the Confused Elderly,* Churchill Livingstone, London.
Isted, C. R. (1979) *Learning to Speak Again after a Stroke,* Kings Fund, London.
Johnson, D. (1972) *Reaching Out,* Prentice-Hall Englewood Cliffs, NJ.
Joseph, D. (1980) Non-verbal communication, in C. C. Hames and D.H. Joseph (eds) *Basic Concepts of Helping: A Holistic Approach,* Appleton-Century-Crofts, New York.
Kastenbaum R. (1979) *Growing Old,* Harper & Row, London.
Kendon, A. (1967) Some functions of gaze direction in social interaction, *Acta Psychologica,* Vol. 28, no. 1, pp. 1–47.
Kenshalo, D. R.(1977) Age changes in touch, vibration, temperature, kinesthesis and pain sensitivity, in I. Birren and K. Schaie (eds) *Handbook of the Psychology of Ageing,* Reinhold, New York.
Knapp, M. (1972) *Non-verbal Communication in Human Interaction,* Holt, Rinehart & Winston, New York.
Leathers, D. G. (1978) *Non-verbal Communication Systems,* Allyn & Bacon, Boston.
Levinson, B. M. (1969) Pets and old age. *Mental Hygiene,* Vol. 58, no. 3. p. 364.
Lewis, G. (1973) *Nurse–patient Communication,* Brown, Dubuque, Iowa.
MacLeod Clark, J. (1981) Communication in nursing: analysing nurse–patient communication, *Nursing Times,* Vol. 77, no. 1, pp. 12–18.
Malan, D. H. (1979) *Individual Psychotherapy and the Science of Psychodynamics,* Butterworths, London.
Melia, K. M. (1982) Tell it as it is – qualitative methodology and nursing research: understanding the student nurse's world, *Journal of Advanced Nursing,* Vol. 7, pp. 327–35.
Menzies, I. E. P. (1960) A case study on the functioning of social systems as a defence against anxiety, *Human Relations,* Vol. 13, no. 2, pp. 95–121.
Miller, E. (1977) *Abnormal Ageing: The Psychology of Senile and Pre-senile Dementia,* Wiley, Chichester.
Mills, R. (1985) The auditory system, in M. S. J. Pathy, *Principles and Practice*

of Geriatric Medicine, Wiley, Chichester.
Mort, M. (1985) *Retraining for the Elderly Disabled,* Croom Helm, Beckenham.
Murphy, K. (1987) Problems of Impaired Hearing, *Geriatric Nursing and Home Care,* Vol. 7, no. 2, pp. 9–11.
Murray, R. and Zentner, J. (1975) *Nursing Concepts for Health Promotion,* Prentice-Hall, Englewood Cliffs, NJ.
Pitt, B. (1982) *Psycho-geriatrics: An Introduction to the Psychiatry of Old Age,* Longman, Harlow.
Porritt, L. (1984) *Communication Choices for Nurses,* Churchill Livingstone, Edinburgh.
Satir, V. (1967) *Conjoint Family Therapy,* Science and Behaviour Books, California.
Silverman, F. H. (1980) *Communication for the Speechless,* Prentice-Hall, Englewood Cliffs, NJ.
Simmons, S. and Brooker, C. (1986) *Community Psychiatric Nursing: A Social Perspective,* Heinemann, London.
Sines, D. and Bicknell, J. (1985) *Nursing the Mentally Handicapped in the Community,* Harper & Row, London.
Stokes, G. (1986) *Screaming and Shouting,* Winslow Press, London.
Sundeen, S., Stuart, E. D., Rankin, E. D. and Cohen, S. P. (1976) *Nurse–Client Interaction,* Mosby, St Louis.
United Kingdom Central Council for Nursing and Midwifery (1986) *Project 2000,* London.
Weber, H. (1980) *Nursing Care of the Elderly,* Reston Publishing, New York.
Wilder-Smith, O. H. G. and Thorpe, T. A. S. (1981) How dangerous are falls in old people at home?, *British Medical Journal,* Vol. 282, pp. 2132–3.
Wilson-Barnett, J. (1981) Communication with patients in general wards, in Bridge and MacLeod Clark (eds) *Communication in Nursing Care,* H.M.&.M., London.
Yurick, A. G., Robb, S. S., Spier, B. E. and Ebert, N. J. (1980) *The Aged Person and the Nursing Process,* Appleton-Century-Crofts, New York.

6. Breathing

Rosemary Webster and David Thompson

INTRODUCTION

The body is dependent on breathing as an integral part of the process of respiration whereby oxygen is supplied to the tissues, carbon dioxide, the waste product of metabolism is eliminated, and the homeostatic acid-base balance is maintained. Breathing is thus necessary for the production of energy for bodily activities. Effective breathing enables efficient carrying out of activities of daily living. In the elderly, breathing problems reflect the effects of both normal ageing and disease processes of the respiratory system. Effective nursing intervention is based on a knowledge of probable causative factors and on an accurate assessment of the extent of the problem.

NORMAL BREATHING

Normal breathing involves the intake of oxygen from the atmosphere on inspiration and the expulsion of carbon dioxide on expiration. The complex interchange of oxygen and carbon dioxide within the lungs, known as pulmonary or external respiration, is dependent on adequate atmospheric oxygen, a functioning respiratory system, and the regulatory effects of muscle, nerve and chemical control. The exchange of gases between the cells and the blood, known as internal respiration, is dependent on the pumping action of the heart, the efficiency of the circulatory system, the oxygen-carrying capacity of the red blood cells and the efficiency of gaseous exchange at cellular level. Reduced functioning of any component of this complex cardiopulmonary system will lead to an impairment in breathing ability.

Change Associated with Old Age

As with any other body system, the respiratory system ages. However, the changes in structure and function that occur are so subtle that, in the absence of acute or chronic disease, the elderly are usually capable of effortless breathing (Krumpe *et al.*, 1985). The lungs have an enormous reserve capacity and are highly efficient, although respiratory failure may develop as a terminal event.

Mechanisms of Breathing

Air is moved in and out of the lungs by movements of the diaphragm and the associated muscles of respiration. Inspiration actively involves contraction of the diaphragm and intercostal muscle and the small neck muscle. The thoracic cavity elongates and the diaphragm distends. The rib cage is lifted up and the volume of the chest cavity is increased. On expiration, the diaphragm ascends, the rib cage falls and because of elasticity the lungs recoil. The abdominal muscles are often utilized for active expiration such as coughing, straining or laboured breathing but are normally relaxed during quiet expiration.

Effects of Ageing on Breathing

With ageing, osteoporosis of the rib cage and vertebrae may cause kyphoscoliosis and chest wall rigidity. The ribs and vertebrae decalcify while the costal cartilages become calcified. Osteoporosis of the spine and kyphoscoliosis appear in about 68 per cent of over 75-year-olds (Edge, Millard and Reid, 1964), and chest wall compliance has been shown to decrease with age (Mittman, Edelman and Norris, 1965).

Reduced elasticity and calcification of the costal cartilages can lead to weakness of the intercostal and accessory muscles of respiration causing impaired functional reserve capacity (the volume of gas left in the lungs after a normal breath, plus the extra that can be expired with effort), especially under stress. Reduced chest wall compliance and resulting reduced mobility of the rib cage accounts for the greater reliance of the elderly on their abdominal and diaphragmatic contribution to breathing (Rizzato and Marozzini, 1970).

The lungs of the elderly appear smaller and flabbier than those of younger persons, and their weight is decreased by about one-fifth. There is stenosis of the bronchi and supporting tissues and degeneration of the mucous glands and bronchial epithelium.

During the ageing process there is a decrease in elastic recoil of lung tissue leading to an increase in residual volume (the volume of gas left in the lungs after maximally filling and expiring fully). This decrease in elastic recoil is due to changes in elastin and collagen. The energy required for breathing necessary to overcome the elastic resistance of the lungs and thoracic cage and the resistance to gas flow in the respiratory passages is normally less than 3 per cent of total energy metabolism but can increase with age.

It appears that increased closure and collapse of narrowed and destabilized membranous bronchioles earlier in the respiratory cycle leads to increased air trapping and hyperinflation in the elderly with an increased amount of anatomical dead space with ageing (Martin Das and Young, 1979).

Lung Volume and Capacity

It is generally agreed (Krumpe *et al.,* 1985) that once growth and maturation are achieved, the minimal change in total lung capacity observed with ageing is probably as a result of diminished maximum inspiratory strength. However, narrowing of the membranous bronchioles with ageing results in a greater resistance to air flow. Residual volume increases with age due to a loss of elastic recoil and continued effort is required to achieve the maximum residual volume at very low lung volumes as expiration appears to be flow limited. Maximum expiration appears limited by the increased airway closure. The end result is a decrease in vital capacity (amount of air able to be expelled from the lungs after maximally filling and expiring fully) with age. Forced expiratory volume in the first second of a forced expiratory vital capacity (FEV_1) decreases by about 29 ml/year in average adult males, though the decrease is height related.

Diffusion of Gases

Oxygen from the pulmonary alveoli diffuses into the blood of the pulmonary capillaries and the carbon dioxide in the pulmonary blood diffuses into the alveoli. Gaseous diffusion occurs as a result of a difference in partial pressure of the gas on either side of the respiratory membrane and is influenced by the blood flow and distribution to the lungs, distribution of inspired gases, gas exchange surface availability, and the resistance to diffusion at alveolar level.

Diffusing capacity decreases with age. The increased residual volume and decreased vital capacity, but a relatively unchanged blood perfusion, mean that there is a decreased ventilation: perfusion ratio leading to alterations in arterial blood gas measurements. There is a decrease in the normal arterial oxygen tension with advancing age. The normal arterial PO_2 in elderly men is about 70 mmHg, compared to a normal adult value of about 100 mmHg.

Regulation of Respiration

Respiration is regulated by chemical, neural and sensory stimulation. Chemical respiratory control is mediated through chemoreceptors located in the carotid artery and aortic arch which respond to changes in the levels of CO_2, O_2 and the pH of the blood and relay this information to the respiratory centre in the medulla which then conveys appropriate information to the relevant repiratory muscles.

Neural signals also enter the medulla. The inflation reflex and pneumotaxic reflexes are important. Receptors in the lungs and thorax detect expansion of the lungs and transmit impulses via the vagus nerve to the respiratory centre to control breathing.

Normal elderly persons at rest breathe with minute ventilations identical to those of younger persons but with faster breathing frequencies and smaller tidal volumes.

Krumpe *et al.* (1985) report that several research studies have shown that the response of elderly persons to low O_2 or high CO_2 levels is blunted. The exact reasons for this are unclear but factors such as a decrease in respiratory neuronal outflow, blunted chemoreceptor drive and decreased ability to perceived changes in mechanical functioning of the lungs are thought to play a part.

Normal elderly subjects have a reduced ability to increase and maintain ventilation at higher levels during periods of increased oxygen demand such as during exercise (Norris, Shock and Yiengst, 1953).

A common disorder of breathing in the elderly is Cheyne–Stokes breathing. This is a regularly recurring cycle of gradually increasing and decreasing tidal volumes. Brandstetter and Kazemi (1983) report that evidence suggests that altered levels of arterial O_2 and CO_2 are not responsible for this disorder. It seems that the elderly may be predisposed to this pattern of breathing as a result of a combination of neurological and circulatory disturbances. It is possible that disease of the cerebral blood vessels with compromise of medullary blood flow and altered perfusion of the respiratory centre contributes to this dysfunction.

Respiratory Protection

Because of direct contact with the external environment the surface area of the lungs is prone to infection. Protective mechanisms include filtration of larger particles by nostril hairs, redirection of inhaled dust, bacteria and spores, etc. by the ciliated tracheal epithelium to the larynx for swallowing and trapping of particles by mucus produced by goblet cells in the trachea and bronchi. Macrophages ingest and destroy invading bacteria.

The elderly are more prone to breathing problems as a result of inhalation and ingestion. They have fewer cilia and the trachea bronchi are less able to recognize the presence of foreign bodies and noxious substances (Pontoppidan and Beecher, 1974). Mucus, bacteria and inhaled material is less easily removed from the lungs. Coughing is less effective in the elderly in terms of volume, force and flow rate. An accumulation of sputum as a result of inefficient clearing can lead to inadequate oxygen entry and inadequate removal of carbon dioxide producing hypoxia and respiratory acidosis. Macrophages become less efficient with ageing as a result of pollutants. Inhalation of foreign material potentially producing major respiratory illness is much more likely to occur in the ageing patient (Krumpe *et al.*, 1985). Ageing results in reduced competence of the lower oesophageal sphincter with increased likelihood of gastro-oesophageal reflux and aspiration for patients with hiatus hernia or oesophageal diverticuli. The elderly are at greater risk from aspiration after anaesthesia. Swallowing may be adversely affected as a result of strokes, muscle weakness or other neurological diseases, increasing the risk of inadvertent aspiration. Hughes *et al.* (1981) report on the incidence of lipid pneumonia occurring as a result of inadvertent aspiration of mineral oil taken as a laxative. Mineral oil can bypass lung defences, failing to incite a cough reflex and impairing the action of macrophages.

Table 6.1 Summary of alterations in lung function associated with normal ageing process

Increased	*Constant*	*Decreased*
Closing volume	Total lung capacity	Vital capacity
Residual volume	Minute volume	FEV_1
Functional residual capacity	$PaCO_2$	Lung recoil pressure
		Diffusing capacity
Use of ancillary muscles to respiration		PaO_2
Breathing frequency		Ciliary function
Anteroposterior chest diameter		Chest wall compliance
		Coughing efficiency

Environmental Factors

Irritants in the environment act on different parts of the respiratory system and produce various problems. In areas of high air pollution there is an increased incidence of coughing, increased or abnormal sputum production and shortness of breath (Bates, 1972). Increased mucus secretion production can occur to soothe inflamed air passages. Hypertrophy of the mucous glands can lead to blockage and increased airway resistance resulting in decreased air circulation and prevention of adequate drainage of secretions thus making infection more likely. The elderly will have had more exposure to environmental pollution. The industrial environment of the past often meant prolonged exposure to coal dust and asbestos leading to progressive fibrosis of the lung. Decreased respiratory protection exacerbates the problem.

The elderly who live in poorly ventilated housing with increased levels of dust and other pollutants are more susceptible to respiratory infection. Inhalation from leaking stoves and fires not properly maintained can cause problems. A change in environment, for instance coming into hospital, which includes central heating, dry air, increased temperature and unusual smells can alter a person's normal breathing activity.

Sleep

Hanning (1986) reports that the normal respiratory responses to hypoxia and hypercarbia are reduced during sleep, particularly REM sleep, as are the cough reflex and the ability to respond to respiratory resistance. Hypoventilation and breathing irregularities are common during sleep (Douglas, 1984): they appear to increase with age in healthy non-complaining individuals. Carskadon and Dement (1981) demonstrated this with elderly women. They found a high prevalence of sleep-related respiratory disturbances in elderly men and women including apnoeas and arousals, and report on the possibility of a worsening of sleep-related respiratory problems when sleeping pills are given. It is thought that awakenings may occur as a mechanism for correcting hypoxia by reducing hyperventilation.

Sleep apnoea syndromes are associated with obstruction to air flow in the upper airways and abnormality in the central regulation of breathing. Both of these disorders may coexist in elderly patients.

BREATHING PROBLEMS IN THE ELDERLY

Acute

Acute breathing problems in the elderly tend to have their origins in disease processes that would cause problems in any age group and their management is similar although drug therapy may be modified in view of increased sensitivity and coexisting disorders. Due to increased susceptibility to infection and a respiratory system already impaired though ageing, acute breathing problems in the elderly are often more disabling and more likely to result in complications than in a younger age group. Pneumonia, pleurisy, influenza, the common cold, pulmonary embolism, anaemia and myocardial infarction, are examples of disease that might lead to short-term breathing problems. Cardiorespiratory arrest is an extreme example in which a breathing problem can be life-threatening and needs to be dealt with immediately. Exacerbations of long-term breathing disorders such as asthma and bronchitis can also produce acute problems with breathing.

Chronic

Chronic breathing problems are common in the elderly and are a major cause of morbidity and mortality in this population group. These problems frequently begin in middle life but increase with age. The severity of the disabling effect of the problem is very variable. In the early stages it may be little more than an inconvenience, progressing to being housebound and dependent at the advanced stage.

Diseases producing chronic breathing difficulties are often grouped together under the heading of chronic obstructive airways disease. This encompasses bronchitis, asthma and emphysema. Although different disease processes are involved they have in common an obstruction to air flow and an association with cigarette smoking, environmental pollution, recurrent infection and bronchial irritation. The elderly may present with more than one of these diseases and thus have multiple symptoms and problems.

Chronic breathing problems add to the existing breathing problems associated with ageing: bronchitis to the consequence of airways obstruction, and emphysema to the loss of elastic recoil. Carcinoma of the lung is a further contributor to chronic breathing problems; especially when the elderly are at increased risk of developing bronchogenic carcinoma.

PSYCHOLOGICAL AND SOCIAL ASPECTS OF BREATHING PROBLEMS

Despite its physiological function, breathing is an integral part of talking, laughing, singing, shouting and many other vocal sounds. It is necessary for communication and maintaining a normal lifestyle (Ashworth, 1979).

An acute breathing problem is frightening, patients often experiencing anxiety, feelings of suffocation and panic. Being admitted to hospital may exacerbate the problem. Anxiety in itself can produce an increased respiratory rate and hyperventilation.

Embarrassment at coughing, wheezing and expectorating may cause some people to suppress these symptoms or avoid company. Anticipated shortness of breath is not only anxiety-provoking but often limits activity, be it sexual, work, leisure or social. Lustig, Haas and Castillo (1972) and Dudley *et al.* (1980) consider that a condition which interferes with normal breathing, reduces vitality and produces progressively severe symptoms is very frequently associated with a loss of self-esteem and dependency. An inability to carry out vocational, social, recreational and sexual activities of living can lead to anger, frustration and depression.

Social isolation and loneliness can result from reduced mobility and limited ability to communicate. This is particularly relevant to the elderly who frequently live alone and may feel too proud to seek help. Chronic breathing difficulties may lead to a deterioration in maintenance of an individual's hygiene and nutrition, and may initiate associated problems of immobility.

The complex area of psychosocial support is extremely important to successful management of breathing problems (McDonald and Hudson, 1982). This is time-consuming and its effectiveness may involve co-ordinating contributions from various health professionals.

NURSING THE ELDERLY PATIENT WITH BREATHING PROBLEMS

Breathing problems in the elderly may be components of various illnesses, acute and chronic. However, the problems these breathing abnormalities produce for the individual concern the nurse. Thus, the provision of nursing is directed towards achieving comfort and relief from symptoms, and maintaining or aiming for an optimal quality of life, be it in hospital or the community.

Nursing Assessment

Rokosky (1981) considers that the two major goals for in-depth respiratory assessment by nurses are (1) the recognition of changes in symptoms that require nursing attention, and (2) determining ways in which respiratory dysfunction is interfering with an individual's daily living activies. Nursing assessment of the elderly patient with breathing problems needs to incorporate the following:

Skin

- Colour of mucous membranes, lips, nail beds, body extremities.
- Presence of nicotine stains on fingers.
- Presence of oedema.
- Evidence of dehydration.

Nature and frequency of respirations

- Respiratory rate and rhythm.
- Use of accessory muscles for breathing.
- Presence and nature of pain or discomfort.

Presence of associated symptoms

- Coughing – nature, frequency, precipitating and/or relieving factors.
- Wheezing – as for coughing.
- Sputum – quantity, consistency, colour, presence of blood, etc., any recent changes.
- Pyrexia.

Body posture

- Preference of posture adopted to facilitate ease of breathing.
- Ability to lie flat.
- Presence of chest deformity.
- Splinting and guarding.

Mobility

- Exercise tolerance.
- Limiting factors.

Mental state

- Drowsy, apathetic, confused, disorientated, alert, agitated, restless.

Sleep pattern

- Normal pattern – body posture, use of pillows, number of awakenings, use of sedatives etc., usual sleep-promoting factors.
- Episodes of shortness of breath during sleep.
- Naps during daytime.

Medication

- Usual medication(s) – changes to therapy, efficacy of therapy, compliance, side-effects, knowledge and understanding by patient.

Nursing history

- Background to present episode – aggravating factors, presence of other relevant disorders, e.g. pulmonary or cardiovascular problems, allergies, etc.
- Normal coping mechanisms; social and family support; usual activity levels; home circumstances – stairs etc.

Knowledge and understanding

- Patient and family assessment.
- Sources of advice and support.
- Utilization of knowledge and support.

Attitude to the problem

- Acceptance, resignation or denial.
- Positive or negative attributes, e.g. motivation.
- Evidence of anxiety and/or depression.
- Attitude of family, especially spouse.

Clinical observations

- Respirations.
- Temperature.
- Pulse.
- Blood pressure.
- Height.
- Weight.
- Urinalysis.
- Peak expiratory flow.

Nursing Management

Nursing management will be based on the assessment (objective and subjective) of the individual patient problems and will usually involve liaison with other members of the health care team, including the physician, physiotherapist, and social worker, as well as the patient and the family. Effective management involves minimizing existing breathing problems and preventing potential ones. Sjoberg (1983) identifies four problems from nursing diagnosis literature for a patient with chronic breathing problems:

(1) Activity intolerance related to actual or anticipated shortness of breath.
(2) Sleep pattern disturbance related to shortness of breath, treatment regime, anxiety or sleep environment.
(3) Non-compliance related to lack of information, impaired thought processes, or lack of physical or financial resources.
(4) Ineffective individual and/or family coping related to role change, denial of disease or other psychological or physical factors.

Some Nursing Considerations

The following considerations are based upon the Roper model of nursing (Roper, Logan and Tierney, 1985):

Maintaining a safe environment

- Advise about dangers of smoking near oxygen.
- Protect from dust and smoke.
- Limit cross-infection by encouraging use of disposable sputum pots and wipes.
- Be aware of possible drug reactions.

Communication

- Alleviate shortness of breath.
- Be aware of diminished ability to communicate when using oxygen mask and encourage use of nasal cannulae where possible.
- Provide a buzzer for summoning aid.
- Encourage use of newspapers, television and radio.
- Be aware of social isolation in the elderly with breathing problems.

Breathing

- Maintain a clear airway and prevent aspiration.
- Administer appropriate medications, oxygen, etc. designed to improve breathing and monitor their effect.
- Limit respiratory tract infection by preventing aspiration, mobilizing secretions and keeping mouth clean (Shell, 1980).
- Ensure careful and comfortable positioning for optimum breathing.
- Provide relief from pain or discomfort.

- Teach breathing exercises and coughing techniques.
- Assist with diagnostic measures, for example peak flow recording and sputum collection.
- Educate about medications, investigations, etc.
- Be aware of potential breathing problems following surgery.
- Advise about the effects of smoking, keeping of pets and avoidance of pollutants, etc.

Eating and drinking

- Ensure adequate fluid intake, dietary supplements if malnourished, unrushed meal-times, and oxygen via nasal cannulae whilst eating.
- Make regular weight recordings, for example daily pre-breakfast recordings if oedematous, weekly recordings if trying to lose weight.
- Advise about losing weight if obese.
- Determine whether 'meals on wheels' service is required following discharge.

Personal cleansing and dressing

- Provide mouth-washes for dry mouth and minimize upper respiratory tract organisms.
- Assist with washing and dressing if necessary, but encourage independence and gradual increase in self-care.
- Provide comfortably fitting clothes that do not impede movement, breathing, etc.
- Encourage use of breathing techniques whilst carrying out hygiene activities.
- Educate about measures to minimize energy expenditure.
- Consider nursing support on discharge home.
- Encourage family involvement in hospital.

Control of body temperature

- Control environmental temperature.
- Ensure adequate ventilation.
- Provide heating or cooling aids if required, e.g. blankets, fan, etc.

Mobilizing

- Devise an activity plan with the patient which incorporates an increase in exercise tolerance with realistic short-term goals, spacing out and timing of activites and planned rest periods.
- Advise about potential mobility aids, e.g. walking frame, bath rails etc.

- Be aware of possible needs following discharge, e.g. 'home help', rehousing or modification of existing home, and refer to appropriate sources.

Working and playing

- Provide a stimulating environment for patient that does not aggravate breathing.
- Advise about modifying leisure interests so that they can be performed within limits of disability.
- Encourage new leisure interests.
- Involve family.

Expressing sexuality

- Discuss potential and actual sexual problems with patient and spouse.
- Provide medical advice and sexual counselling if required.

Sleeping

- Be aware of changes in sleep pattern with ageing and breathing problems.
- Encourage patient to adopt a posture that ensures maximum comfort and sleep.
- Be aware of possible dangers of giving sleeping tablets to the elderly with breathing problems.
- Encourage methods of rest and sleep promotion, e.g. hot drinks, relaxation etc.
- Discourage activity immediately prior to bedtime.
- Maintain normal bedtime and sleeping routines where possible.

Dying

- Continue to maintain optimum comfort.
- Remove sputum and aspirations (this may require airway and suction).
- Provide counselling and support (including liaison with spiritual leader).
- Involve family.

Administration of Oxygen

Hypoxia, signifying a reduced amount of oxygen in the lungs or tissues, can be caused by obstruction of the passage of oxygen across the alveolar membrane (as occurs in pneumonia, emphysema or chronic bronchitis) as a result of reduced blood flow (as in heart failure) or from anaemia.

Hypoxia occurs long before cyanosis becomes apparent. Low levels of oxygen in the blood, hypoxaemia, recognized by tachycardia, high blood pressure, cool extremities, anxiety and tremor, is often corrected by administering oxygen. Wheeler (1980) gives normal blood gas results for a 70-year-old man as being: PaO_2 = 80 mmHg and $PaCO_2$ = less than 50 mmHg. Reichel (1978) considers that the elderly require admission to hospital for respiratory disorder if their $PaCO_2$ is above 50 mmHg and/or the PaO_2 is below 50 mmHg and the situation has developed acutely.

The lowest inspired oxygen concentration which produces adequate arterial oxygen concentration needs to be administered. Care has to be taken in giving oxygen to elderly patients with chronic obstructive breathing problems. Often these individuals lose the ability to increase their total ventilation in response to a rise in $PaCO_2$. They have an abnormally high $PaCO_2$ at all times and increase their ventilation only in response to a fall in PaO_2. If inspired oxygen is increased considerably above 21 per cent in order to treat hypoxia the hypoxic drive is depressed and total ventilation decreases. This leads to an increase in $PaCO_2$ and can result in a respiratory arrest. The inspired oxygen concentration for these patients should not exceed 28 per cent. Promisloff (1980) recommends that a patient should be given oxygen whenever blood gas results show a PaO_2 below 50 mmHg. The cyanotic or dyspnoeic patient may need oxygen before blood gas studies have been performed. Fuchs (1980) considers that most patients with chronic respiratory disease can tolerate a nasal cannula at 2 litres/minute until blood gas levels are known.

Nasal cannulae can deliver between 21 and 100 per cent oxygen, depending on the amount of room air inspired with each breath. The greater the room air inspired the lower the functional inspired oxygen concentration. Because the concentration of oxygen delivered via nasal cannulae is not constant, and may be too high, this method of oxygen administration may be dangerous for patients with irregular breathing pattern or chronic respiratory disease. It appears unimportant whether the patient is mouth or nose breathing (Fuchs, 1980).

Simple face masks at 6–10 litres/minute deliver 35–60 per cent oxygen dilution by room air preventing 100% oxygen being inhaled. With these masks the inspired oxygen level is variable being dependent on the patient's peak respiratory demand and minute volume. Simple masks need a flow rate of at least 6 litres/minute to flush CO_2 from the mask (Fuchs, 1980).

The most accurate way of giving oxygen is via a Venturi mask which delivers precise oxygen concentrations through variable orifice size connectors. The smaller the orifice size the lower the concentration of inspired oxygen.

All face-masks can produce problems of discomfort, irritation, sweating and feelings of claustrophobia. They also inhibit eating, drinking and normal conversation. It is important that air entry ports controlling the amount of room air that is inspired do not become blocked by bedclothes or the patient lying on them, or the percentage of oxygen received will be higher than that prescribed. Unconscious or drowsy patients need to be observed for vomiting and aspiration within the mask. All patients need to be aware of the reasons for and the importance of their oxygen therapy, and can perhaps use nasal cannulae for short periods whilst eating and receiving visitors.

Oxygen should be humidified as this prevents drying of the mucous membranes of the upper airways and helps decrease mucus viscosity. Direct respiratory humidification carries the risk of bacterial contamination and bronchospasm. Sterile solutions need to be used for humidification and Acee (1984) recommends cleaning or sterilizing the equipment at least every twenty-four hours.

Some patients with chronic breathing problems resulting in right heart hypertrophy and/or failure due to lung diseases are prescribed oxygen at home. McDonald and Hudson (1982) report that continuous oxygen therapy in these patients reduces the mean pulmonary vascular resistance, and the chronic symptoms of right heart failure. Three types of systems exist for home use: traditional tank oxygen with regulator; liquid oxygen; and oxygen concentrators. The choice of system will depend on the activity level of the patient. Howard (1983) considers concentrators to be the most convenient.

Safe and appropriate use of oxygen is essential and will be achieved by patient and family education, support and continued follow-up. Some areas are developing community respiratory health workers to help patients in the community with breathing problems (Heslop, 1985).

Inhaler Therapy

Drugs need to be administered by the most effective and acceptable route for the patient. However, careful review and monitoring of any treatment is essential as patients do not respond uniformly.

Breathing problems are often treated with fixed dose inhalers in pressurized aerosol containers designed to target directly to the bronchial mucosa. This method of administration provides rapid and efficient relief with small doses of a drug. Only minute amounts of the drug escape into the systemic circulation. The main groups of agents administered in this way include bronchodilators, e.g. salbutamol, and corticosteroids, e.g. beclomethasone. The former group are given to reduce bronchospasm which produces wheezing caused by air being forced at high velocity through an airway narrowed by mucosal oedema and increased mucus secretion. By easing bronchospasm, bronchodilators help reduce the work of breathing. Peak flow meters are often used to assess the effectiveness of bronchodilators. These measure the ability to expel explosively air from the lungs after maximal inspiration and will depend on the ability to contract the respiratory muscles as well as the degree of bronchodilation. The value is expressed in litres per minute, the normal range being 4–6 litres/minute. Corticosteroids reduce the overall mucosal inflammatory reaction by reducing oedema and secretion of mucus. Elderly patients usually have initial difficulty in using their inhalers, especially when fine co-ordination is further minimized by shortness of breath and panic. Careful demonstration and advice regarding the use of inhalers is required. Practical advice should include the need to breathe slowly and hold the breath as long as is comfortably possible whilst releasing the drug. The bronchodilator should be taken prior to the corticosteroid to ensure that the latter is able to penetrate deeper into the lungs. Dunlap and Marchionno (1983) recommend waiting ten mintes in between inhalations to allow the second dose to penetrate further into the lungs (as a result of the bronchodilatory effect of the first).

Despite such preparation, some patients are unable to co-ordinate their breathing with aerosol release and these individuals may find the dry powder inhalers such as Ventolin Rotacaps easier to use.

In cases of acute severe bronchospasm, aerosol inhalers no longer deliver the drug effectively to the airways and aqueous nebulized administration has proved more effective. Administered in this way the drug is easy to inhale and is given over a period of 15–20 minutes. Side-effects are more likely as larger doses of the drug are given.

Steam inhalations such as tincture of benzoin or menthol, designed to keep the air passages moist, are sometimes prescribed to ease breathing. These need to be given with caution to the elderly. The water has to be almost at boiling point to prevent vaporization of irritant substances and there is grave danger of patients being scalded either by the water or the steam.

Breathing Exercises

Breathing exercises need to be taught to the elderly in accordance with the extent of their problem and their ability and motivation to perform them.

Deep breathing exercises help dislodge secretions and move them up the trachea so that they can be expectorated. Surfactant, a secretion released by the alveolar cells and which decreases surface tension, is released with each deep breath. Obesity and osteoporosis of the rib cage encourage shallow breathing and pneumonia, fibrosis and pulmonary oedema inhibit deep breathing by decreasing lung tissue compliance. Shallow breathing is often a feature of impaired respiratory function and patients with chronic obstructive airways disease require greater effort to move air in and out of the lungs. Patients who are inactive or who are in pain also tend to take shallow breaths. Shallow breathing minimizes surfactant production (surfactant increases the elasticicity of the lung tissue and facilitates gaseous exchange). Deep breathing helps minimize infection as organisms are most likely to grow in poorly ventilated areas of the lung. Deep breathing exercises need to be performed three or four times a day for two or three minutes at a time by patients with a chest infection or excessive sputum production. Timing of such activity needs to be planned to minimize exertion and maximize effectiveness.

Coughing is a normal physiological response to the presence of excessive mucus or other irritants in the respiratory passages. It is an attempt to clear these passages and improve ventilation. Efficient coughing does not tire the patient. Acee (1984) recommends that efficient coughing should be reinforced two hourly whilst the patient is awake.

Expectoration is a secondary concern for patients with chronic obstructive airways disease as the effect of coughing can aggravate bronchospasm and increase shortness of breath. For effective coughing patients need to be taught to take a slow deep inspiration to open the trachea and adequately inflate the lungs. A quick tight closure of the glottis increases intrathoracic and intra-abdominal pressure thus ensuring sufficient force to expel the mucus. Finally, contraction of the intercostal and abdominal muscles compresses the thoracic and abdominal cavities to produce the cough. In the elderly there is a decrease in the strength and speed of the contraction of the skeletal muscles needed to produce a forceful cough. Effective coughing can be encouraged by sips of water or changing position as in turning or ambulation. Elderly patients who have undergone abdominal surgery may benefit from supporting the wound with a hand or a pillow whilst coughing. Thompson (1984) recommends the use of a forced expiratory technique for dislodging secretions from the upper chest that are proving difficult to expectorate. This technique, when used in conjunction with breathing exercises, clears bronchial secretions without causing or increasing bronchospasm. It involves one or two forced expirations from the mid-lungs, a period of relaxation and deep breathing, followed by a cough at high volume to clear secretions moved into large airways.

Sputum specimens are best collected early in the morning because deep secretions collect in the bronchi at night and are more easily expectorated. In addition, early morning specimens usually contain the most organisms and leucocytes. Normal respiratory secretions are clear, mucoid and colourless. Sputum tends to be sticky and tenacious in acute conditions and less viscous in long-term conditions. Green-yellow sputum is indicative of pus being present, and purulence indicates infection. Frothy pink copious sputum suggests pulmonary oedema and small amounts of sticky rusty pink sputum pneumococcal pneumonia. Patients need to be encouraged to use a disposable sputum pot and handkerchiefs to minimize the risk of infection and to expectorate rather than swallow.

Patients with chronic breathing problems may have been using their lungs inappropriately for some time and need to be advised to breathe with the base rather than the apex of their lungs, breathing in around the lower ribs and diaphragm and relaxing on expiration to make breathing out a passive movement. Kim (1984) advocates the use of respiratory muscle training for patients with chronic obstructive airways disease to prevent respiratory failure.

Breathing in through the nose and then out through pursed lips may help rid the lungs of stagnant trapped air by maintaining a raised pressure in the bronchioles and preventing early bronchiole collapsing. Patients should breathe in normally through the nose and then exhale slowly and unforcefully out through the mouth, pursing the lips whilst doing so for at least twice as long as they have inhaled. This exercise usually takes a while to perfect but is useful during exercise or when short of breath.

Patients need to be advised not to hold their breath when carrying out heavy lifting and other strenuous activity because their impaired respiratory reserve will result in shortness of breath after the activity has been performed. Advising to inhale before performing such activity and the exhaling whilst actually doing it may be helpful.

Body Posture

Maintaining a body posture that allows the chest wall and diaphragm to move freely is an important aid to breathing. Patients with breathing problems tend to adopt positions that ease their breathing.

Sitting upright in bed or chair aids the full expansion of the lungs, increases the volume of lung available for oxygen absorption, and facilitates expectoration by allowing the bronchioles to open. It also improves gaseous exchange (Craig *et al.,* 1971). Lying down decreases both the amount of air that is moved with each breath (tidal volume) and the vital capacity, because it increases intrathoracic blood volume and the abdominal viscera press upwards on the diaphragm limiting the range of movement.

Lateral positioning of the comatosed or paralysed patient provides drainage for pooled oral secretions thus preventing aspiration. Side-to-side positioning about every two hours also deters the accumulation of secretions in different areas of the lung (Shell, 1980), which minimizes the risk of infection and facilitates gaseous exchange. Grosmaire (1983) reports that frequent turning of patients results in decreased arteriovenous shunting consequently increasing the PaO_2 value, but that some patients with particular pulmonary dysfunction may benefit from being placed in a specific position with regard to the site of their lung disease rather than being turned routinely from side to side. Careful positioning is necessary after nasogastric feeding to prevent aspiration should vomiting occur.

Postural drainage which utilizes gravity to enhance drainage of mucus may be inappropriate for the elderly who may find the position uncomfortable. Procedures need to be adapted in liaison with the physiotherapist and the patient.

Patients with chronic breathing problems will require advice for discharge home, including the adoption of a suitable body posture which permits relaxation, expansion of the chest and minimization of muscle energy needed to support themselves. Rifas (1980) recommends three positions to ease breathlessness:

(1) Sitting resting forward on a table removes the weight of the arms and gives better lateral chest expansion.
(2) Sitting in a chair with feet apart, leaning forward resting elbows on the knees allows unneeded muscles to relax.
(3) If breathlessness occurs on walking leaning the back and hips against a wall with the feet 12 inches away, slumping the shoulders forward and dangling the arms, allows the chest to expand fully while relaxing the other muscles and giving time to regain control of breathing.

Exercise

The disabling effect of breathing problems in the elderly is often superimposed on the effects of other disorders such as rheumatism, arthritis and ischaemic heart disease.

Shortness of breath limits exercise tolerance. Partridge (1984) grades exercise tolerance into five categories:

(1) Normal.
(2) Able to walk with healthy people of his/her own age and sex on the level but unable to keep up on hills and stairs.
(3) Unable to keep up with healthy people on the level but can walk long distances at his own pace.
(4) Unable to walk more than 100 yards on the level before being stopped by breathlessness.
(5) Unable to walk more than a few steps without dyspnoea and becomes breathless on walking and dressing.

Ordinarily, exercise tolerance increases with repetition of an activity over time. Unger, Moser and Hansen (1980) and Cockroft, Saunders and Berry (1981) recommend a well-planned programme of graded exercises for patients with chronic obstructive airways disease to improve their capacity for exercise. Unger, Moser and Hansen (1980) consider that the exercise level needs to be safe and acceptable for the patient but at the same time be sufficient to promote an improvement in exercise tolerance. Increased activity has a number of beneficial effects including an improvement in respiratory rate and depth, greater expansion for the lungs and more efficient coughing. Inactivity aggravates breathing problems.

Patients need to be given the confidence and motivation to gradually increase their level of activity. As independence increases so does morale. Care needs to be taken not to exhaust patients. In our culture daily exercise usually decreases with advancing age. Thus, a gradual increase in exercise needs to be aimed at that takes into account the capabilities and needs of the individual. Partridge (1984) advocates the use of visual analogue scales to monitor changes in exercise tolerance over a period of time.

Thoughtful planning of activity around drug therapy and breathing exercises with sufficient rest periods will help increase exercise tolerance. Optimum activity and independence needs to be maintained in hospital to equip for discharge home.

Case study

Mr Bradshaw had difficulty breathing because of his long-standing chest problem, which became worse from time to time. During these exacerbations, brought on by a superimposed chest infection, he would become very weak, cyanosed and breathless with the least exertion. To reduce his breathlessness and help restore a normal breathing pattern and meet body oxygen needs, the main points of care were considered:

- Help him adopt a suitable position to reduce breathlessness, for example the orthopnoeic position in bed/chair well supported with adequate pillows behind (sometimes he prefers to remain in a chair during the night).
- Use at least two nurses to assist, to minimize his exertion.
- Keep locker/bedtable/personal items within hand reach to prevent over-exertion.
- Use of suction equipment if appropriate to help clear sticky secretions, teach him to do this himself.
- Assist/teach him in breathing exercises to reduce effort if breathless.
- Administer humidified oxygen as prescribed.
- Check need for eye/oral toilet whilst on oxygen.
- Record observations of respiratory function – degree of cyanosis, respiration rate and report changes and abnormalities.
- Check peak flow rate before and after inhalers.
- Administer drugs as prescribed. Check for effectiveness with patient and review with medical staff.
- Describe and record abnormalities in sputum production.

- Establish an exercise pattern within his capabilities by
  recording how far he can walk without becoming breathless;
  planned increased daily mobility (see Chapter 9); and consider administration of medicines before exercising etc.
- Teach self-medication/management of problem, involve him fully in his care, keep him up to date with progress with positive outlook.
- Assist with activities (see other problems) as required and give time to complete activities at own pace.
- Stay with him if he is particularly breathless, until the problem is relieved and help alleviate his anxiety (see Chapter 5).

Hydration and Nutrition

Adequate hydration is essential for efficient respiration. Water is required to warm and humidify inspired air, and much is contained in the mucosa of the trachea and bronchi. According to Acee (1984) 1 litre of water per day is used for normal respiration together with skin losses. Dehydration may ensue if fluid loss is increased by fever or diaphoresis, or if intake is inadequate. As dehydration develops pulmonary secretions thicken and become difficult to clear, increasing the risk of infection.

Weight loss is sometimes a problem for the elderly with chronic respiratory disease. Tissue hypoxia; increased energy expediture on breathing, coughing and expectorating; depression; anxiety; and anorexia may all contribute to malnutrition (McDonald and Hudson, 1982).

In obese patients, losing weight may be of help in the elderly with chronic respiratory problems (Luce, 1980). Obesity leads to an excessive accumulation of fat which results in a higher than normal oxygen consumption and carbon dioxide production at rest. Due to a decreased chest wall compliance as a result of fat accumulation around the ribs, diaphragm and abdomen, extra energy is required to move the chest during breathing.

Advice about dietary habit change will need to be realistic and should involve the patient and family. Short-term goal-setting will make successful weight loss more likely.

Cigarette Smoking

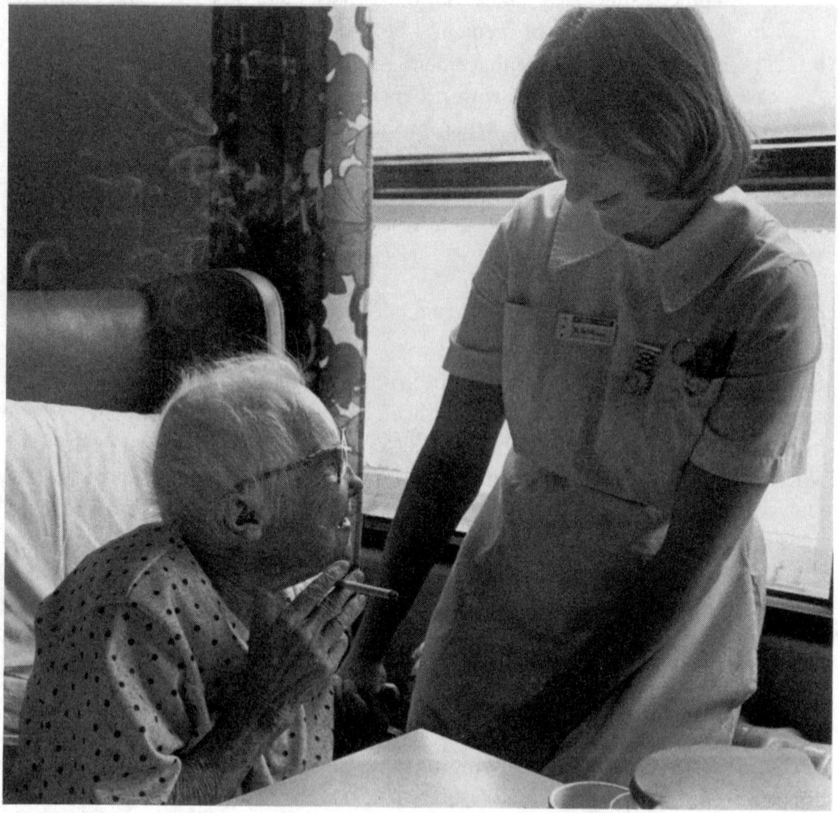

Smoking is thought to be a contributory factor to the majority of respiratory diseases. Cigarette smoke irritates the airways, deposits tar and nicotine and impedes the ability to cough effectively. The degree of irritation is related to the type of cigarette smoked and the depth to which it is inhaled.

The elderly who smoke and have breathing problems need to be aware of the probable exacerbation caused by their smoking. However, the moral and ethical issues behind nursing interventions aimed at discouraging people from a lifetime of smoking need to be considered and discussed. Certainly patients need to be presented with the available information to make a realistic decision for themselves.

Patients receiving oxygen therapy should be warned of the dangers associated with smoking.

Education, Support and Counselling

Patients will require information and advice on all aspects of their illness and its management so that they are aware of their role and have realistic plans and expectations. Whilst in hospital they will need information about investigations and drug therapy, etc. In addition, they may require more considerate help in view of the factors associated with ageing, for example help to hold and use the peak flow meter, or physical support whilst positioning for a chest X-ray. They will need advice on methods to maximize their breathing capabilities bearing in mind a possible reluctance to change and adopt new life-styles with advancing years. Impaired memory and learning capacity may necessitate extra time being invested in reinforcing specific information. Involvement of the family, especially the spouse, is usually essential if this is to be accomplished properly.

Psychosocial support, a most important concern of the nurse, has already been discussed. Awareness of potential problems of depression and social isolation in this group of patients is essential and care plans should be formulated with this in mind. These problems will manifest themselves after discharge home and it is important that provision for follow-up is arranged with community nursing services.

REFERENCES

Acee, S. (1984) Helping patients breathe more easily, *Geriatric Nursing,* Vol. 5, pp. 230–3.

Ashworth, P. (1979) Psychological and social aspects of respiratory care, *Nursing*. Vol. 7, pp. 295–9.

Bates, D. V. (1972) Air pollutants and the human lung, *American Review of Respiratory Disease,* Vol. 105, pp. 1–13.

Brandstetter, R. D. and Kazemi, H. (1983) Aging and the respiratory system, *Medical Clinics of North America,* Vol. 62, pp. 419–31.

Carskadon, M. A. and Dement, W. (1981) Respiration during sleep in the aged human, *Journal of Gerontology,* Vol. 36, pp. 420–3.

Cockroft, A. E. Saunders, M. J. and Berry, G. (1981) Randomized controlled trial of rehabilitation in respiratory disability, *Thorax,* Vol. 36, pp. 200–3.

Craig, D. B., Wahba, W. M., Don, H. F., Couture, J. G. and Becklake, M. R. (1971) 'Closing volume' and its relationship to gas exchange in seated and

supine positions, *Journal of Applied Physiology,* Vol. 31, pp. 717–21.
Douglas, N. J. (1984) Control of breathing during sleep, *Clinical Science,* Vol. 67, pp. 465–71.
Dudley, D. L., Glaser, E. M., Jorgenson, B. N. and Logan, D. L. (1980) Psychological concomitants to rehabilitation in chronic obstructive pulmonary disease: Part 1, Psychosocial and psychological considerations, *Chest,* Vol. 77, pp. 413–20.
Dunlap, C. I. and Marchionno, P. (1983) Help your COPD patient take a better breath – with inhalers, *Nursing,* Vol. 13, no. 5, pp. 42–3.
Edge, J. R., Millard, F. J and Reid, L. (1964) The radiographic appearance of the chest in persons of advanced age, *British Journal of Radiology,* Vol. 37, pp. 767–74.
Fuchs, P. L. (1980) Getting the best out of oxygen delivery systems, *Nursing,* Vol. 10, no. 6, pp. 34–41.
Grosmaire, E. K. (1983) Use of patient positioning to improve PaO_2. A review, *Heart and Lung,* Vol. 12, pp. 650–3.
Hanning, C. D. (1986) Sleep and breathing, *Intensive Care Nursing,* Vol. 2, pp. 8–15.
Heslop. A (1985) Community respiratory health workers, *Nursing Mirror,* Vol. 160, no. 15, pp. 37–8.
Howard, P. (1983) Oxygen in the home, *Thorax,* Vol. 38, pp. 161–4.
Hughes, R. L., Freilich, R. A., Bytell, D. E., Craig, R. M. and Moran, J. M. (1981) Aspiration and occult esophogeal disorders, *Chest,* Vol. 80, pp. 489–95.
Kim, M. J. (1984) Respiratory muscle training, *Heart and Lung,* Vol. 13, pp. 333–40.
Krumpe, P. E., Knudson, R. J., Parsons, G. and Reiser, K. (1985) The aging respiratory system, *Clinics in Geriatric Medicine,* Vol. 1, pp. 143–75.
Luce, J. M. (1980) Respiratory complications of obesity, *Chest,* Vol. 78, pp. 626–31.
Lustig, F. M., Haas, A. and Castillo, R. (1972) Clinical rehabilitation regime in patients with COPD, *Archives of Physical Medicine and Rehabilitation,* Vol. 53, pp. 315–22.
Martin, C. J., Das, S. and Young, A. C. (1979) Measurement of the dead space volume, *Journal of Applied Physiology,* Vol. 47, pp. 319–24.
McDonald, G. J. and Hudson, L. D. (1982) Important aspects of pulmonary rehabilitation, *Geriatrics,* Vol. 37, pp. 127–34.
Mittman, C., Edelman, N. H. and Norris, A. M. (1965) Relationship between chest wall and pulmonary compliance with age, *Journal of Applied Physiology,* Vol. 20, pp. 1211–16.
Norris, A. H., Shock, N. W. and Yiengst, M. J. (1953) Age differences in ventilation and gas exchange responses in graded exercise in males, *Journal of Gerontology,* Vol. 10, pp. 145–55.
Partridge, M. (1984) Difficulty in breathing, *British Journal of Hospital Medicine,* Vol. 31, pp. 288–91.
Pontoppidan, H. H. and Beecher. H. K. (1974) Progressive loss of protective reflexes in the airway with the advance of age, *Journal of American Medical Association,* Vol. 60, pp. 2209–13.
Promisloff, D. O. (1980) Administering oxygen safely. When, why, how, *Nursing,* Vol. 10, no. 10, pp. 54–6.

Reichel, J. (1978) Pulmonary problems in the elderly, in W. R. Reichel (ed.), *Clinical Aspects of Aging,* Williams & Wilkins, Baltimore, pp. 85–90.

Rifas, E. M. (1980) How you and your patient can manage dyspnoea, *Nursing,* Vol. 10, no. 6, pp. 34–41.

Rizzato, G. and Marozzini, L. (1970) Thoraco-abdominal mechanics in elderly man, *Journal of Applied Physiology,* Vol. 28, pp. 457-60.

Rokosky, J. S. (1981) Assessment of persons with altered respiratory function, *Nursing Clinics of North America,* Vol. 16, pp. 195–209.

Roper, N., Logan, W. W. and Tierney, A. J. (1985) *Elements of Nursing,* 2nd edn, Churchill Livingstone, Edinburgh.

Shell, G. (1980) Upper and lower respiratory tract infections – nursing intervention, *Nursing Clinics of North America,* Vol. 15, pp. 715–27.

Sjoberg, E. L. (1983) Nursing diagnosis and the COPD patient, *American Journal of Nursing,* Vol. 83, pp. 245–48.

Thompson, M. C. (1984) Physiotherapy – the essentials of care, *Nursing,* Vol. 27, pp. 797–80.

Unger, K. M., Moser, K. M. and Hansen, P (1980) Selection of an exercise program for patients with chronic obstructive pulmonary disease, *Heart and Lung,* Vol. 9, pp. 68–76.

Wheeler, H. H. (1980) A patient with chronic bronchitis, emphysema, cor pulmonale and pulmonary embolism, *Nursing Times,* Vol. 76, pp. 1339–45.

7. Maintaining Normal Body Temperature

Steve Wright

The capacity to maintain a stable deep body temperature (homeothermy), enables the person to have a controlled 'core' temperature, while the superficial 'shell' of the body acts as a variable insulator. The heart and circulation provide the heat exchange system between the two. In a warm environment, the blood flow to the skin is increased to promote the transfer of heat to the body surface and its loss, for example through sweating. In cooler conditions, the blood flow to the periphery is reduced to retain heat in the core. In more extremes of cold this heat retention may be further aided, by shivering, since its rapid muscular contractions generate heat (Exton-Smith 1985), by increasing activity or by adding extra clothing.

Core body temperature, which in the younger patient is usually 37°C, is lower in the aged and may normally be as low as 35°C (Herbert, 1986). Thus, the individual whose normal temperature is 35°C may be febrile at 37°C, but the patient is not identified as such because the temperature is within the normal range for the general population (Eliopoulos, 1980). For every 0.6°C increase in body temperature the pulse rises by about 710 beats per minute, and a delay in recognizing temperature changes in the elderly new therefore delay changes in metabolic, respiratory and pulse rates being recognized, which can have serious implications, for example strain on the cardiovascular system.

The lower body temperature can also cause infectious processes to go unnoticed. Manney (1975) suggests that the healing process is generally slower, wounds taking 31 days to heal in a 20-year-old, take 55 days in a 40-year-old and 100 days in a 60-year-old.

ENDOGENOUS FACTORS

Most elderly persons are as capable as a younger person of keeping a deep body temperature at their normal level, and as able to use their cardiovascular and other mechanisms described above effectively to maintain it. Exposure to extremes of heat and cold can produce difficulties (hypothermia and hyperthermia) for any age group. The elderly, however, are more susceptible for a number of important internal, physiological or *endogenous reasons.*

Responses to Higher Temperatures

In older people, sweating activity is diminished and the sweat threshold (i.e. the temperature at which sweating will begin) is raised. The ability to lose heat is therefore less and is especially marked in women as compared to men (Foster *et al.*, 1976).

Ellis (1976) has indicated that the elderly are particularly at risk when exposed to higher temperatures (e.g. during heatwaves or with infections) because of the prevalence of underlying cardiovascular and cerebrovascular disease. Therefore the physiological stresses accompanying higher temperature increase vulnerability to cerebrovascular accident or cardiac failure. Similar risks occur with illnesses where more heat is produced, such as infections.

Responses to Lower Temperatures

MacMillan *et al.* (1967) suggest that the elderly have a poor vasoconstrictor response to cooling. The reduced efficiency of the cardiovascular mechanism to conserve heat leads to an increased vulnerability to heat loss in extremes of cold.

Heat production is adversely affected (Herbert, 1986) because the basal metabolic rate falls because of a reduction in the number of active cells in the body.

The shivering response may diminish with age, it is often less intense and the heat production therefore reduced (Collins *et al.*, 1980).

Certain drugs (e.g. the phenothiazines) may have a hypothermic effect, enhancing the risk of for those elderly persons in whom other factors are present (Exton-Smith, 1985).

Many older persons have diminished sensitivity to cold. Collins *et al.*

(1977) indicate that younger people can perceive changes in temperature of 0.8°C while the elderly may not recognize changes of 2.5°C and some in the study could not detect changes of 5°C or more. In addition, when given the responsibility for controlling their own environmental temperature, many elderly people had difficulty in making precise adjustments to produce the optimum temperature for thermal comfort (Collins and Hornville, 1981).

A number of other diseases appear to have hypothermic effects including hypothyroidism or myxoedema, hypopituitarism (Exton-Smith, 1985) and diabetes mellitus (Gale and Tattershall, 1978). A fall and resulting immobility after a stroke may expose the older person to hypothermia. Parkinson's disease is believed to have both an autonomic effect as well as reducing activity, with consequent reduction in heat production. Patients who are disorientated may be unaware of environmental hazards and there is evidence of temperature impairment with dementia. In addition, cardiac and pulmonary diseases may derange the thermoregulation mechanism (Exton-Smith, 1985).

Many drugs prescribed for the elderly (e.g. chlorpromazine, barbiturates, as well as alcohol) interfere with normal temperature regulation mechanisms (Herbert, 1986). Herbert also notes how alcohol should not be used to warm up someone who is cold because it causes increased vasodilation to the skin (and hence further heat loss).

Problems, such as arthritis, may reduce not only the ability to produce heat through activity, but may also restrict the ability to adjust environmental temperatures, for example by adjusting heating controls or changing clothing (Oliver, 1983).

EXOGENOUS FACTORS

The above internal factors are significant in the elderly person's control of body temperature. However, they represent only a part of the whole picture. The physiological and a pathological process associated with ageing are not the sole determinants in problems associated with temperature regulation problems. *External or exogenous factors* play an equally significant role.

External Heat

Climatic changes where environmental temperature increases, especially associated with heatwaves, has been shown in many countries to produce a rise in the death rate among the elderly, mainly due to cardiovascular and cerebrovascular disease (Exton-Smith, 1985). Similar effects have been observed in the UK (OPCS, 1975, 1976).

External Cold

Exposure to cold is the overriding cause of hypothermia in the elderly. Yurick *et al.* (1980) cite a Royal College of Physicians' survey in 1975. It indicated that 3.6 per cent of all old people admitted to hsopital were hypothermic (deep body temperature below 35°C). There was a significant correlation between exposure to cold prior to coming into hospital and low body temperature. The survey also showed that in a random sample of 1,000 people over the age of 65, 754 cases (75 per cent) were living in room temperatures at or below 18.3°C, the minimum recommended by the Parker–Morris report on council housing.

MacLean and Emslie-Smith's (1977) survey reported that 85 of the 100 consecutive cases of hypothermia were over the age of 60 years. About half of these patients were found lying on the floor after a fall due either an accident or illness. One or more underlying disorders were present in one-fifth of the patients.

Many elderly people living at home who develop hypothermia have some common characteristics, namely they usually live alone, under cold conditions and their homes lack basic amenities. Often they have impaired mobility, nocturia, insomnia and liability to falls (Exton-Smith, 1985). A fall at home, while living alone, may lead to the elderly person lying on the floor unattended for many hours and result in prolonged exposure to cold.

Oliver (1983) and Wicks (1978) argue that one of the main problems is financial. Elderly people on low incomes may fear the debts that can arise with heating costs and so minimize the heating of their homes. An Age Concern (1983) campaign suggested that up to a million elderly people are at risk from hypothermia, especially in winter, because of the combination of bodily changes associated with the ageing process and the effects of low incomes.

Oliver (1983) further cites a Research Institute for Consumer Affairs report which indicated that 87 per cent of elderly people had never seen any pamphlet or leaflet about keeping warm or heating problems. Nor do many elderly people claim benefit to which they are entitled to supplement their incomes. There appears therefore to be an underlying lack of awareness in many elderly people of the dangers to themselves and of the means of help available. At times of severe weather, such as the winter of 1986/7, efforts to increase public awareness were demonstrated in massive leaflet and poster campaigns and considerable coverage in the media.

Both economic and social factors therefore appear to contribute significantly to the problem of hypothermia in the elderly. Lack of money, insufficient clothing, lack of warm food and drink and lack of fuel conspire with the physiological changes of ageing and the psychological effects (loneliness, apathy, lack of visitors, pride in rejecting help, disorientation) to produce a category of high risk elderly people who may succumb to this problem.

HYPOTHERMIA

The term accidental hypothermia is used to imply that 'the lowering of deep body temperature is unintentional and it has to be distinguished from hypothermia which is induced therapeutically' (Exton-Smith, 1985). Herbert (1986) defines hypothermia as a state of subnormal body temperature in which the deep body temperature falls below 35°C.

Prevention of the problem is preferable to curing it. However, some aspects, such as the debate over the adequacy of the size of the pension, are matters over which nurses as individuals have little direct control. Oliver (1983), however, identifies a number of strategies based on the work of Age Concern in which nurses, particularly those working in the community, can participate. Certainly there is needs for a considerable degree of teamwork involved between doctors, nurses, social workers, health visitors and voluntary agencies if those at risk are to be identified and helped before the problem arises. According Oliver (1983), Saddington (1983), Tinker (1984) and Exton-Smith (1985) the following main points should be considered:

- In cold weather, bedrooms need to be kept heated and windows closed at night. The bed needs to be moved away from an outside wall and perhaps into a living room, so that at least one room of the house can be kept heated at all times. Perhaps a commode can be provided for the room to save trips to the toilet. Rooms and passageways need to be well lit, with even floors to minimize the risk of falls. A couple of blankets and pillows kept on the floor can be available for use if the fall does occur, while awaiting help.

- Advice needs to be given on claiming fuel allowances, easy payment methods for bills and social security benefits for fuel, clothing and bedding.
- A system of regular visits needs to be co-ordinated, perhaps involving neighbours and friends and relatives, as well as the professionals. Thus every old person, especially the housebound and alone, can have visits to check their safety several times each day – especially during extremely cold weather.
- Oral temperatures can be checked routinely, and may need to be checked rectally by the nurse if it falls below 35°C. A rectal temperature of 35°C should be regarded as the danger point below which the patient's temperature should not fall.
- Clothing should be worn in several layers, with more natural materials, e.g. wool and cotton, than made-made fibres. Heat loss is greatest through the head, so some form of head cover is advisable, with added gloves, bed-socks and extra bed-jacket or pullover to cover the shoulders.
- A telephone needs to be kept at the bedside, and preferably low down so that it can be reached in the event of a fall. In addition, a stick to bang on a wall or window, alarm bell or buzzer should be on hand to attract help.
- A room thermometer will help to monitor temperature. It should not fall below 25°C.
- A store of food needs to be kept available, with the possibility of having both meals (e.g. meals on wheels) and food supplies delivered. This has the added advantage of ensuring extra checking visits. Foods which can be easily prepared (but avoiding tinned stuffs if the person has difficulty opening them) should be kept available, including supplies of milk, eggs, cheese, bread (preferably wholemeal) and soup.
- Advice on diet selection, types of food and drink and meal preparation needs to be offered. At least one hot meal a day needs to be taken with regular warm drinks throughout the day, including first thing in the morning and last thing at night.
- Caution needs to be exercised when enlisting the help of friends, neighbours and relatives. They may have commitments of their own. They need to know where to contact the nurse if necessary. A method of indicating that the old person needs help can be agreed,

for example curtains drawn or a duster held at the window.

- Supplies of candles, matches and a torch need to be kept available.
- The older person needs to be advised on personal safety, checking points about the home which might be hazards, for example mats which slip, damaged stair rails, etc. An opportunity can be taken to ensure that the older person feels secure, making the house as burglar proof as possible. The crime prevention officer, contactable at the local police station, provides advice free of charge on anti-burglar equipment. Many simple measures can be achieved quite cheaply, e.g. window locks or door safety chains. The elderly should be asked to check that callers to the house, when not known to them, possess valid identification documents before admitting them.
- Advice on simple exercise patterns can be given. Even if not leaving the house for walks, then simple exercises in the home can be carried out. These can be so much more enjoyable if performed with somebody – and many television and radio programmes now include fitness sessions which are aimed at or can be easily modified for the elderly person.
- Spending the time of day with the older patient, just in general conversation, especially with those who live alone, can be as beneficial as a period of giving practical advice. Time spent in chatting or sharing a cup of tea can do much to remove the sense of isolation and loneliness.

The Features of Hypothermia

The core body temperature of 35°C (taken rectally using a low-reading thermometer) is the defining factor, but the nurse should be aware of other features that will help in assessing the patient. This is especially so if they provide advance warning that the patient is becoming hypothermic. These features are:

- A full background social history, including details of accommodation and life-style. There may be many features here which place the patient at 'risk' (see notes above).
- The skin feels cold to the touch all over the body and there is a mixture of pallor and cyanosis.
- The patient first becomes confused, then becomes progressively drowsy. Three-quarters of patients with rectal temperatures below

27°C are unconscious (Rosin and Exton-Smith, 1964). Shivering is not usually present, and muscles and limbs may appear rigid. The heart rate and respiratory rate falls, while bronchopneumonia may be present without any obvious symptoms. Gastric dilation can lead to aspiration of the stomach contents and haematemesis can occur (Exton-Smith, 1985). Oliguria usually occurs, and occasionally so does profound hypoglycaemia (Mills, 1973).

Once the patient has reached the profoundly hypothermic state, then the probability of recovery diminishes. Goldman *et al.* (1977) suggest that the lower the core temperature, the greater the chances of death occurring.

Restoring Normal Temperature – the Nurse's Role

Providing warmth in the home and hot food and drinks, together with close supervision, can reverse the trend towards a continously lowering body temperature. This can alleviate the difficulty and remove the necessity for admission to hospital.

If the stage had been reached where the patient is very drowsy, and possibly comatose, then emergency action to restore temperature is necessary. The main features of care are summarized as (after Exton-Smith, 1985; Thomas, 1985):

- Nurse the patient in a warm, well-ventilated but draught-free room. The temperature should be around 25–30°C.
- Rapid active surface re-warming is dangerous because of the stress placed on the cardiovascular system. Exton-Smith (1985) recommends a warm room with light clothing over the body and a gradual rise in core temperature of 0.5–1.0°C per hour. However, it has to be recognized that warming is extremely difficult to maintain and control. Concurrent blood pressure and pulse checks may give a more accurate guideline as to how safely the warming up procedure is proceeding.
- Check temperature and pulse at least quarter-hourly at first. Temperature needs to be checked rectally, using a probe to provide continuous monitoring if possible (this also reduces disturbance to bed-clothes).
- Give warm, but not hot, fluids if conscious.
- Give foods that will supply heat and energy (carbohydrates) if the

patient is able to take them. An intravenous infusion may be prescribed by the doctor and needs to be given as planned.

- If the patient is critically ill, relatives and friends need to be kept up to date with what is happening and given appropriate advice and support.
- Talk to the patient, explain everything that is going on and give positive words of encouragement - even if he/she is confused or comatose.
- Oxygen therapy (see Chapter 6 on breathing) may be given as prescribed by the doctor. Drugs such as antibiotics will also often be required and should be given as prescribed.
- Pulse and blood pressure should be monitored along with temperature. A fall in blood pressure means that the warming up is occurring too quickly.
- Other measures, such as changes of position, need to be carried out to prevent the complications of immobility (see Chapter 9).
- Along with an intravenous régime, the doctor may also carry out a variety of blood tests to detect dehydration and electrolyte imbalance. A urinary catheter may have to be passed to measure urine output accurately, with consequent management of catheter care required (see Chapter 12).
- Bed-clothing should be light and the use of a thermal or 'space' blanket may be prescribed. The patient needs to be lightly covered, with as little of the body exposed as possible. The thermal blanket, if used, needs to be next to the patient's skin shiny surface innermost. Generally, the patient should be disturbed and exposed as little as possible. The folds of the blankets, for example, can be placed along the patient's buttocks, necessitating minimal uncovering when checking temperature. Essential washing should be carried out only if the patient is very soiled, for example has been incontinent. It should be carried out quickly, using warm water (35°C) and followed by thorough drying.
- As the patient recovers, a thorough background history needs to be obtained. Reference to relevant other members of the team (e.g. social services, community nurses, health visitors) needs to be made to provide home support. All members of the team, especially the nurse, need to participate in a programme of patient education to provide help at home, promote awareness of the dangers and prevent a recurrence of the problem.

Case study

In the winter of 1986 Mr Abbot was admitted unconscious with a rectal temperature of 28°C. Immediate life-preserving measures to gradually restore his body temperature to normal (use of a 'space blanket', intravenous infusion, maintenance of his airway, etc.). His successful recovery through this stage led to a reappraisal of the reasons for his hypothermic state.

It transpired that he lived alone - and felt lonely. Both his children lived with their families several hundred miles away. His terraced house was cold because central heating system was out of action, partly due to lack of use, as he was afraid of the cost of heating bills. A number of initial actions were decided upon:

- Nurses and dietician to advise on dietary intake and to plan simple, cheap, nutritious meals for him which he could prepare easily himself at home.
- A meals-on-wheels service was applied for.
- Through social services, applications were made to review his pension, supplementary benefits and heating allowance claims.
- Approaches were made to several neighbours, who agreed to call upon him in rotation every few days to check that he was well, and to seek help if he did not respond to their calls, especially during the winter months.
- The health visitor would continue follow-up visits at home.
- The family were contacted and the situation explained to them. They offered to help with costs of repairs to the heating system and one son paid for a telephone to be installed so that they could remain in contact.
- As part of his teaching plan, Mr Abbot was given written information about preventing hypothermia and nurses and the health visitor spent time with him explaining the dangers and how to avoid them.

HYPERTHERMIA AND PYREXIA

The effects of a high temperature in the elderly are as serious as hypothermia. Hyperthermia or 'heat stroke' is usually referred to as high temperature states brought on by high environmental temperatures. In the UK, because of climatic conditions, this is relatively rare (Lyster, 1976) except at time of 'heatwaves'.

Heat stroke in the elderly, however, manifests itself differently than in younger age groups. Levine's (1976) study on a group of patients whose temperature exceeded 41.3°C rectally showed them to be more prone to developing severe dehydration, breathing problems due to pulmonary congestion and coma. Exton-Smith (1985) suggests that the effects can be reversed and deep body cooling achieved, but that the prognosis is poor. Cold water sponges and iced baths can be helpful, but need to be accompanied by vigorous massage to the skin to counteract reflex vasoconstriction. The skin may be cooled by the ice baths, but the core temperature may be otherwise unaffected because of the vasoconstriction. Ellis (1976) has suggested that the stress of heat stroke in the elderly has a poorer outlook because of the degenerative changes in the cardiovascular system in later years. The heatwave in Greece during the summer of 1987 was a major cause in the rise in mortality rates, especially among the elderly.

More commonly encountered by nurses in the UK is a raised body temperature (pyrexia) due to underlying disease processes, such as infection. Apart from dealing with the underlying cause (e.g. helping to treat the chest infection) for the special reasons mentioned above, the nurse needs to be aware of the dangers to the elderly of a high body temperature and to be able to reduce it safely. Even low grade pyrexias can have serious consequences, and Eliopoulos's (1980) points cited earlier in this chapter needs to be borne in mind. A pyrexia of 38°C for a young adult, whose normal body temperature is 37°C, is of differing significance to the elderly person with a temperature of 38°C when normal body temperature is 35°C.

Like hypothermia, prevention is better than cure, and the nurse has an important role to play (especially those in daily contact with the elderly in the community) as a health educator. Those at risk in times of high temperature can be advised on means of keeping cool – remaining in the shade, taking cool drinks during the day and using cooling aids such as fans. Light, loose-fitting clothing in natural fibres such as cotton assists heat loss as does a cool wash, or shower/bath at regular intervals during the day.

Cooling the patient with a high temperature needs, like managing hypothermia, to be carried out gradually in view of the potential stress on the cardiovascular system and resulting dangers. The patient who simply feels hot and uncomfortable can be offered cooling washes and drinks during the day, with changes of bed-clothing especially if sweating. Bed-clothing needs to be light and non-restricting.

Pyrexias in excess of 39°C need more nursing intervention, and possibly the use of tepid sponging techniques to reduce temperature to safe levels (Campbell, 1984; Royal Marsden, 1985). A cool, well-ventilated room is necessary, perhaps assisted by the use of a fan, and drinks need to be provided to maintain an intake of at least 3 litres in twenty-four hours (cool not hot, and avoiding stimulants). Patients will feel hot, uncomfortable and frightened, and need the nurse to be with them to give information, comfort and reassurance. Much of this can be carried out on a continuous basis while dealing with other activities, such as temperature monitoring, while the efforts to produce cooling are taking place.

The main aim is to reduce body tempeature to normal and, concomitantly, reduce the raised pulse, respiration and blood pressure rates that accompany it. Because of cardiovascular risks, a similar rate of cooling needs to be provided as with warming in hypothermia (0.5–1.0°C per hour [Exton-Smith, 1985]). However, in reality temperature cooling is difficult to monitor and control strictly. Pulse and blood pressure need to be checked concurrently as a rise in both may be a more accurate indication of potential changes in the patient.

Patients, also need to feel comfortable by attending to their general comfort in bed (offering cool washes, a cool moist cloth to the forehead, changing of sheets and bed-clothing) as well as to psychological comfort. Staying with them, teaching and explaining and using the various verbal and non-verbal techniques suggested in Chapter 5 also need to be employed as an equally important part their care.

REFERENCES

Age Concern (1983) *Help Warm up Winter*, London.

Campbell, C. (1984) *Nursing Diagnosis and Intervention*, Wiley, New York.

Collins, K. J., Dore, C., Exton-Smith, A. N., Fox, R. H., MacDonald, I. C. and Woodward, P. M. (1977) Accidental hypothermia and impaired temperature homeostasis in the elderly, *British Medical Journal*, Vol. 1, pp. 353–6.

Collins, K. J., Exton-Smith, A. N., James, H. M. and Oliver, D. J. (1980) Functional changes in the autonomic nervous responses with ageing. *Age Ageing*, Vol. 9, pp. 17–24.

Collins, K. J. and Hornville, E. (1981) Temperature requirement in old age, *Building Services Engineering Research and Technology*, Vol. 1, pp. 165–72.

Eliopoulos, C. (1980) *Geriatric Nursing,* Harper & Row, London.

Ellis, F. P. (1976) Heat waves and drugs affecting temperature regulation, *British Medical Journal*, Vol. 3, p. 474.

Exton-Smith, A. N. (1985) *The Autonomic Nervous System*, in M. S. J. Pathy *Principles and Practice of Geriatric Medicine,* Wiley, Chichester.

Foster, K. G., Ellis, F. P., Dore, C., Exton-Smith, A. N. and Weiner, J. S. (1976) Sweat responses in the aged, *Age Ageing*, Vol. 5, pp. 91–101.

Gale, E. M. and Tattershall, R. B. (1978) Hypothermia in a complication of diabetic keto-acidosis, *British Medical Journal*, Vol. 2, p. 1387.

Goldman, A., Exton-Smith, A. N., Francis G. and O'Brien, A. (1977) Report of a study of low temperature in old people admitted to hospital, *Journal of the Royal College of Physicians,* Vol. 11, pp. 291-306.

Herbert, R. (1986) The biology of ageing: body temperature regulation, *Geriatric Nursing*, July/August, pp. 16-18.

Levine, J. A. (1976) Heat stroke in the aged, *American Journal of Medicine*, Vol. 47, pp. 251-7.

Lyster W. R. (1976) Death in summer, *Lancet*, Vol. 2, p. 469.

MacLean, D. and Emslie-Smith, D. (1977) *Accidental Hypothermia*, Blackwell, Oxford.

MacMillan, A. L., Corbett, J. L., Johnson, R. U., Crompton-Smith, A., Spalding, J. M. K. and Wollner, L. (1967) Temperature regulation in survivors of accidental hypothermia of the elderly, *Lancet*, Vol. 2, pp. 165-9.

Manney, J. R. (1975) *Ageing in American Society,* University of Michigan.

Mills, G. L. (1973) Accidental hypothermia in the elderly, *British Journal of Hospital Medicine*, Vol. 10, pp. 691-9.

Office of Population Censuses and Surveys (1975, 1976) *Monitor*, London.

Oliver, C. (1983) Old and cold, *Nursing Times*, 26 October, pp. 8-10.

Rosin, A. and Exton-Smith, A. N. (1964) Clinical features accidental hypothermia with observations on thyroid function, *British Medical Journal,* Vol. 1, pp. 16-19.

Royal Marsden Hospital (1985) *Manual of Clinical Nursing Policies and Procedures*, Harper & Row, London.

Saddington, N. (1983) Winter of discontent, *Nursing Times*, 26 October, pp. 10-11.

Thomas, L. (1985) *Learning to Care for Elderly People*, Hodder & Stoughton, London.

Tinker, A. (1984) *Staying at Home: Helping Elderly People*, HMSO, London.

Wicks, M. (1978) *Old and Cold; Hypothermia and Social Policy*, Heinemann, London.

Yurick, A. G., Robb, S. S., Spier, B. E. and Ebert, N. J. (1980) *The Aged Person and the Nursing Process*, Appleton-Century-Crofts, New York.

8. Personal Hygiene, Dressing and Undressing

Paul Mangan

HYGIENE IN THEORY AND PRACTICE

One of the greatest tragedies to have fallen on modern nursing is the gap which has grown between nursing theory and so many practitioners (Briggs, 1972; RCN, 1985). Forests have been turned into libraries in an effort to influence nursing practice and yet still so much of what passes for nursing care is mere routine, carried out in the time-honoured and long outmoded name of 'we've always done things this way'.

With the possible exception of their treatment of pressure sores, a topic generally seen as being different to prevention, the greatest affront to staff is to question their approach towards maintaining and improving a patient's hygiene. Sadly the ritualized, institutional approach prevails in many settings to this day (Millar and Gwynne, 1972; Wells, 1980; Fielding, 1986).

'Hygiene' is something that many nurses do, with little if any thought. 'Getting through the work' becomes a dominant theme (Clarke, 1987). It features highly in break-time conversations: 'I've washed six before breakfast and twelve more before lunch', and confers prestige and reputation as a good worker on those who manage more of it than others. Such success has left me baffled on many occasions. I have wondered how, when receiving a lunch-time handover, they managed to do so much in so short a time, when I knew how long such feats would have taken me. I was left wondering if I was not pulling my weight in the battle against grime on the ward. This worried me so much that I once asked a 'good worker' how on earth she got through so much work. 'It's a question of getting in and getting on until it's time to get off,' she told me. Strange to relate a surprising number of patients who had had 'hygiene' looked untouched. The men were, by and large, left unshaved and the women's hair was unkempt. Both sexes had dirty, uncut nails and, judging by their breath, uncleaned teeth. They had had little more than immersion in a bath or a bed-bath consisting of a flannel passed over face, chest, legs and back. This is the secret of the good worker's high output. This is the performance carried out on the dependent category of patient, those who need this done for them. Then there is the assisted wash, in which patients do what they can for themselves, which may be augmented by the good worker; lastly, there are self-caring patients, who are left to their own devices with little or no supervision.

There are reasons for this state of affairs, and not all of them are the fault of individual nurses failing to provide adequate care for those in their charge. The worst such nurses can be charged with is a lack of imagination in performing their duty. What they really lack is leadership helping them to set standards of care, rather than expecting them just to get on with it. They are trapped inside nursing's self-imposed hierarchy which stamps routine and fear of deviation upon anybody who does not want to carry out the ritual way of doing things. The nurses involved do not know what it is they are really supposed to be doing nor why they should be doing it, just that it needs doing, and that they must fulfil their allotted task.

Ward routine is to get patients up before breakfast, wash them, breakfast them, make beds, do dressings and many other relatively simple but time-consuming tasks. All of these tasks must be performed in order to receive the accolade 'good worker'. Failure to perform these tasks means an inability to cope. Good workers cope (Salvage, 1985). This absurdly simplistic approach means the nurse has no time to deal with the patients as individuals or some of the other tasks would be left undone. By reducing her morning's work into bite-sized chunks, she also reduces her patients into collections of work which have higher and lower priorities (Pearson and Vaugham, 1986). An immersion counts as a bath in this scheme, whereas, for example, mouth care would count as a detail, something which can be left to be done later if there is time. What counts is what can be seen at first glance, and what needs more investigation to uncover is left. Thus large tasks are done daily, small tasks go undone. Baths are given, mouths left undone; beds are made, sputum pots left for days beside the locker. Patients become work units, and work can be managed because it is routine. In such a system, what price individual nursing care, as anything other than the ravings of educationalists and speakers at conferences?

If nurses had the time to wait the matter could perhaps be left there as a further call to back up that of Briggs (1972) for nursing to become a research-based profession and thus sweep away thoughtless procedures. It would seem, though, that nurses do not have this time, and that many patients are being neglected by professionals who believe that what they are doing is 'adequate'. It is difficult to define what a 'good standard' of care is on this issue because the whole question of hygiene is one that can cause great personal upset as it is fraught with subjectivity and based on past practice and socialization (Williamson, 1987; RCN, 1987). People brought up in age of relative prosperity and inside plumbing may well feel that a daily bath is essential, whilst others, remembering times when a zinc bath had to be filled using kettles of boiling water might be excused for feeling that one per week, or even one per month, is more than adequate.

There are aspects of hygiene, though, that apply almost universally. It is these that tend to be ignored and that the rest of the chapter will consider.

OFFERING A CHOICE

A recent King's Fund report (1982) details the risks of institutionalization when the older person comes into the hands of carers:

> Washing, bathing, going to the lavatory are everyday events which we all take for granted. Most of us have access to baths, hot water, and lavatories, whether at home or at work, which we can use how and when we wish. We choose how often we wash, how hot the water, and what time of day.
>
> How different this becomes when we have to depend on other people to help us, or to provide these ordinary facilities for us in an institution which has a set of routine procedures by which everyone has to abide. Instead of the usual early morning clatter of bowls, with the lukewarm flannel around the face, could not the residents choose when they wash? It is necessary for everyone to have a wash and bed made by a pre-ordained time which may have been decided upon many years ago? Must there always be a set day for taking a bath?
>
> (King's Fund, 1982)

A key point here is that nurses must offer real alternatives and 'choice' in care (Williamson, 1987). The nurse should be acting as an adviser and enable to help patients make realistic choice in a non-ritualistic, non-dictatorial manner.

Case study

Mrs Heath had difficulty maintaining personal hygiene independently because of weakness of the limbs on the left side of her body. To help maintain hygiene to her own standard and restore maximum self-care, a number of features were identified, with the intention that she should eventually be able to wash hands and face and clean her teeth herself.

- Offer a bed-bath/general bath as desired (used to bath every two to three days at home).
- Offer equipment for washes especially after meals etc.; assist where needed in promoting independence where possible. Give praise for attempts made.
- Teach Mr Heath how to help her, involve him in care as both prefer.
- Check eyes/ears/mouth and review for help with hygiene.
- Provide equipment for cleaning dentures.
- Help with hair and make-up as she prefers.
- Use of ambulift (two nurses to assist) with bathing.
- Help to sit at wash-basin to attend to own hygiene – help with equipment. Give time to attempt hygiene at own pace and intervene only when essential.
- Ensure privacy.
- Give praise to encourage her when she achieves independent activity, no matter how small. Tell her when she has 'done well' or is 'looking good'.

BENEFITS OF HYGIENE

The benefits of adequate hygiene range from the correct functioning of tissue and protection from corrosive agent such as dirt, sweat and tears, to the feeling of psychological well-being resulting from feeling clean. This is particularly so if nurses can avoid ritualized and routinized approachs.

Cleanliness serves a secondary sexual role. Clean people are more attractive to be with if for no other reason than they feel good about themselves. Attention paid to the hair of an elderly person is of more value than any amount of platitudes about how nice the weather is outside. It is an essential as other aspects of hygiene to provide a non-institutionalized hair-style. Elderly men are of a generation who have undergone national service. To leave such people looking and feeling ill-kept and neglected is surely a gross dereliction of duty.

Nurses have specific duties in relation to people in these circumstances which fit into Henderson's (1966) view of the role of the nurse. This is to help the patient to do those things they would do unaided if illness or incapacity did not prevent them. Therefore, arranging a hairdressing appointment is not just a nice thing to do when the nurse gets around to it, but should be an integral part of the patient's care. The importance of this cannot be over-emphasized. Neglect of it is akin to telling an anaemic patient that 'We will throw up a unit of blood later if we get the chance'. Male patients, unless they express a desire to grow a beard, should be able to expect a shave daily or more frequently. Shaving is a skill nurses should learn, in order to be able to perform without cutting their patients too often. It would seem that this puts many nurses off shaving men. It is just a matter of practice, however, and it should not be forgotten that most shavers cut themselves from time to time and come to no harm. Anyway, the new safety razors reduce the size of most cuts to nicks that can be easily managed with a little tissue paper. Electric razors are often not as effective in removing facial hair and may be unacceptable to many elderly men, especially if they are seen to be used on other patients as well. Razors designed for theatre preparation should not be used as they are unsuited to be used on a man's face. Any ward with elderly male patients can be adequately stocked with supplies of disposable safety razors. It is worth remembering that some of these men fought their way across battle-torn Europe carrying shaving equipment with them! As a student nurse once pointed out to me, 'If the Jerries could not stop them shaving, why on earth should Geris?' It seems that 'geriatric nurses' can be more effective in stopping the patient shaving than the privations of war!

CONTINENCE

Hand-washing after using the toilet is seen as a basic requirement, and most of use would certainly complain if such facilities did not exist in a restaurant. It seems a pity that this facility is often not extended to hospital patients. And it is not only hand-washing that is often overlooked, but hygiene too after episodes of urinary or faecal incontinence.

Quite often the response to incontinence is to have the patient wear a pad and knickers which are designed to prevent urine and faeces from leaking out and staining clothes and sheets (see Chapter 12). These items are excellent in what they do. Unfortunately they do their job almost too well in that they save laundry by keeping the urine and faeces next to the skin. Unless a patient's skin is cleaned after every episode of soiling they risk developing skin problems including painful and irritating rashes and ulcers. Perhaps this risk is overlooked because it is so basic, but so often patients are at risk because of it. It is not enough merely to change incontinence pads or to put the patient into clean pyjamas or nightdress. Sadly time or the lack of it is often used as an excuse for neglecting to wash incontinent patients, as if other things were important. Incontinence is a personal tragedy, and if dealing with its after-effects is not seen as being a job worthy of the nurse's time, then I would suggest the nurse has her priorities wrong.

CLEANLINESS HEAD TO TOE

The skin should be cleaned when the patient is sweating otherwise the patient is left feeling uncomfortable, perhaps smelling unpleasantly and at risk of irritation and rash. It should be remembered that dehydration is a major problem for many elderly sick people. A combination of dehydration and poor elasticity may leave the skin more prone to damage by certain soaps and so emollient creams may be prescribed, The obese patient, particularly, is at great risk at the hands of the provider of the cursory wash. Unwashed sweat under folds of skin can lead to excoriation which may not be noticed until the time for 'basic hygiene' is past and more drastic and time-consuming means need to be employed.

Patients should have the opportunity to have at least a basic hand-wash before meals. The hands are used to convey food to the mouth, as well as to rub, scratch and pick, however unconsciously, those areas that might be better left unrubbed, unscratched and unpicked. This is of more importance in the case of a debilitated patient whose natural resistance to infection is compromised but it is also a basic social nicety for most people.

Nails need not always be kept short, but attention should be paid regularly to them as a scratch with dirty fingernails, with their ability to accumulate bacteria from all over the body is about as good a way to introduce germs into the bloodstream as any I have yet come across.

The eyes also need special attention as they are not only the windows of the soul but also just about the best culture medium outside of a Petri dish. Any form of discharge from the eyes should be reported and a swab sent for culture and sensitivity. The eyes may also be damaged by drying, again more so in the case of the debilitated. A common cause, often overlooked, is the positioning of a fan used to cool a patient with a pyrexia. Patients whose eyes have been left unnaturally open for any reason, after a stroke, or when unconscious, because they lack the normal bath of tears are in danger of corneal damage. Eyes may be gently closed against dirt and draughts, topical lotions may be prescribed and the eye bathed in sterile saline. The eyes should be treated separately to prevent the risk of cross-infection.

The care of the feet is a topic many nurses, who have to spend a great part of the day walking and standing, may well feel sympathetic about. The revulsion that neglected feet inspires, however, is one of the reasons why foot care is seen as a distasteful job which can be left to somebody else. The feet should be washed daily and nails kept short. They should be checked regularly for signs of damage. Most foot problems cause a great deal of discomfort and lead to difficulty with mobility. However, if dealt with promptly these can be kept to a minimum. As an example, athlete's foot can be dealt with by regular cleaning, adequate drying with separate towels and the use of anti-fungal powder. A myth seems to have grown that only the chiropodist should cut an elderly person's toenails. There is no reason whatsoever why nurses should not cut toenails. However, a chiropodist should be called in if the nails are painful or ingrowing or badly overgrown. Special care should be taken in the education of the patient with diabetes because of the risk of vascular damage.

Case study

In the home, Mrs Jackson regularly complained of aching feet and, because of her limited mobility, had little opportunity to exercise or attend to her own foot care. Using a pair of strong nail clippers, cutting directly across the nail and avoiding the skins of the toes, her nurse kept Mrs Jackson's toenails trimmed regularly. Every few days she enjoyed soaking her feet for a few minutes in warm soapy water followed by thorough drying. A few minutes massage with olive oil further relieved her discomfort.

ORAL HYGIENE

Jones, in the RCN research paper *Food for Thought* (1975) quotes the adage 'the condition of the patient's mouth is the most reliable indicator of the kind of nursing care being given to the patient'. Certainly the poorer the patient's condition, the more reliant he is on the nurse to keep his mouth clean and moist 'within the prescribed limits'. A large number of problems can arise due to poor oral hygiene, and again all are treatable, or at least, and perhaps more importantly, preventable (Walker, 1985).

The major problems associated with the neglected mouth are infections of the mouth itself and surrounding structures, and unpleasant taste leading to loss of appetite, bad breath, dryness and cracking of lips. All of these are complications of dehydration, to which the elderly sick may become particularly prone for a number of reasons. There may be an insufficient oral intake of fluids because these are not offered, or are left out of reach and not readily available, or not encouraged when the patient is difficult or very passive. Sweating, due to pyrexia, can lead to dehydration as can excessive mouth breathing. Saliva production may be reduced by either the lack of stimulation, when for example food is not taken, by drugs such as atropine and in anxiety due to the overaction of the sympathetic nervous system.

Most texts on practical nursing contain details of the precise methods of oral hygiene but the main points are: adequate oral fluids, antiseptic mouth-washes and citrus fruits which stimulate the salivary glands. Two further points need to be borne in mind: firstly, that unswallowed food should be removed from the mouth; and secondly, that dentures need to be removed and cleaned regularly as debris can be trapped under the plates.

SHOWERS AND BATHS

So far the emphasis has been on perceived hygiene problems and reasonable nursing responses to them. It should be remembered though that the goal of any nurse is that people themselves should be able to deal with all the activities of daily living, within the limits of their own individual problems. It is therefore not a successful ward that has completely clean patients, if all that cleanliness is accomplished by the good worker technique. A good ward may be measured by the number of 'dirty – but getting there' patients it contains!

The way many people deal with hygiene is by having a bath or a shower. A warm bath, a long luxurious soak, with bubble bath or cologne may be seen as the highlight of a day, the prelude to a romantic evening or a solace and escape from the trials of life. For many elderly people living at home alone a bath can be a potentially dangerous and frightening ordeal. Socialized into the idea that cleanliness is next to godliness and yet physically unable to get in and perhaps more importantly to get out of the bath, they are faced with the alternative of a strip wash balanced on a towel. One of the few luxuries of coming into hospital or residential home is the possibility of a soak in the tub with the aid of nurses and the mechanical aids in a specially designed safe bathroom. Unfortunately, too often this event is marked by the loss of all privacy. A bath becomes a hurried event in a busy (nurse's) day, in a room with a door that is not locked, but is a public thoroughfare for seekers after gossip, talcum powder and truth (Kings Fund, 1982).

CLOTHING

Mention must be made of clothing. It is all very well for good workers to bathe someone every day and then re-dress them in clothes that (if boiled) would produce a reasonable soup. Good leadership and planning would allow nurses to expect an adequate supply of suitable clothing to be available each day. A ward whose patients are dressed in second-hand institutional clothing, or without underwear, tights and socks, is as open to criticism as one where there are no syringes and needles. The special needs of elderly patients for laundry and clothing facilities must be taken into account in the planning and provision of care, both in the long stay and acute setting (Ruston, 1977; Wilshere, 1981).

Case study

Mrs Heath also had difficulty dressing and undressing and she was to be helped with a view to enabling her to carry this out independently:

- Help with choice of own suitable clothing and advise on suitable garments, methods of fastening, etc.
- Give positive reinforcement for attempts made.
- Use of clothing with velcro/other fastenings.
- Liaise with occupational therapist and physiotherapist where appropriate and co-ordinate plan of care.
- Maintain privacy when dressing/undressing.

- Give time to attempt self-care and intervene only when essential.
- One nurse needed to assist.
- Keep record of progress made.
- Involve husband in care and teach him how to help without reducing attempts at self-care.

Barton (1966) first identified 'institutional neurosis' in the hospital population at a time when elderly women wore uniform crossover aprons and 'pudding-basin' haircuts and men wore shapeless and colourless suits and shaven heads. Many settings today still have inadequate provision for providing personal clothing that is the patient's own, labelled, fitted and cleaned to suit his or her personal needs.

However, as the King's Fund report (1982) points out, there cannot be many settings 'where the mere mention of the word laundry does not produce a groan of despair among nurses'. It is often an inevitable effect of bulk purchase of clothes which can stand up to harsh cleaning in hospital laundries that the choice for the patient is reduced. However, there has been an increase in many health settings of the provision of 'personalised clothing' systems. Smaller units can make better use of launderettes and automatic washer services, or give patients an opportunity to wash their own clothing. The use of imagination by nurses as well as applying continual pressure for change within the system can do much to bring about improvement, where the organization fails to meet the patient's right to choice (Raphael and Manderville, 1979).

KEY POINTS FOR PERSONAL HYGIENE AND DRESSING

The following summarize the practices recommended in this chapter (after Raphael and Manderville, 1979; King's Fund, 1975, 1982):

(1) Provide privacy for dealing with hygiene and dressing, for example drawing curtains around beds, toilet doors which lock (safety locks can be fitted which can be opened from the outside in emergency), screens around wash-basins.

(2) Allow patients to help each other and involve relatives as well if they wish to do so. (Nurses should help with teaching appropriate skills.)

(3) Provide adequate shelves, hooks and handrails within the patient's reach.
(4) Provide facilities so that the patient can sit at the wash-basin if necessary.
(5) Ensure mirrors are available, both fixed and mobile to suit the patients' height.
(6) Offer the use of the toilet whenever possible and use bedpans and urinals as a last resort.
(7) Ensure patients have the opportunity to use separate facilities in mixed sex areas if they prefer, for example segregated wash-rooms, toilets and bedroom areas.
(8) Ensure patients' problems related to hygiene, bowels, etc. are discussed in private with them and to avoid patients and others nearby overhearing.
(9) Ensure that patients have a choice of clothing suited to their needs with well-fitting shoes and slippers. Clothing should be measured and fitted to personal sizes and choice, be labelled and the institute should provide a personalized clothing system that ensures their safe return in good condition.
(10) Provide facilities on wards, in homes for prompt washing of clothing and enable patients to continue washing their own clothing if desired.

A dirty person has the right to remain dirty, and would probably do so in spite of nursing efforts, but somebody who is not normally dirty or unshaven should never be made to become so because of old age or admission to a hospital or other institution.

We should always be aware of what nursing is about. It is as Virginia Henderson (1966) states, those things that the patient would do unaided if able, and not imposing views of cleanliness that are not based on research or knowledge.

REFERENCES

Barton, R. (1966) *Institutional Neurosis*, Wright, Bristol.
Briggs, A. (Chairman) (1972) *The Report of the Committee on Nursing*, HMSO, London.
Clarke, M. (1978) Getting through the work, in R. Dingwall and J. McIntosh (eds.) *Readings in the Sociology of Nursing*, Churchill Livingstone, Edinburgh.
Fielding, P. (1986) *Attitides Revisited*, RCN, London.

Henderson, V. (1966) *The Nature of Nursing*, Macmillan, New York.
Jones, B. (1975) *Food for Thought*, RCN, London.
King's Fund (1975) *Catalogue of Garments for the Handicapped and Disabled*, Kings Fund , London.
Kings Fund (1982) *Living in Hospital*, Kings Fund, London.
Millar, E. J. and Gwynne, G. V. (1972) *A Life Apart,* Tavistock, London.
Pearson, A. and Vaugham, B. (1986) *Models for Practice*, Heinemann, London.
Raphael, W. and Mandeville, J. (1979) *Old People in Hospital*, Kings Fund, London.
Royal College of Nursing (1985) *The Education of Nurses: A New Dispensation*, RCN, London.
Royal College of Nursing (1987) in collaboration with British Geriatrics Society and the Royal College of Psychiatrists, *Improving Care of Elderly People in Hospital*, RCN, London.
Ruston, R. (1977) *Dressing for Disabled People: A Manual for Nurses and Others*, Disabled Living Foundation, London.
Salvage, J. (1985) *The Politics of Nursing*, Heinemann, London.
Walker, D. M. (1985) Oral disease, in M. S. J. Pathy, *Principles and Practice of Geriatric Medicine,* Wiley, Chichester.
Wells, T. (1980) *Problems in Geriatric Nursing*, Churchill Livingstone, Edinburgh.
Williamson, C. (1987) *Reviewing the Quality of Care in the NHS*, NAHA, Birmingham.
Wilshere, E. R. (ed.) (1981) *Clothing and Dressing for Adults*, Oxfordshire Area Health Authority, Oxford.

9. Mobilizing

Lesley Wade

IMAGES OF MOBILITY

Dr Bronowski (1979) tells us that the ascent of man began, in a parched African landscape, when man first put his foot to the ground. 'By this simple act the human made a commitment to a new integration of life'.

The freedom and independence that mobility gave is as highly valuable now as it was to the first nomadic tribes. Early humanity's attitudes to those that were not as mobile differ little from today's – if you could not keep up you were left behind. The transition to old age involves the loss of many attributes that are highly valued in society. In the nineteenth century this derisory comment was made of the elderly's attempt to mobilize: 'They set off, and hobbled along, nearly even with each other for some time yet frequently and to the inexpressible division of the company, they stumbled and tottered' (*Evelina* by Francis Burnley).

The image today however is slightly different. Len Rolls, a 75-year-old, was recently interviewed by the Sunday papers. He has won the over-70s national fun run four times. 'He trains daily, and last July won two silver medals and a bronze, in the European Veterans' Championship in Sweden' (Harris, 1986). About his active life he states,

> I keep pondering on whether it is inevitable to deteriorate. I'd like to think it isn't. One of the chaps has worked out exactly how much slower your time becomes each year, but I don't accept that. I'd like to see if I can

> manage to improve each year. When I taught a keep-fit class I used to ask, what's the difference between a young and an old person? I replied, it was only the spring in your step.

In less than 100 years therefore, human experience has varied to the degree that the elderly runner is more to be applauded than derided. Yet, just like past generations we know that mobility is not just a question of the ability to move. Mobility is a matter of purpose, an activity, since without this ability and the resources to be mobile the individual cannot participate in social life (Barker and Bury, 1983). Mobility amongst the elderly must therefore take account of the cultural and social structures that individuals live in, as well as the medical and physical factors.

SLOWING DOWN

Ageing does not start at any one time, but the gradual accumulation of cellular and tissue changes have external signs and affects that become increasingly self-evident. These changes occur within and without the cell. In particular, many organs lose their reserve capacity, and cell division slows down altering function. Outside the cell the amount and quality of collagen is affected. Collagen is a long chain of protein that forms an imporatnt part of all connective tissue. In tissue such as lungs and heart, not normally rich in this material, there is an increase. The lens of the eye and the skin, for example, become thicker and less elastic. Bones become thinner and less impregnated with calcium salts. Degenerative changes and disease affect arteries, building up atheroma, and joints, and produces changes in the brain. There is an increased incidence of cancer, and of acquiring auto-immune disease. The acquisition of disease and the chronic nature of it means that the older patient tends to collect disease. Older people may have several disorders at the same time and suffer from 'multiple pathology' (Pathy, 1985). As health is usually assessed by the presence or absence of disease, it is often best to estimate the health of the elderly in terms of *functional abilities,* that is whether or not everyday tasks can be performed.

Ninety per cent of men and 80 per cent of women are able to get out and about without assistance, but the amount of help required increases with age (Tables 9.1).

Table 9.1 Relationship of mobility problems to age

Age group	*Permanently bed-fast (%)*	*Permanently housebound (%)*	*Requiring assistance (%)*
65–69	0.0	1.1	3.2
70–74	0.0	2.5	6.6
75–79	0.4	4.9	9.6
80–84	1.0	9.7	12.5
85+	1.9	17.7	26.8

Source: Hunt, 1978.

Hunt suggests there is a variation in mobility between the male and female elderly population. These differences are a direct consequence of the higher proportion of arthritis and rheumatism in the elderly females (Table 9.2).

Table 9.2 Cause of loss of mobility or of being bed-fast or house bound

	%
Arthritis/rheumatism	36.2
Pulmonary conditions	17.2
Strokes/paralysis	14.9
Blindness/failing sight	14.4
Circulatory conditions	13.8
Cardiac conditions/blood pressure	13.2
Effects of accidents	9.8
Nervous conditions	4.6
Other specific illness or condition	29.9
Old age/other vague descriptions	6.9

Source: Hunt, 1978.

The environment outside the home, also produces mobility difficulties for the elderly (Table 9.3).

Table 9.3 Mobility problems outside the home

Environmental challenge	*% of all elderly*	*% of elderly with arthritis*
Hills and ramps	31	68
Traffic and road crossing	23	48
Uneven pavements	16	73
Steps and kerbs	4	59
No problems	40	not recorded

Source: Age Concern, 1978.

The above figures illustrate the immense difficulties that can occur for those elderly people for whom mobility is reduced in old age. Hunt (1978) goes on to show how reduced mobility affects large numbers of people in their ability to complete even the most simple activities of living. For example over 50 per cent of the over-85s needed help with bathing or cutting toenails. Household chores such as gardening/cleaning floors for more than half of this age group are severely restricted or impossible to achieve alone.

Bradfield and Leeming (1978 personal communication, cited in Barker and Bury, 1983) analysed the mobility of the elderly in a Manchester group practice. Out of 365 over-75-year-olds they found 107 housebound. Of this number the health visitor assessed that half were unsafe to cross the road in heavy traffic, a third were too breathless and the remaining third did not have access to shops within a quarter of an hour's walk.

Therefore, not only do the elderly have inherent problems, but the very environment creates restrictions and barriers to freedom and independence. From a sociological perspective the influence inner city decay, slum clearance and high rise flats have on all the population can clearly be seen. To elderly town dwellers the destruction of the inner city is the quintessence of past life and experiences. Shopping becomes a major problem. When the corner shop is replaced by the hypermarket a distance away it is costly both in time and effort in obtaining transport. Distance is not the only problem of access. Lifts, escalators, uneven surfaces, and unfamiliar signs are alien. Centralizing doctors' clinics and chemists are not totally to the benefit of the elderly. The walk for the pension may be much longer due to the reduction of community sub-post offices; with this there is the added risk of carrying of pension money. Because of the availability of bus passes, public transport appears more accessible. However, frail elderly people often have difficulty manoeuvring on and off this type of transport. New town planning has altered the elderly's perspective of the place they used to live in. Flyovers and subways may appear frightening (Elder, 1977).

Case history

A few years ago Emily, 88, decided to go Christmas shopping for her granddaughter. She managed the changes of bus, arrived at the new bus station and walked into the new shopping precinct where she ventured into a boutique. However, on returning home she became totally lost in the subway. She wandered for three-quarters of an hour in this subterranean passage until two teenagers approached and guided her out. Emily never went back into the old town she once knew. Like many individuals she retreated into her own world, becoming a passive member of the community. Thinking to herself, 'I'll stay at home, there I know I can control my own world,' she became housebound.

Many of the elderly do not have the choice of withdrawing voluntarily from the community, because they have become victims of the disease process. Disorders of the heart and the lungs have a great effect on mobility. Chronic bronchitis leads to breathlessness, particularly when climbing stairs, but also when simply gently walking. Heart failure may make such demands on the individual's narrowed coronary artery that pain ensues from walking. Some of these problems may be treatable, but often it would take a good detective to unravel the causes of impediments to mobility.

Case history
In appearance Bert is rather obese and neglected. He has recently been widowed and lives in a stone cottage. He tells the nurse that his problem is at the top of his legs but it is worse when he walks up the stairs. When he does manage the stairs it takes him fifteen minutes, resting on each step. The mystery of Bert's mobility problems can be unravelled by the skilled assessor. The pain in the hip may well be due to osteo-arthritis. The breathlessness is due to mild heart failure. The physical assessment clearly tells us that Bert is overweight; close examination may show oedema of the lower limbs and overgrown toenails. It is a combination of all these problems that contribute to Bert's immobility and they are further complicated by his two-storey house and upstairs toilet. Bert's multiple pathology, degenerative changes and social problems alone have not fully contributed to this state. Bert's loneliness and depression due to his recent bereavement may also contribute. Nursing needs to use a holistic assessment perspective before it can start to provide care for the elderly immobile.

GOING OFF MY LEGS

Many elderly people describe their problems of immobility by stating, 'I'm going off my legs.' To find out why people go off their legs, logically we should examine the nature of falls. Sheldon (1960) looked extensively at the nature of falls and found it was not inevitably a process of ageing. Out of 500 clients interviewed he categorized his findings as follows:

Accidental fall	171
Drop attacks	125
Trips	53
Vertigo	37
Recognizable central nervous system lesions	27
Head back	20
Postural hypotension	18
Weakness in legs	16
Falling out of bed chair	10
Uncertain	23

All but one category had some explanation. Sheldon found that within the accidental fall group the greatest hazards were stairs and poor lighting. Slippery surfaces and seasonal weather also contributed. The problems arising from drop attacks were seen by the length of time it took for the individual to recover or to be found. Sheldon found that many of these attacks were a manifestation of a decrease in postural control. Many of the falls due to trips were precipitated by not lifting feet as high as before. This tendency to reduction in gait had been described as early as 1931 by Critchely. He called it '*marche a petits pas*'. Falls due to vertigo are of a small percentage, the reason being that the development of an attack of vertigo is usually slow enough to allow safety measures. One-tenth of the falls in the sample were due to disease of the central nervous system. A majority of the falls were also due to the individual looking upwards with the head going back; a smaller proportion were due to rapidly standing erect producing postural hypotension. Therefore, a high proportion of causes Sheldon found for the elderly going 'off their legs' were treatable.

Sheldon's findings are not the only reason for the elderly 'going off their legs'. Arthritis literally means joint inflammation but osteo-arthritis is a non-inflammatory disorder that causes cartilage degeneration. On assessment of an elderly person the history may indicate joint pain following exercise, morning stiffness and problems with dressing. Physical assessment may show swollen limbs due to fluid around joints, again producing limited mobility (Pathy, 1985). Since it can be included in many of these problems, the nurse must not forget the hereditary metabolic disease gout. Assessment may show joint inflammation due to excessive urate deposits. A warm, tender joint is often found around the big toe. It is not, as is often thought, just those that enjoy rich living and purine-rich foods who are susceptible to gout. Those who are on long-term diuretic therapy may often aggravate this condition.

A more systemic problem is a disease known as rheumatoid arthritis which effects the connective tissue throughout the body. Reduction of mobility may occur from the incapacity produced by pain, also from the deformed joints that become so acutely inflamed. This prevents the wearing of shoes and makes walking difficult. On assessing the patient the nurse will find not only swollen and painful joints at wrists and fingers but often deformity, and wasting of muscles. Working with other members of the team, planned care may include;

- Cold pack application to reduce joint inflammation.
- Planned rest to reduce joint inflammation.
- Application of appropriate lightweight splints to protect joints.
- Swimming to promote range of movements.

- Medication to reduce joint pain.
- Joint surgery to replace joints immobilized by degenerative changes.

THE TEAM APPROACH

The team approach is not only essential in promoting mobility, but the cross-fertilization of ideas and shared experiences are immensely rewarding. Myree is a physiotherapist working within such a team. The following highlights many of her skills and attitudes:

> For the physiotherapist working with the elderly patient 'mobilizing' is carried out to give that person the physical means and encouragement to act as independently as possible. For instance, this independence could mean not having to wait for help when the need to go to the toilet arises, or it could mean being able to walk quickly enough to cross a busy road safely.
>
> On the ward, often the situation is a stark one. If the elderly patient's mobility is improved or regained, that person can return to his or her former home and life-style; if not, the options of where that person will live are very restricted, for probably the rest of that person's life. The rehabilitation, of an elderly patient must begin from day one, and for twenty-four hours a day in hospital, and mobilization is a key aspect. It continues in the community with both nurse and domiciliary physiotherapist continuing care.

Effective communication between the physiotherapist, the elderly patient and members of staff is essential. This creates a consistent, supportive environment that allows the required progress to take place (Rodgers, 1985). The lines of communication should be many and frequently used. They may be formal, as in a weekly ward meeting, or informal, as when the physiotherapist helps the nurse to transfer a patient from bed to chair, or when the nurse encourages a patient to put on his or her own shoes without help.

This communication must be patient-centred. Patient-centred means firstly that person must be listened to carefully, that both openness and tact are used when setting goals, which must be realistic, and that adequate information and enough time are given to allow that person choices both in day-to-day activities and in the long term.

The physiotherapist must first make a detailed assessment. It is necessary to note how much help, if any, the patients needs to perform

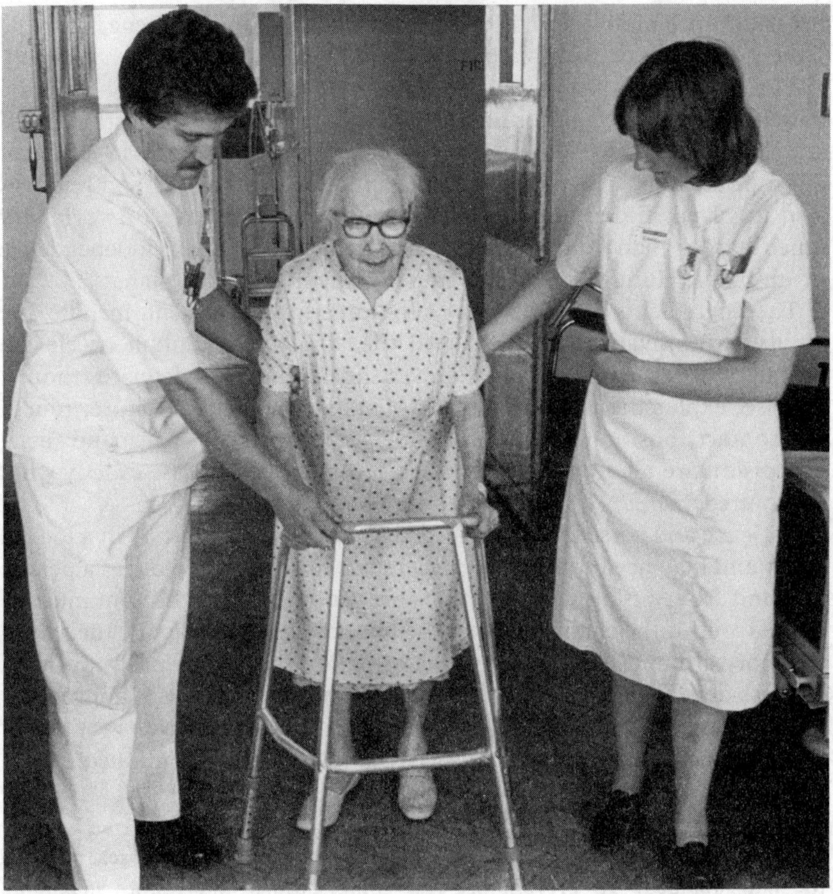

functional activities such as rolling, moving up and down the bed, sitting, transfers, standing, walking, getting up from the floor and stair climbing. Balance, joint mobility, muscle strength and co-ordination are also assessed as they affect mobility. Once this assessment has been done, the information gained should be communicated to other staff members working with the patient. This helps to prevent an over-cautious 'protective' approach, or the demoralization which will occur if the patient is asked to do something physically beyond him/her.

This assessment is essential. The physiotherapy treatment must be planned so that improvement can be evaluated and progression follows in an orderly way. Continuous assessment is also needed when the aims for the future mobility and level of self-care and independence that the patient may achieve are planned.

The physiotherapist must also liaise with all staff working with the patient, not forgetting those in the community, such as the district nurse and domiciliary physiotherapist, in planning care and the selection of appropriate aids. The patient's home situation is discussed and relatives also involved. Elderly patients need more time and have to work very much harder than younger patients to achieve maximum independence of mobility (Hunt, 1978). They must be involved in the plan.

The ingredients of successful physiotherapy treatment include the ability to motivate the patient and the ability to maintain or elevate morale and self-confidence, whatever the condition. Adequate, though concise, explanations and instructions should be given. Gesture, touch, eye contact, positioning of both helpers and furniture, voice and facial expression are all very important and must clearly indicate exactly what is required.

Patience and persistence are needed as instructions must be in a logical order and may need to be frequently repeated. For example, for a person to stand from sitting several actions are required. Their bottom must be at the front of the chair, their feet well back and slightly apart, their head well forward and they must use the arms of the chair to push up from. Success depends greatly upon repetition, and upon the team approach – teaching, advising, helping – and praising the patient as even very minor goals are achieved to reinforce success and encourage continued effort.

Case study

Mrs Cesno had great difficulty moving herself in bed and could not get from bed to chair unaided. To prevent bed-rest complications and restore maximum independence and mobility, at least to the point where she could get to the toilet unaided, a gradual plan of mobilization was devised.

- Provide hoist over bed.
- Help with position changes in bed at least every two hours with two nurses to assist.
- Use of full-length sheepskin.
- Help with chest and limb exercises. Teach these to her so she can maintain them independently.
- Refer to physiotherapy, and liaise with, to co-ordinate exercises.
- Help with lifting from bed to chair and back again (two nurses).
- Use of footboards in bed for support and 'push-up' cushion on chair to aid standing.

- Use upright armchair.
- Help with positioning limbs in good alignment.
- Help with walking (two nurses to support with frame) around bed or bed to chair at least twice daily for the first week.
- Gradually increase distance walked within her level of comfort until she is able to walk full length of ward with walking frame.
- Give praise to encourage her as mobility improves.

There must also be an orderly sequence of progression from assistance to supervision, to maximum independence. Returning abilities must be immediately utilized in daily activities. Therefore the physiotherapist and nurse must constantly work together to keep up to date on what levels of functional ability the patient has, so that the treatment is reinforced by practice.

Often physiotherapists will give advice about what equipment or walking aid is needed. To change the height of a person's chair sometimes is a very simple but effective means of improving mobility, and all those working with the patient must be made aware of this, if it is changed, for example by keeping up-to-date records in a care plan. Walking aids, such as sticks or frames, must be checked to see that they are not defective, are of the correct height and are suitable for use in the patient's home. Again, improvement in mobility is much quicker if all staff helping the elderly patient to walk use the same walking aid and give instructions in the same manner. Referrals to social services, voluntary organizations (see appendix of addresses on p.304 and local authorities may be necessary to provide practical help and financial assistance if rehousing or rearrangement of the home is necessary.

MEETING NEEDS

In helping the immobile patient, especially those with hemiplegia, Adams (1967) states that there are four vital elements. He emphasizes the team approach, with its variety of skill mixture (see also Chapter 3). Also needed is that team working as a cohesive body. He also states that although these immobile individuals need speical facilities, they need not be expensive. Space and equipment must be used judiciously. What the hemiplegic patient needs is time, both in terms of attention with each session as well as the weeks and months needed to allow the individual to adjust to their disability. Emphasis should be given to the need for after-care whether at home, in day centres or in day hospitals. Planning for after-care is a natural progression of the care given to a patient who has suffered a cerebrovascular accident or any restriction to mobility requiring continuous support. The patient's progression was noted by Adams (1967) to be not so much influenced by physical disability; more often progression was impeded by the patients being unaware of their own shortcomings and the facilities available to help them.

BARRIERS

Loss of body awareness, due to cerebrovascular accidents, can produce many barriers. These include disorders of special senses, problems of defective comprehension, like loss of reasoning and memory, as well as loss of sensation. Those caring, which includes both professionals as well as friends and relatives, must be able to recognize these barriers and the problems that can ensue. Helping the patient with a mobility problem requires a multidisciplinary approach and including education for non-professional carers in the best way to help. Some special difficulties to consider (Gould, 1987) include the following.

Sight

Defective vision may be resolved by wearing glasses or even eye surgery. Hemianopia may resolve in time but often non-dominant hemisphere lesions with parietal lobe involvement leads to individuals ignoring and often disowning not only the affected side but also the surroundings on that side. Mobility is interfered with, as a patient cannot appreciate anything to do with this field of vision. Many activities of daily living are altered. Half-dressed, or even half-eaten meals may be a consequence. Space blindness means that the patient cannot assess the relationship of objects in space to his own body image – the world is no longer a three-dimensional one. Often this means bumping into things. This is often seen when such a patient approaches an object, like a chair. Clumsy fumbling will occur as the patient tries to bring the right part of the anatomy in proper relationship with the chair. More often than not, the patient may end up sitting on the floor.

Hearing

The perceptive nurse will remove excessive wax or apply hearing aids for her patient. Deafness, however, takes various forms. Perceptual deafness causes distortion of quality with intolerance amplification. Difficulties in communication often tax both the patients and carer's tolerance, making it more difficult for the patient to follow the nurse's teaching (see Chapter 5).

Intellectual Barriers

Intellectual barriers can be due to defective comprehension and impaired interpretation. Often, responses are inappropriate as the instructions have been received without proper grasp of meaning. Individuals may often give a response which would have been more appropriate to the previous instruction. This term is known as preservation and can produce much frustration. Inattentiveness is often due to sheer exhaustion but may be also one of the first signs of oncoming depression. Drug therapy which elevates mood may prove beneficial, but needs to be seen as a second resort, to be used with the teaching and therapeutic communication skills (Chapter 5) of the nurse.

Learning

The loss of ability to perform a previously learnt skill is known as apraxia. This may lead the individual in thinking that rehabilitation is futile.

In meeting the needs of the immobile patient, consideration of the individuality of the person is integral to his care. Adams (1967) found that many problems that inhibit mobility produce bed-fast patients, 'For no better reason than the loss of confidence and initiative induced by too frequent falls.' He stated that many actually acquire a new 'postural set' and find it difficult to stand upright.

CREATIVE PLANNING

Loss of confidence within the patient may also be a symptom displayed.

The following serves to illustrate how this may be overcome, not least by the use of a sense of humour:

Case study

Two nurses helped Jimmy to attend his grand-daughter's twenty-first. Jimmy had eight weeks previously suffered a cerebrovascular accident and had a left-sided hemiplegia. Despite great efforts the best-made plans of mice and men do not always go according to plan. All three gave an hilarious account of unexpected problems. One of the situations they had to explain themselves out of was their accompanying of Jimmy to the male toilets. There Jean and Alice stood supporting Jimmy, shoulder to shoulder with other male guests. How do you begin to explain! The situation was rationalized by many of the company with the aid of alcohol consumption.

Many other practical problems affect the ability of the elderly to mobilize. One of the greatest, as suggested earlier, is the inability of the elderly to cut toenails (Hunt, 1978). Caring for feet includes advice and actual treatment. Many signs of serious illness may manifest themselves in the feet and legs. Problems with toenails are often associated with poor eyesight and the presence of other conditions like arthritis, making it difficult to bend. Eye changes make focussing difficult, arthritic fingers make it difficult to grasp scissors. Those with good eyesight and reasonable mobility should continue to cut their own toenails provided they have not grown too thick or deformed. Otherwise, the services of the chiropodist are necessary. On assessing the lower limbs the nurse should be aware of many things. Inappropriate footwear must be avoided, ill-fitting shoes and socks or stockings may cause back pressure on the foot creating pain, tissue damage and eventful deformity. The nurse should always make careful assessment for the presence of oedema and the possibility of pressure sores. Certain aims must be kept in mind in promoting footcare and mobility for the elderly. They are:

- Keep the individual as mobile and independent as possible.
- Refer any problems with nail-beds or corns to a chiropodist.
- Observe carefully for signs of impending deterioration in lower limbs and act upon it, e.g. swelling, redness, bruising or cracking of skin, undercurving of toenails or blackened areas of nail-beds or skin.

USING KNOWLEDGE AND RESEARCH

If mobility is not promoted eventually there may be problems with pressure sores. The elderly are more at risk due to the risks of becoming chair and bed-bound, and with the possible problems of continence. The cost of treating pressure sores, not including discomfort and pain, is thought to be more than £150 million and to affect 5 out of every 100 patients admitted to hospital (Livesey, 1985).

One of the many criticisms made of nursing has been in its poor ability to disseminate research findings. Over twenty years ago Norton (Norton, McLaren and Exton-Smith, 1962) devised a simple scoring system based on levels of activity; Goldstone and Goldstone (1982) still found this predictive system of anticipating pressure sores beneficial. Yet despite the quantity of research into this area there still appears to be as many opinions about treating pressure sores as there are nurses (Chapman and Chapman, 1986). David (1982) made a comprehensive literature review into the treatment of pressure sores producing much clarity on the subject. Within her paper she concluded that problems of treating these sores rests mainly on remembering the individuality of the patient. No dogmatic approach should be taken because the sores vary with age, prognosis and physical state. What is important is a knowledge of the healing process, establishing what is realistic to achieve, and determining what might impede this achievement.

MOBILITY RESTRICTION AND THE PRESSURE SORE

Any form of restraint or restriction that could further hinder the mobility of the elderly adds to the risk of developing pressure sores along with other potential complication of bed-rests. The elderly are particularly at risk of developing pressure sores for a variety of reasons associated with the ageing process. These include the following problems according to Barton (1976):

- Loss of subcutaneous tissue.
- Loss of skin elasticity.
- Loss of sensation.
- Poor nutrition.
- Advancing senility.

Unplanned tissue breakdown of any kind is traumatic. Pressure sores develop when there is a sustained pressure greater than the mean capillary pressure of 25 mmHg. This may result in ischaemia and death of tissue from anoxia.

There are four different types of pressure known to lead to pressure sore formation. These include the following (Colquhon, 1983):

- Pressure from compression – namely skin squeezed between a bony prominence and a hard exterior surface, e.g. a chair.
- Pressure from shearing force – underlying blood vessels damaged as overlying skin is dragged across them.
- Direct disruption – injury to skin affecting blood supply.
- Friction – damage to skin by objects rubbing the surface.

Removal or reduction of pressure requires good assessment skills. Lowthian (1979) suggests that as a priority the patient should be encouraged to do this him/herself; if not able, a schedule for turning high risk patients should be introduced.

In searching for aids to help to relieve pressure, there appears to be no universal item. Research at the tissue viability centre at Northwick Park Hospital (Crow, 1979) obtained these results from aids tested:

- Synthetic sheepskins – raised pressure
- Heel pads – reduced pressure
- Real sheepskins – reduced pressure
- Para pads – raised pressure
- Feather pillows – most effective

From the information gathered it can be seen that many aids used could aggravate the problems of pressure sores.

Lifting and moving the patient in order to reduce and relieve pressure is one of the most effective measures in preventing tissue damage. Those involved in lifting the elderly patient should be taught to do so in order to maximize comfort and safety. Poor lifting technique and excessive use of pillows may further aggravate the situation.

Recent research and knowledge has altered a great deal of practice once based on myth in dealing with pressure sores. It has long been recognized that massaging the skin to promote better circulation is unhelpful. Excessive cleansing of the skin can cause loss of natural oils, and the alkalis in soap can lead to epidermal damage (Dyson, 1978). It has also been found that using protective plastic sheeting on beds is not recommended it increases the skin's temperature, preventing evaporation of sweat (Norton, McLaren and Exton-Smith, 1962).

The complexity of the skills needed in caring for the elderly at risk of developing pressure sores, requires a systematic, scientific approach.

Early assessment is essential, and assessment tools like the Norton Scale are often underused.

The Norton Scale

The Norton Scale is used as a means of assessing the patient's risk of developing pressure sores when in hospital. The following factors are used to work out the score:

	A	B	C	D	E
Factor	*Physical condition*	*Mental condition*	*Activity*	*Mobility*	*Incontinence*
4	Good	Alert	Ambulant	Full	Not
3	Fair	Apathetic	Walk/help	Slightly limited	Occasionally
2	Poor	Confused	Chairbound	Very limited	Usually urine
1	Very bad	Stuporous	Bed-fast	Immobile	Doubly

Identify the most appropriate description of the patient and total the results from columns A to E. For example, a patient in poor physical condition (score 2) who is confused (2), bed-fast (1), with limited mobility (2) and doubly incontinent (1) has a total score of 8. A score of 14 or below denotes a need for intensive pressure area care, for example a half-hourly position change and use of pressure-relieving aids.

Note: If sacral oedema is present, even if the score is above 14, it may still indicate a risk of sores.

(Norton, McLaren and Exton-Smith, 1962)

Assessment includes the skill of accurate history taking and the application of practical skills, like touch, smell and observation.

Information gained in this way allows the nurse to plan and implement strategies. These should involve:

- Assessment of nutritional states. It may be necessary to increase protein and vitamin C, as both are known to contribute to tissue growth and repair (Winter, 1976).
- Assessment for oedema which may impede the micro-circulation interfering with the healing process.

Attention should be paid to the lower limbs, especially the heels, as this is one of the most difficult areas of care (Norton, McLaren and Exton-Smith, 1962). Problems with pressure on heels are found not only on orthopaedic wards due to fractures of femur, but through badly designed, ill-fitting chairs. Heel pressures often exceed the mean capillary pressure, and any pressure above 30 mmHg can cause damage. Regular accurate assessment is needed to detect early tissue breakdown. If this is seen the nurse must take action and plan care according to how developed the pressure sore has become.

The skin may present in different stages:

Type 1 – The skin discoloured, especially around areas known as pressure points, for example the sacrum, heels and elbows. The area may appear raised, red, blistered or black.
Type 2 – The skin is broken. However, there is only epithelial damage. The area looks grazed.
Type 3 – Damage extends through full thickness of the skin.
Type 4 – Tissue other than skin is involved and often a cavity forms.

If there is tissue damage the aim is to create optimal conditions in which cellular activity and wound contraction takes place. In order to promote healing the nurse should remember these points (Winter, 1976):

- Wound swabs must be taken if infection is suspected.
- The wound should be treated as any other asceptic dressing.
- Caution needs to be exercised when removing dressings, for further damage to the wound may occur. If removal may cause trauma, the dressing should be soaked beforehand with saline.
- The choice of dressing is dependent on the needs of each individual patient. It is known that epidermal regeneration is enhanced by a moist wound surface. Application of a permeable occlusive dressing prevents dehydration and promotes healing.

Teaching patients at risk to help themselves is perhaps one of the most effective ways of preventing pressure sore formation in the elderly. The learning needs of the elderly include advice on the following (Francis Jones, 1979):

- *Clothing*. Emphasis should be placed on wearing loose-fitting cotton/wool clothing and correctly fitted shoes.
- *Avoidance of pressure*. Relatives and patients may need to be taught about lifting and the correct use of aids.
- *Self-care*. A mirror is a good way of allowing patients to monitor care of the skin themselves. Patients should also be helped to become more responsible for their own weight control.

Research from the tissue viability team at Northwick Park indicates that often inappropriate care is given due to the lack of evaluation in dealing with this problem. Constant inquiry and reassessment is essential in preventing and promoting care of pressure sores.

The consequence of immobility not only affects the patient but the safety of those providing care. Back pain can affect both relatives and carers alike. Rodgers (1985) showed that a positive environment incorporating teaching of nurses and other carers, within a ward enhanced better lifting. This was achieved by good staff relationships, a powerful role model in the sister and a comprehensive policy on lifting that was both taught and practised. Selection of the correct lift depends on assessing the individual, again no one dogmatic approach can be taken. The critia is what is safe for the patient and carer and what is comfortable for both.

Based on the RCN and the Back Pain Association's guidelines (1987), the nurses in one clinical area drew up the following advice on good lifting technique for use on their ward:

- The weight to be lifted or moved (pushed/pulled) must be within the competence of the individual concerned with the activity.
- The period of time that the operator has to sustain the lift or movement should be as short as possible. Prolonged lifting or moving activity increases the risk of back strain. This may mean that a series of short lifts may be required to reach the objective.
- Never lift alone. Two or more nurses must lift patients, selecting the most appropriate technique.
- The weight to be moved must be held as close to the operator's trunk as possible, and the back should always be held straight. The knees

should be flexed, this ensures that the power for the lift comes from the strong muscles of the legs, and not the weak back muscles.

- Trunk rotation must be avoided. If one needs to turn whilst supporting a weight, walk round in a small circle.
- Clothing must allow freedom of movement. Tight skirts prevents movement of the legs. High heels or platform shoes make the ankles unstable and thus increase the risk to the spine.
- The lifting environment must be safe. Floors should be free from obstruction and there must be room for the lift. Planning of the lift or move must be made before the action is implemented.
- Nurses lifting together must nominate a 'leader' to say when to lift and should lift simultaneously.
- Lifts and movements should be carried out steadily and smoothly. Jerking considerably increases the compression on the spine.
- Always consider the aim and overall objective to be served by every task. *Never* lift a patient unless you have to. Given the correct equipment decide whether the patient could move him/herself.
- Assess the patient's needs and physical condition. Use lifting or moving devices whenever possible.
- Explain to the patient exactly *what* you are going to do and *when* you are going to do it so that he/she and you are prepared and the patient can help and not be panicked into uncontrolled activity.
- Ensure that firm contact exists between nurses and patients, e.g. arms well under thighs, shoulders or hips, and between nurse and nurse, e.g. good wrist or handgrips.
- Ensure brakes on beds, trolleys, chairs are in the *on* position before commencing lift. Also, if the bed is adjustable, ensure you select correct height. Bedding should not restrict lift.

RETURNING HOME

Mobility is one of the all important criteria in being able to return home. The team planning discharge must ask themselves many questions before that patient goes home:

- Does the patient get in and out of the bed unaided, if not how many people are needed to help?
- Can the patient get out of the chair unaided or is help required?
- Can the patient walk unaided and if so how far?
- Do they need aids and can these be provided and used at home?

Planning for home involves establishing a link which is seen as a continuation of care. This involves a great deal of teaching for both patients and relatives (see Chapter 10). Often, the day hospital, nursing home or community nurse and physiotherapist must continue aspects of enabling and fulfilling the individual's maximum potential, despite the difficulties.

There is wide range of labels and categories given to the elderly with problems of mobility. It has repeatedly been shown that the whole person, their abilities, life-style, anxieties and aspirations play the most important part. The commitment to an active life is central in order to promote mobility. It can be seen that mobility is the key to making participation in life a reality.

REFERENCES

Adams, G. F. (1967) Hemiplegia and immobility, *Gerontology Clinicia,* Vol. 2, pp. 285–94.

Age Concern (1978) *Problems of the Elderly,* Age Concern, London, Vol. 6, pp. 7–8.

Barker, J. and Bury, M. (1983) *An Ageing Population,* Open University Press, Milton Keynes.

Barton, A. A. (1976) Pathogenesis of the skin wounds due to pressure bed sore biomechanics, in R. M. Kenedi, I. M. Cowden and J. D. Scales (eds), *Bed Sore Biomechanics,* Macmillan, London.

Bronowski, J. (1973) *The Ascent of Man,* BBC, London.

Chapman, E. J. and Chapman, R. (1986) Treatment of pressure sores: The state of the art, in A. J. Tierney (ed.) (1986) *Clinical Nursing Practice,* Churchill Livingstone, Edinburgh.

Colquhon M. B. (1983) Nursing management of pressure sores, *Nursing,* Vol. 2 no. 11, pp. 320–22.

Crow, R. (1979) *The Prevention of Pressure Sores,* DHSS, London.

David, J. A. (1982) Pressure sore treatment, a literature review, *International Journal of Nursing Studies,* Vol. 9, no. 4, pp. 183–91.

Dyson, R. (1978) The injuries hospital staff inflict on patients, *Nursing Mirror,* Vol. 146, pp. 30–2.

Elder, G. (1977) *The Alienated: Growing Old Today,* Writers and Readers Publishing Co-operative, London.

Francis Jones, H. W. (1979) Teaching and equipping the patient at risk, Proceedings of a conference on the prevention of pressure sores, Oswestry, 1979.

Goldstone, L. and Goldstone J. (1982) The Norton Scale – an early warning of pressure sores? *Journal of Advanced Nursing*, Vol. 7, no. 5, pp. 419–26.

Gould, D. (1987) The biology of ageing – the special senses, *Geriatric Nursing and Home Care,* Vol. no. 2, pp. 15–19.
Harris, I. (1986) *Sunday Times Publication,* 17 August.
Hunt, A. (1978) *The Elderly at Home,* HMSO, London
Livesey, B. (1985) Airways take the pressure, *Nursing Times,* 23 January.
Lowthian, P. T. (1979) Turning clock systems to prevent pressure sores, *Nursing Mirror,* 24 May 1979, pp. 30–1.
Norton, D., McLaren, R. and Exton-Smith, A. N. (1962) *An Investigation of Geriatric Nursing Problems in Hospital,* Churchill Livingstone, Edinburgh.
Pathy, M. (1985) *Principles and Practice of Geriatric Medicine,* Wiley, Chichester.
Rodgers, S. (1985) Positive lifting, *Nursing Times,* 23 January.
Royal College of Nursing (1987) *Handling Patients – A Guide for Nurse Managers,* RCN, London.
Sheldon, J. H. (1960) Natural History of Falls in Old Age, *British Medical Journal,* Vol. 11, pp. 1685–90.
Winter G. D, (1976) Some factors affecting skin and wound healing, in R. M. Kenedi, J. M. Cowden and J. T. Scales (eds), *Bed Sore Biomechanics,* Macmillan Press, London.

10. Learning

Betty Kershaw

THE NURSE AS EDUCATOR

In order for patients to manage their own care, and thus control their life-style, they need knowledge about, and insight into, their health difficulties. Nurses must remember that patients, their families and their friends are quite able to understand disease processes, treatments, nursing interventions, prognosis and alternatives available. In fact most patients are capable of understanding much about their disease and the intervention necessary and are therefore as able as the professionals to make rational choices. They are also capable of understanding what they must do to maintain health and to improve it provided they are adequately and professionally taught. The Nurses Rules laid down in the Nurses' Act (1979) state that the nurse is the most important health educator in the multidisciplinary team and that she has a duty to develop this aspect of her role.

Although the ability to learn new subjects deteriorates with age (Baski *et al.,* 1983) it does not vanish. Frequently the press report on old-age pensioners who obtain O-level examination passes, A-levels and degrees. A small, but significant number of Open University students are pensioners, as may be witnessed at any Open University degree ceremony, whilst most local authorities provide day-time academic classes especially for pensioners. Education should be an opportunity for the elderly too (Midwinter, 1982).

Wilson-Barnett (1983) emphasizes that all patients benefit from understanding their disease and treatment and by having explanations given as to how they can best co-operate with the nursing care plan. The inclusion of patient (and relatives and friends) in education should be an integral part of any care plan, whether the patients are being cared for in hospital or in their own homes, and whether the attitude and behavioural changes one seeks to achieve through education are temporary or permanent.

Like any other aspect of nursing assessment, the nurse needs to discover her patients' abilities to achieve realistic health goals. It is necessary to ascertain their willingness and readiness to learn, and also discover when they last made an attempt to learn anything new.

If the nurse is to plan a teaching programme she must be experienced in the information-giving process, and fully understand all aspects of intervention (Redman, 1980). Nurses need to communicate with patients in an appropriate language, which causes problems when the patients come from countries other than the UK. Also, there are enormous variables within the UK, both locally and regionally, in language and culture, class and values. The nurse also needs to empathize with the patients, to understand that the elderly do not learn as quickly as the younger person, and be interested in helping patients achieve their goals of self-care through education. Fears of being watched have to be overcome, since any patient who has relatives or friends who are involved with their care need to be taught as well. They are often the ones who ask the awkward quesions. Also to be considered are the factors that affect the patient's learning ability. Both Wilson-Barnett (1983) and Redman (1980) give considerable guidance on factors that affect learning ability. Age has already been mentioned as one, and any physiology text-book will support this statement. Among the factors they mention as affecting learning are arterio-sclerotic changes that reduce oxygen circulation in the brain as well as glucose up-take, and the failure of brain cells to replace themselves.

Ley and Spelman (1967) were the first researchers to demonstrate that patients learn best when the teacher (in their research study, the doctors) reinforces what the patients wish to hear or what they have already decided for themselves. Also, the nurse must remember that not everyone wishes to learn to care for themselves or to accept responsibility for their own care. All too often relatives do not wish to learn skills either, since many people who are caring for relatives, as well as the patients, still believe it is the nurse's job to care and that those who need care have a right to receive care from a nurse.

The nurse needs to develop an open and friendly relationship with patients and their friends and relatives. Trust is an integral part of the teacher/learner relationship regardless of who the student is.

In order to help people learn, the teacher needs to convince them of the benefits of learning new skills and a new way of life. Education may enable them to enjoy a social life again, to perhaps take a voluntary or part-time job, or to enjoy a sexual relationship in old age.

But no one learns if they are anxious, stressed, in pain, confused by drugs or sleep or if they are worried about their present situation. Part of the nursing assessment should be aimed at identifying any such problems and priority nursing intervention must aim to reduce or resolve them so learning potential can be maximized (see also Chapter 5).

Sometimes topics being taught can be embarrassing - care of a stoma, meeting changing sexual needs, coping with a prosthesis for example, and the nurse needs to ensure teaching takes place in private. It is also important to check before including relatives or friends in any teaching that this is what the patient wants. Patients, like many people, may wish to keep body image problems private, and they, and they alone, have the right to choose what friends and relatives are told.

A few simple measures must be remembered. Check that hearing aids are switched on, working and correctly tuned, for example. Patients require the appropriate glasses for looking at supportive literature or slides/video, and it helps the patients' speech if dentures are in place. Finally comfortable seating and privacy are essential.

The next step is to check what the patient already knows. Howard and Erlanger (1983) writing in Wilson-Barnett's book, document the use of a questionnaire for patients who have had a myocardial infarction. The questionnaire is used as a pre-test and again after instruction using a planned teaching programme to assess the learning that has taken place. Similar methods of assessment were advocated in the 1970s and early 1980s by the then Joint Board of Clinical Nursing Studies (1973–84) who were responsible for validating continuing education courses for nurses.

Once the patient's learning abilities have been assessed and the learning needs identified by observation, conversation and more formal methods if appropriate, the nurse can begin to plan care and set learning objectives. In other words the next stage is to prepare the teaching plan. This needs to be planned carefully, taking into account the objectives (or goals) the patient wants to achieve, and remembering that most people have a learning attention span of no more than 15–20 minutes.

In the beginning it is important to reinforce the knowledge the patient already has, provided of course that nurse and patient are satisfied that that knowledge is accurate. The easy aspects can be considered first, then the more complicated. Visual aids can be used in the form of slides, posters, videos or appliances. It is so much easier to show patients how to change their stoma bags visually than to do it by words. Remember the value of diagrams to illustrate the spoken word. The teaching programme should be pursued one step at a time, and, as with the implementation of any care plan, with evaluation of understanding of each step (i.e. objective achieved) before moving on further.

Once patients have gone through the teaching plan, let them demonstrate the skill, or explain what they have learned. This will give confidence in their own ability for self-care, but will also help the nurse identify areas where learning is not yet fully achieved and further teaching is needed.

The teaching process is very similar to the nursing process, especially if it is viewed as a spiral in which the steps intermingle and the outcomes are also part of one another. It is easier to view the teaching process as a spiral since teaching is never completed. The achievement of one outcome merely leads to the setting of another goal until the student

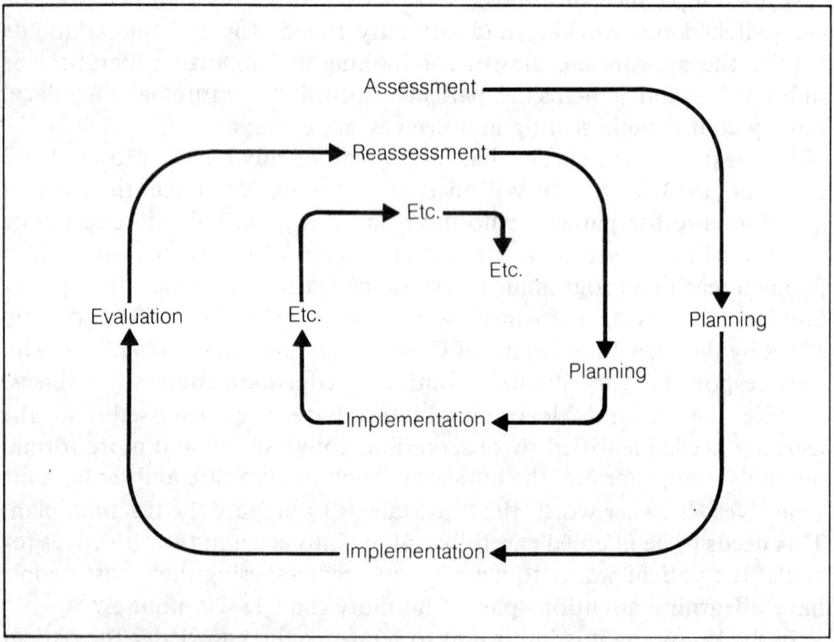

Figure 10.1 The educational spiral.

(patient) can progress to setting their own educational goals based on the ability to identify their own learning difficulty (Figure 10.1).

As has been seen, the nursing assessment needs to involve patients from the beginning, and friends and relatives if they agree. However, the nurse planning the education programme does need to consider other aspects of care. If patients are to be discharged home it will be necessary to assess their home environments. The nurse needs to be aware of the services that are available to support patients since it is pointless teaching patients to use facilities and services (perhaps a soiled dressing collection) that some local authorities do not provide. It is equally essential that those that are provided are adequately explained to patient and relatives.

Implementation needs step-by-step staged planning to meet the individual patient's specific learning ability, building gradually from a sound knowledge base. So plan - implement - evaluate - replan - through a cyclical process which goes on until the patient can take over responsibility for identifying learning needs and the help he/she requires to meet them.

One way in which patients can be helped to set and achieve their own learning goals is through self-help groups such as BACUP (British Association of Cancer United Patients), BDA (British Diabetic Association) local groups and telephone link lines like Cancerlink. Groups of patients and carers can be brought together in ward or community for mutual support. Such groups provide up-to-date information on new treatments and care, give advice on diet, provide social contacts in a reassuring environment and provide support to relatives and other carers as well. Sometimes people who feel stigmatized gain security from discussing their worries with those who share the same problem. Often this voluntary, frank discussion can be facilitated by a nurse or social worker who can direct the discussion towards the areas of concern and then tactfully withdraw.

A nurse who is working with a self-help or peer group teaching meeting, should undertake further training in communication and counselling skills. It is essential to know how to encourage communication and to direct and manipulate the expression of anxieties without being seen to be either 'bossy' or 'in control of the group' (see Chapter 5). Even more important, the nurse must be able to take a back seat when the time comes although the good group teacher will be ready to respond with supportive help if requested. Some determination may be needed to encourage the shyer, older patient to participate fully in a group discussion and it can take time for them to feel comfortable especially among younger strangers.

But peer groups are not only of value for the teaching opportunities they provide. They also are used for valuable socialization: outings, dances, cookery demonstrations, especially appropriate for the lonely elderly who need social rehabilitation as well as physical. There is little point in learning to walk with an artificial leg if there is nowhere to go. Often day care centres can provide the beginnings of friendships over and above those normally accessible to the housebound.

The Diabetic Patient

One area where patient education for the elderly has been shown to be effective is in the field of diabetic care. The British Diabetic Association has a well-established patient education programme which has been instrumental in concentrating the skills of all members of the multidisciplinary team into positive and successful education programmes.

Many authors, like Brook (1977), Millar *et al.* (1978), Regensburg (1982), have shown that the diabetic patients' knowledge of their condition is not only poor but is often also inaccurate. Millar further suggested that knowledge needs to be reassessed at regular intervals both for evaluation and because a regular check-up aids retention. This is particularly true in the elderly.

Connors, writing in Baski *et al.* (1983) is one of the few authors to demonstrate – as opposed to hypothesize – that patient education is cost-effective. Using evidence from a Swiss study he relates the cost of below-knee amputation to nursing salaries, and emphasizes that six below-knee amputations cost £6,843 (his 1982 prices) which was £700 more than the then ward sister's yearly salary. So the prevention of only six below-knee amputations (caused by diabetic gangrene) which occurred as the result of poor control would save a ward sister's salary or make one more nurse available for patient education.

There are two groups of elderly diabetic patients who need teaching:

- The insulin-dependent diabetic who has been a diabetic for many years and who is affected by changing metabolic needs as he or she ages. These ageing changes are common to all: for the diabetic patient it means adjustment to insulin doses, to diet and to exercise patterns, all of which need relearning (or even learning).
- The newly diagnosed elderly diabetic who is most likely to be controlled by diet or drugs (or both). If stabilization is to be

> achieved and life-style habits maintained, patients must learn to accept responsibility for their care. It is just as important as if they were on insulin. Connors has already identified that unstable diabetics are at risk of developing diabetic complications such as gangrene, and careful adherence to treatment routines are vital if this (and other) complications are to be prevented.

Lawrence and Cheeley (1980) identify many reasons why elderly diabetic patients have difficulty in learning or remembering necessary skills and knowledge. They quote 'constantly changing practice, misunderstanding, laxity, forgetfulness, diminishing eyesight, arthritis and the effects of stress'. Add to this list hearing loss and the multiplicity of advice offered by well-meaning neighbours and friends, and it is easy to see how confusion occurs.

They again advise periodic assessment and re-assessment of knowledge and skills and advise that, following initial teaching, the nurse holds six-monthly revision sessions.

This advice is surely applicable for all those who aim to help their elderly patients learn. The teaching programme they advocate is informal, taking place in a one-to-one nurse–patient relationship but including relatives and friends if this is the patient's wish. The patient has a list of objectives (similar principles can be applied to the teaching on any problem) to be achieved and these are covered systematically. Take *urine testing*, for example. The patient

- Names and describes tests.
- Selects appropriate equipment.
- States testing time correctly.
- Stores items properly.
- Carries out procedure accurately.
- Records results correctly.
- Keeps records and brings them to clinic.

Similar lists exist for insulin/drug therapy, diet and coping with (or preventing) hypoglycaemia. Follow-up teaching sessions identified that the causes of error were often the result of memory or dexterity loss, which resulted in omitting to test at the correct time, or failing to follow a procedure correctly because of inability to handle the equipment.

Brook (1977) documents a similar study in which she identified learning deficits by questionnaire and then provided supportive teaching to meet individual learning needs. She used a basic check-list which took under ten minutes to administer and shared her teaching role with community and clinic nurses who were involved in regular care. She emphasized that patients remember teaching better if they have been involved in practising and demonstrating their newly acquired skill rather than 'just being talked to'.

Baski *et al*. (1983) includes a substantial check-list covering the total management of diabetes. If the patient acquires all the knowledge on the list he is likely to surpass that of his carers, but it is most interesting to see what this doctor, one of the most experienced diabetic teachers in the UK, expects his patients to know.

Regensburg (1982) makes valuable suggestions concerning education of the elderly:

- Reinforce teaching with written information.
- Spend time in a one-to-one conversation and discussion.
- Encourage questions.
- Do not do all the talking.
- Supervise the practice of necessary skills from time to time, for example fitting stoma bags, urine testing.
- Consider group teaching. Time is especially valuable when demonstrating new menus or when you have gone to the expense of hiring a video or film.
- Invite a visiting speaker on a subject that will interest the patients.
- Involve community nurses and general practitioners. In this way, they will know what is going on and understand the reasons behind it.
- Follow up the teaching regularly.

All authors constantly advise on the need to plan teaching within a structured programme based on patients' identified needs (Figure 10.2).

This may remind the reader that earlier in this chapter the educational spiral was identified - a constant process by which new knowledge deficits are always being identified - eventually, it is hoped, by the patient rather than the teacher.

ASSESSMENT

Nurses need initially to assess their own ability to carry out the teaching programme. Is there a knowledge deficit which must be rectified? Can it be rectified by reading, by using a distance learning package, by

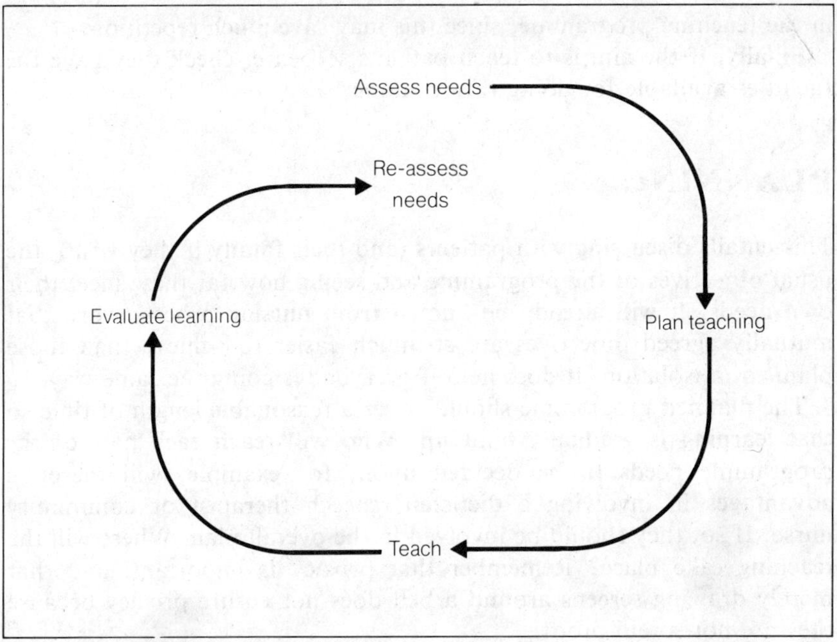

Figure 10.2 The structure of teaching.

attending a course or conference or by visiting another nurse who is experienced in a particular aspect of care? (see list of addresses on p. 304). Has recent literature been reviewed to ensure up-to-date knowledge of what is appropriate at this point? It can be very harmful to teach 'old knowledge'.

Secondly, it is necessary to assess the patient's

- *Previous knowledge.* It is useful or harmful?
- *Ability to learn.* Is he/she pain-free? Does he/she have a hearing or visual problem which needs correction? Is the environment free of distractions?
- *Interest in learning.* Will he/she be alert and inquiring?

Nurses are also advised by Redman (1980) to consider how patients will best learn. This involved assessing their usual method of acquiring new knowledge (do they read, watch television, like to be told what to do?), and making some judgement on their levels of understanding. It is also wise to check from the outset if the patient wishes to involve others in the teaching programme, since this may save much repetition.

Finally, if the aim is to teach patients self-care, check they have the facilities available for doing this at home.

PLANNING

This entails discussing with patients (and their family if they wish), the usual objectives of the programme and seeing how far these meet their own needs. It will already be known from nursing process work that mutually agreed objectives are so much easier to achieve than those planned in isolation. It does help if everyone is going the same way.

The planned programme should cover a reasonable length of time so that learning is gradually built up. Who will teach each part of the programme needs to be decided upon; for example, will there be advantages in involving a dietician, speech therapist or community nurse. If so, they should be involved in the overall plan. Where will the teaching take place? Remember that privacy is important, and that merely drawing screens around a bed does not ensure privacy because they are not sound-proof.

Any tapes, slides, videos or film programmes that are available should be considered, and the nurse education centre often has a list of those in stock and those that can be rented for a reasonable fee. Organizations such as Age Concern and the Royal National Institute for the Blind produce material of use to nurse educators, and teaching booklets, such as those produced by the Royal Marsden Hospital can be very helpful.

Finally, remember that the teaching needs to be documented and follow-up sessions planned as appropriate to the patient's needs.

IMPLEMENTATION

This is best carried out when the patient is rested, perhaps in the afternoon. Unless relatives are involved, it should be checked that the patient is not expecting callers. It is most irritating to be half-way through a session and to have to break it off because the door bell rings. It must be remembered that no one learns readily if their mind is on other things, so the time for the teaching must be decided with the patient. It is a good idea to check any equipment being used – that it is available and that it works.

The programme should be pursued in a logical sequence – clean the stoma first, put a clean bag on, then dispose of the old one. Jumping from one part of the task to another should be avoided. Anyone else involved needs to know when to turn up, or when the patient is due to visit them. Nothing is more confusing for all the team, especially the older person, than a failure to adhere to an agreed plan.

Any supportive booklets should be included. This gives the opportunity to offer advice on what he/she should concentrate on reading first, or to recommend a section which supports the teaching that day. The booklet should be left with the patient to read later, although questions should not always be expected. Wilson-Barnett's (1983) work reminds us it may be better for sensitive issues, like sexual problems, to be read about first, and discussed after if the patient wishes.

It is also necessary to allow time to read since it often takes longer than anticipated. Nurses who carry bleeps should leave them somewhere else to minimize disturbances.

EVALUATION

This needs to take place in two stages, on-going and follow-up. There are three main ways of doing this: (1) by the pre- and post-test (Howard and Erlanger, 1983), (2) by asking a patient to review the previous session verbally, or (3) by observing the practice of a skill (Baski *et al.,* 1983). Like everything else, variety is all-important, as is positive reinforcement, and the impression should never be given that the patient is slow. Don't forget he needs praise for things remembered.

Evaluation also means checking how well the nurse did the teaching, so ask the patients how they felt the session went. It is possible to use an evaluation check-list (Baski *et al.,* 1983), especially for the follow-up evaluation weeks after. And, since the process approach is being used, it will be necessary to check back to see that individual objectives have been met.

The following case history outlines the teaching process.

Case history

Mrs Simons, aged 67, is admitted to your ward for removal of breast lumps and auxiliary nodes. The lumps in her right breast are malignant but the body scan shows no metastases so she is to have follow-up radiotherapy treatment - thirty sessions of half an hour each over a six-week period.

Assessment

On admission Mrs Simons is very anxious about both her diagnosis and her operation. She is concerned that lumpectomy rather than mastectomy is advised and is asking why her breast is not being removed.

She lives locally with her husband and, apart from this recent problem, both are fit and well and have no financial anxieties. She has a daughter who visits their home at least weekly and a son and grandchildren nearby. She works part-time as a voluntary librarian for the RNB. Before she retired she worked in the local public library. Her husband is an accountant.

You assess her readiness to learn as follows: interested, intellectually inquisitive (admits to reading about cancer in library books) but very anxious.

Planning

In discussion she states a preference for one-to-one teaching. She doesn't want to involve her husband in 'private matters' though she recognizes he needs to know and asks you to tell him for her. She also wishes someone to see her daughter and advise her daughter about her mother's need for regular breast examination. Together you plan:

(1) To discuss the research data demonstrating that lumpectomy results are as encouraging as mastectomy ones and much less likely to cause lymphoedema. This should reassure her and thereby reduce her anxiety.
(2) To explain the operative procedure to her.
(3) To demonstrate post-operative arm exercises and ensure she can do them.
(4) To explain radiotherapy and the treatment required.
(5) To advise on the management of side-effects.
(6) To discuss follow-up after-care including breast self-examination.

Implementation

The first three topics must be covered pre-operatively, but the rest can wait until she has recovered from the immediate effects of surgery. With the aid of a patient who had a lumpectomy three years ago you manage to convince her of the reasons for this approach to treatment and its success. You leave an education booklet with her and suggest she might find a follow-up visit from the Mastectomy Association helpful on return home.

Immediately after the operation you are able to visit Mrs Simons to reassure her all is well and thus reduce her natural anxiety.

Once she has recovered you implement the rest of your programme, involving her radiographer in the teaching. Since much of her treatment is planned on an out-patient basis you remember to ensure that her GP is aware of progress to date.

Evaluation

Five days after the operation Mrs Simons goes home. Thanks to your teaching she is considerably less anxious, her exercises are reducing the risk of lymphoedema and she understands the staging of the radiotherapy treatment that will begin in four weeks' time. You make an appointment to see her as an out-patient, since you still have to teach her (and ensure she can demonstrate) self-examination.

Nurses are important health and patient educators. They have unique skill, and a unique understanding of the person that makes them especially suited to teach the elderly, who do not always find learning easy (Baski *et al.,* 1983). They are in close contact with patients and families and are seen by them as knowledgeable and able to provide accurate information. For the nurse there is considerable satisfaction in watching a patient achieve self-care goals through education.

Further Training

You may feel unable to teach patients because of an inadequate knowledge base or lack of teaching skills. Your nurse education department and nurse managers will be able to advise on courses run by the National Boards that will provide knowledge on care of the elderly and on teaching skills, or you may wish to write to the Open University or the other distance learning centres. The Nurse Adviser on Care of the Elderly at the Royal College of Nursing can also give details of courses and conferences. Enquiring is well worth doing since well-educated patients, of whatever age, have a greatly improved life-style (Baski *et al.,* 1983; Wilson-Barnett, 1983; Redman, 1980). And remember, if courses are to the advantage of patient care, authorities can give assistance with time off and fees. Useful addresses for many of the above aspects can be found at the end of the text on p. 304.

REFERENCES

Baski, A. K. *et al.* (1983) *Diabetes Education,* Wiley, Chichester.

Brook, P. A. (1977) Diabetic patients' understanding of their disease and its treatment, *Nursing Times*, 21 July, pp. 1117–19.

Howard, V. A. and Erlanger, H. (1983) Teaching methods for coronary patients, in J. Wilson-Barnett (ed.) *Patient Teaching,* Churchill Livingstone, Edinburgh.

Joint Board of Clinical Nursing Studies publications on Assessive Competence (1973–84) London (obtainable through the English National Board).

Lawrence, P. A. and Cheeley, J. (1980) Deterioration of diabetic patients' knowledge and management skills as determined during outpatients' visits, *Diabetes Care*, Vol. 3, no. 2, pp. 214–18.

Ley, P. and Spelman, M. (1967) *Communicating with the Patient*, Staples Press, London.

Midwinter, E. (1982) *Age Is Opportunity*, Centre for Policy on Ageing, London.

Millar, L. V. *et al.* (1978) Evaluation of patients' knowledge of diabetes self-care, *Diabetes Care*, Vol. 1, no. 5, pp. 275–80.

Redman, B. (1980) *The Process of Patient Teaching in Nursing*, C. V. Mosby, London.

Regensburg, D. J. (1982) Education of the elderly mature onset diabetic, *Geriatric Nursing*, June 1982, pp. 14–17.

The Nurses, Midwives and Health Visitors Act (1979) HMSO, London.

Wilson-Barnett, J. (1983) *Patient Teaching*, Churchill Livingstone, Edinburgh.

11. Eating and Drinking

Steve Wright

CHANGES ASSOCIATED WITH AGEING

A number of age-related changes may affect the older person's ability to maintain normal nutritional balance. Decreases in the senses of taste and smell with ageing may lead to an increased use of salt, sugar and other condiments to enhance flavour of foods (Yurick *et al.*, 1980), and there may be a shift from bland to spicier foods. Many special diets prescribed for the elderly may therefore not be complied with, especially if they require modifying salt intake or include unpalatable low calorie foods.

An ability to maintain a normal diet is also closely linked to the social and psychological changes associated with old age (Janes, 1980). Living alone may be a disincentive to prepare a full nourishing meal, and changing economic circumstances (for example, dependence on a lower pension instead of a larger income derived from work) may inhibit the selection of foods to produce a balanced diet. In addition, declining physical abilities, to operate the fittings of a cooker, for instance, may further diminish the desire to give attention to preparing food. Particularly at risk, according to Janes are

- those living alone,
- the handicapped (blind, deaf, i.e. the socially isolated),
- recently bereaved people, especially widowers,

- the very old (over 85 years),
- the ill,
- the housebound,
- those in institutions, and
- individuals living on low incomes.

Older adults who may have lower incomes, or are lonely, or have other problems that affect their ability and incentive both to get access to and to prepare food are therefore at higher risk of malnutrition problems. Vousden (1986) had identified a number of significant problems affecting eating ability:

- Poor seating posture.
- Weakened grip and arm strength.
- Tremor, as in Parkinson's disease.
- Poor hand–eye co-ordination.
- Perceptual disturbance.
- Paralysis of the mouth.
- Poor tongue control.
- Lack of swallow reflex.
- Poor dentition.
- Chewing and swallowing difficulties.
- Carrying food in the mouth.
- Difficulty in locating food on the plate.

The elderly patient in an institution may often face rigid meal patterns and limited choice of foods. While the dish offered may be well balanced, the older patient may face malnourishment if certain foods are disliked and alternatives are not available. The institutional environment may further affect eating habits – disrupting a lifetime of settled patterns for meals or being forced to sit with others who may inhibit the desire to eat.

DENTAL CARE

The wearing of dentures in themselves may not influence the nutritional status of the elderly, unless they are ill-fitting or associated with mouth ulcers (Todhunter, 1976). Some elderly people may remove dentures in order to eat, and this may lead some to increase consumption of softer carbohydrate foods.

Poor dental care earlier in life coupled with poor nutrition has lead most elderly people to be edentulous (Beal and Dowell, 1977). Once dentures are fitted, the elderly person may assume that no further visits to the dentist are necessary, which can lead later to ill-fitting dentures and mouth sores (Walker, 1985). Williams (1981) has noted that early detection of oral cancer is diminished in the elderly. One of the major roles of the nurse seeking to help people with eating and drinking problems is therefore to develop thorough assessment techniques to identify difficulties and potential dangers (Ebert, 1980), such as cancers, mouth ulcers and loose and painful teeth.

Nursing also has an important role to play in education in relation to dental hygiene and it needs to be emphasized that ageing alone does not necessarily mean a loss of teeth. The use of a toothbrush is more effective in removing debris and improving gingival tissue than swabs or other soft devices (Harris, 1980). However, this needs great care as the oral tissues of the elderly are more sensitive and prone to injury (Miles, 1972). Dental problems need to be attended to promptly as they can affect virtually every system in the body.

THE EFFECT OF DRUGS

Many drugs being taken for illnesses may suppress rather than stimulate the appetite, and may in addition lead to a dry and sore mouth (Todd, 1982). Because the older body is slower to metabolize them, the effects of diuretics may be delayed, so that if they are taken late in the day, or even if taken earlier, the patient may have to 'get up several times in the night and consequently feels tired all day' (Janes, 1980). This may increase disinclination to prepare meals.

INDIGESTION, FOOD INTOLERANCE AND DIETARY NEEDS

Indigestion and food intolerance are more common in the elderly. Gastric secretion, motility and emptying time are reduced (Steen, 1985). Small meals more frequently and less fried foods are necessary (Ebert, 1980). The nutrients most at risk in the elderly are iron, vitamin C and folate (B_{12}) and vitamin B_1. The last of these in particular is associated with confusion and unsteadiness (Janes, 1980) and is sometimes a cause of cardiac disorders. Confusion, breathlessness or unsteadiness may therefore have their origins in vitamin deficiency. Constipation due to lack of fibre and/or fluids in the diet may also be linked to confusion, and other difficulties such as urinary retention (Luker, 1980).

There appears to be no great difference in the dietary needs of the elderly from the middle-aged adult. Many studies suggest (Debry, Bleyer and Martin, 1977; Steen, 1985) that, with the exception of calories, the requirements for most nutrients are the same for the older as the middle-aged adult. The need for calories is largely determined by the activity levels – an active elderly person will require the same levels as an active younger person. Monitoring of the patient's weight is therefore one means of determining nutritional status. Weight gain over a period of months or years may indicated that calorie intake has increased, or remained the same while activity levels have declined.

DHSS guidelines (1969) recommend the following daily intakes (Table 11.1).

Different diets are necessary for certain specific culture groups. Nurses in the UK are now far more likely to encounter a wider variety of dietary requirements among their patients. The multicultural nature of society, plus increasing emphasis on 'healthy eating' (Health Education Council, 1986) may bring the nurse into contact with patients who have specific religious requirements (Shukla, 1980; see also Surman's chapter on worshipping later in the text) or who have adopted vegetarian, non-meat, low fat or wholefood dietary habits.

DIABETES MELLITUS

Another common dietary issue the nurse will encouter is diabetes mellitus. Although a universal health problem, it has become a major problem in some countries (West, 1978). In Western Europe, the disease now affects about 16 per cent of those over 65 years. Jackson (1985) notes that, with demographic changes associated with ageing, the size of the diabetic population is likely to double over fifteen years. The management of this problem is essentially a team responsibility. Chapter 10 drew attention to the nurse's role as an educator in this field.

Most importantly, nurses must work closely with patients, relatives, dieticians and catering departments to ensure that the patient's dietary requirements are fulfilled. Many patients (and nurses) have found help and advice from organizations such as the British Diabetic Association (see addresses on p. 304). It must be remembered however that in

Table 11.1 Recommended daily intakes of energy and nutrients for the UK

Assuming a sedentary life	*Men 65-75*	*Men over 75*	*Women 55-75*	*Women over 75*
Energy (kcal)	2350	2100	2050	1900
Protein (g)	59	53	51	48
Thiamine (mg)	0.9	0.8	0.8	0.7
Riboflavine (mg)	1.7	1.7	1.3	1.3
Nicotine acid (mg equivalent)	18	18	15	15
Vitamin C (mg)	30	30	30	30
Vitamin A 9 (retinol equivalents)	750	750	750	750
Vitamin D 9	2.5	2.5	2.5	2.5
Calcium (mg)	500	500	500	500
Iron (mg)	10	10	10	10

Source: DHSS, 1969.

assisting the elderly diabetic, the patient's and carer's ability to understand and comply with his/her diet and treatment are important factors to consider. In addition adequate finance and home cooking facilities may also determine whether or not a patient is able to comply with the requirements of his/her diet.

FLUIDS

The fluid consumption of older adults should range between 2,500 and 3,000 ml daily, including drinks, the fluid content of foods and that produced by metabolism (Davidson *et al.*, 1975). Achieving this level may be hindered if the older person lacks motivation, has problems with nocturia, frequency incontinence (may avoid drinking to minimize urine output) or an inability to obtain drinks independently (Willington, 1980).

The risk of dehydration is compounded by the age-related changes affecting the renal system (see also Chapter 12). Saxon and Etton (1978) note three main elements:

(1) A decrease in the number of nephrons, which implies a decrease in the filtration rate.
(2) A reduction of excretory and reabsorptive functions.
(3) A more easily disrupted acid-base balance.

Thus any loss of fluid, as by vomiting or diarrhoea or by simply not drinking enough, impairs renal function and leads to dehydration (Luker, 1980).

The social aspects of drinking also need to be considered. In hospital or nursing home it may not be possible to prepare a drink as preferred, or use a favourite cup. The extra time to communicate with the older patient may lead the nurse to make decisions for him/her - putting the sugar or milk in the tea without asking the patient's preference, for example. Without the choice, the conversation and the companionship associated with drinking the patient's interest in and willingness to take fluids may decline.

The choice of container for the drink is also important, as Luker (1980) succinctly notes:

> People with arthritis of the hands or failing vision may use a mug at home since this does not need to be replaced on a saucer and so reduces the likelihood of drinks being spilled. In hospital there is often very little

choice about drinking receptacles and patients given a cup and saucer may be reluctant to drink that second cup of tea in case they disgrace themselves by spilling it. For patients who have this difficulty a plastic feeding beaker with a spout may be the answer and can give them greater independence; for others a feeding beaker may be totally unacceptable and a deterrent to drinking. As always, it is only by consulting with the patient that the most satisfactory solution can be found.

Giving the patient a drink of choice may be difficult within the limitations on offer in hospital or other institution. Taking alcohol as beer or spirits plays an important social fuction in Western cultures. The local 'pub' may not be as accessible as it always was (see Chapter 13) because of reduced mobility or perhaps there are fewer friends or companions around to make it worthwhile. Eliopoulos (1980) notes how moderate amounts of alcohol can prove an important aid to stimulating the appetite or promoting sleep (in preference to drugs). Nurses or relatives and friends may be able to take patients to the 'local' for drinks, or may develop innovative schemes to provide a pub-like service in the hospital or nursing home. Quick and Maddocks (1984) showed how it is possible to provide an atmosphere where fluid intake is combined with social pleasure: 'The patients sit round in wheelchairs playing darts or dominoes and the hemiplegics cope well with their specially made card-stands, all enjoying a beer at the same time.'

AIDS TO EATING AND DRINKING

The social aspects of eating and drinking that nurses need to exercise care in the choice of suitable available aids when feeding difficulties arise. Hospitals and nursing homes can produce problems for those who are unused to eating in large groups or at set times. Aids for feeding, such as specially designed cutlery for those with limited mobility, may help with the eating, but undermine the patient's sense of dignity and independence.

Vousden (1986) lists a number of available aids and adaptations, which nurses need to use discriminatingly if they are to benefit the patient. Once again, close liaison with occupational therapist, physiotherapist and dietician are essential. Some possibilities include:

- Provide heated plates so that food does not go cold if more time is needed to eat.

- Liquidize selected foods.
- Lightweight cutlery.
- Long-handled cutlery for those with limited wrist elbow movement.
- Straps to fasten cutlery to hands.
- Large-handled utensils.
- Rubazote tubing to extend the patient's own cultery.
- Rocking-knife for single-handed use or combined knife/fork/spoon.
- Special plates with lips and plate guards to keep food on the plate/assist getting it on the spoon or fork.
- Suction base for egg cup/plates or non-stick mats.
- Lightweight beakers, handles designed to fit disabled or deformed hands, and arm supports for weakened limbs.

Other measures, such as nasogastric feeding or intravenous infusions, not only undermine the social elements but may also remove the pleasures of the taste and smell of food and drink. 'Eating is not only a physiological necessity, but is also a social and emotional experience' (Royal Marsden, 1986). If necessary to restrict normal methods of eating, the nurse should not lose sight of the effects for it may 'dramatically alter the patient's attitude to food'. The nurse plays a vital role in helping patients to understand the chosen method of feeding. 'The nurse can make it pleasant and relaxed or it can become a distressing affair, guaranteed to destroy the patient's confidence. The outcome is, therefore, dependent on the nurse's attitude and clinical knowledge' (Royal Marsden, 1986).

HELPING THE PATIENT EAT AND DRINK

Suggestions offered by Kastenbaum (1979), Ebert (1980), Parsonage (1980) and Steen (1985) offer many guidelines for nurses helping the older patient with an eating or drinking problem. There are a number of main points to consider.

Firstly, the patient and other carers must be involved whenever possible in all decisions about dietary choice. Close liaison is necessary with the dietician when special diets are needed. Realistic diets that take account of the patient's special wishes and ability to comply need to be chosen.

The patient needs to help maintain good dental hygiene, with referral to a dentist if necessary. Dentures need to be clearly labelled where patients must mingle in large groups. Education of the patient may be necessary in denture care and oral hygiene and in the importance of regular dental check-ups. The nurse also has a role as teacher adviser to help the patient select a well-balanced diet containing adequate protein, fat, carbohydrate, water, vitamin and minerals and fibre (see also Chapter 10).

Providing a choice of foods at meal-times and offering alternatives to meet the patient's wishes is essential. Relatives and friends can be involved in providing special requests for patients or help in preparing and supplying food at home. Liaison with social services, for example, can help to provide a 'meals on wheels' service. Relatives, friends and other voluntary organizations can help to provide meals at home for the housebound or transport to pensioners' clubs etc.

Privacy with meals might be essential for some patients, while others will expect the nurse to provide facilities for sharing drinks and meals with friends, relatives or other patients. Patients' individual preferences will have to be assessed so that their needs can be met as far as possible. Nutritional status, through regular health checks that include weight, haemoglobin levels, etc. should be monitored. The patients themselves should be taught these techniques where possible, and, especially where weight loss is desirable, the group competition can be an important motivator to success.

Food should be presented attractively, in portions the patient can manage, with choices of condiments and drinks to stimulate the appetite (e.g. fresh fruit juices, sherry, wine, beer). Extra drinks, small meals or snacks can be offered during the day as preferred, and especially before sleeping at night or where the patient is unable to tolerate a full meal. The serving of meals should include offering choices, talking with the patient and reinforcing it as a social occasion. Once the meal or drink is presented, patients need to be allowed time to take them at their own place. If hurrying the patients is avoided (for example by indicating that they must finish more quickly by collecting dishes too quickly) they will be more inclined to complete the meal. Offering meals as closely as possible to the patient's usual meal-times is preferable, although nurses might have to 'bend the rules', for example by keeping food and serving it later to comply with the patient's wishes.

Sitting with patients if they need help with feeding/drinking and appearing unhurried and relaxed indicates that they can take their time. Testing the temperature of food or drink can be done first by tasting a small sample. The selection of feeding/drinking aids needs to be appropriate to the patient's abilities and take account of individual wishes. It is essential that the patient is helped into a comfortable (sitting upright) position for feeding and that normal utensils, chairs, tables, etc. are provided whenever possible, with the food at elbow level to minimize the distance travelled. At the same time background noise and fuss must be minimized to provide a quiet, relaxing environment for meal-times. Other factors which may diminish appetite must be dealt with as priority, e.g. pain control, relief of anxiety. The patient who is unhappy, nauseated or uncomfortable will have little incentive to enjoy or complete a meal.

Case study

Because of her deformed hands, and the weakness of her grip, Miss Ellis had difficulty feeding/drinking herself. To ensure an adequate nutritional intake was maintained and to enable her to do as much for herself as possible, her nurse decided to

- Offer help with serving of meals, cutting food and feeding as she wishes. Give foods of choice and ask family to provide any special preferred foods/drinks from home.
- Advise her where necessary in the selection of a balanced diet and the choice of suitable foods.
- Ensure she drinks at least 2 litres of fluid daily – keep drinks within hand reach.
- Check her weight each week.
- Offer alternatives (e.g. 'Build-up', diet drinks, etc.) where meals are not taken.
- Provide feeding aids as appropriate: doubled-handled light beaker, angled utensils with thickened handles, non-slip mat under plates, plate ring.
- Check position suitable for feeding/drinking.
- Give time to take meals at own pace and intervene only when essential.

Written information on diet plans can be provided and the nurse should be prepared to teach and explain the contents. It is important to be ready to answer his/her questions about selecting foods, and to be able to offer realistic economic choices and suggest sources for purchase. Referral to appropriate agencies, for benefits, will be necessary if the income to provide a nutritious diet is inadequate. Medical and dietary prescriptions need to be followed closely, especially with special nasogastric or intravenous feeding regimes.

Providing an aesthetically pleasing setting for eating and drinking – comfortable furniture, tablecloths, clean utensils, pictures, flowers, and so on - and an opportunity where possible to smell the food being prepared all help to motivate the patient towards taking food and drink.

The above factors are a summary of the major points for nursing consideration when helping the older patient who has an eating and drinking problem. Providing good nutrition is a complex issue, with the nurse often closely involved in balancing the social, psychological and physical needs of the patient. As with many themes throughout this book, the involvement of the team in promoting healthy eating - dietician, doctor, physiotherapist, and so on - as well as the nurse, the patient and other carers is of great importance in meeting the older patient's needs.

REFERENCES

Beal, J. F. and Dowell T. B. (1977) Edentulous and attendance patterns in England and Wales 1968-1977, *British Dental Journal*, Vol. 143, pp. 203–7.

British Diabetic Association (1982) *Report of the Medical Advisory Committee*, London.

Davidson, S., Passmore, R., Brook, J. F. and Truswell, A. S. (1975) *Human Nutrition and Dietetics*, Churchill Livingstone, Edinburgh.

Debry, G., Bleyer, R. and Martin, J. M. (1977) Nutrition of the elderly, *Journal of Human Nutrition*, Vol. 31, pp. 63–83.

DHSS (1969) *Recommended Daily Intakes of Energy and Nutrients for the Elderly in the UK,* HMSO, London.

Ebert, N. J. (1980) *Nutrition and Elimination in the Aged and the Nursing Process* in A. G. Yurick *et al.* (eds) *The Aged Person and the Nursing Process*, Appleton-Century-Crofts, New York.

Eliopoulos, C. (1980) *Geriatric Nursing*, Harper and Row, London.

Harris, M. D. (1980) Tools for mouth care, *Nursing Times*, Vol. 76, pp. 340–2.

Health Education Council (1986) *Eating for Health*, London.

Jackson, R. A. (1985) *Diabetes*, in M. S. J. Pathy (ed) *Principles and Practice of Geriatric Medicine,* Wiley, Chichester.

Janes, E. (1980) Nutrition in the elderly, *Nursing*, Vol. 12, pp. 511–17.

Kastenbaum, R. (1979) *Growing Old: The Years of Fulfilment*, Harper & Row, London.

Luker, K. (1980) The elderly, *Nursing*, Vol. 13, pp. 576–7.

Miles, A. E. W. (1972) 'Sans teeth' - changes in the oral tissues with advancing age, *Journal of the Royal Society of Medicine.*, Vol. 65, pp. 801–6.

Parsonage, S. (1980) There's more to eating than food, *Nursing*, Vol. 11, pp. 471–2.

Pathy, M. S. J. (1985) *Principles and Practice of Geriatric Medicine*, Wiley, Chichester.

Quick, K. and Maddocks, S. (1984) Do drop inn!, *Nursing Times*, 18 April, pp. 52–3.

Royal Marsden Hospital (1986) *Manual of Clinical Nursing Policies and Procedures*, Harper & Row, London.
Saxon, V. S. and Etton, J. E. (1978) *Physical Change and Ageing: A Guide for the Helping Professions*, Tiresias Press, New York.
Shukla, K. (1980) Diet and culture, *Nursing*, Vol. 12, pp. 523–4.
Steen, B. (1985) *Nutrition*, in M. S. J. Pathy (ed) *Principles and Practice of Geriatric Medicine,* Wiley, Chichester.
Todd, B. (1982) Drugs and the elderly: dry mouth – causes and cures, *Geriatric Nursing*, Vol. 3, no. 2, pp. 122–3.
Todhunter, E. N. (1976) Life style and nutritional intake in the elderly, in M. Winick, (ed.) *Nutrition and Ageing*, Wiley, New York.
Vousden, M. A. (1986), Problems with eating, *Geriatric Nursing and Home Care*, Vol. 6, no. 6, pp. 28–30.
Walker, D. M. (1985) Oral disease, in M. S. J. Pathy (ed.) *Principles and Practice of Geriatric Medicine,* Wiley, Chichester.
West, K. M. (1978) *Epidemiology of Diabetes and its Vascular Complications*, Elsevier, New York.
Williams, R. G. (1981) The elderly diagnosis of carcinoma of the mouth, *Annals of the Royal College of Surgeons*, Vol. 63, pp. 423–5.
Willington, F. L. (1980) *Incontinence in the Elderly*, Academic Press, London.
Yurick, A. G., Robb, S. S., Spier, B. E. and Ebert, N. J. (1980) *The Aged Person and the Nursing Process*, Appleton-Century-Crofts, New York.

12. Eliminating

Anne Kennedy

Each individual has a slightly different pattern of elimination but correct or 'normal' behaviour in getting rid of our bodily wastes is something we are all taught from a very early age. We learn there is a normal place to void – the toilet – and that we are expected to be able to go for three to four hours between visits; it is also expected we will be able to sleep through a night without needing to empty our bladders. 'Normal' behaviour also includes a daily evacuation of the bowels.

THE BLADDER

The capacity of the bladder is about 500 ml, but a strong desire to void is felt at a volume something below this (varying from person to person). As the bladder fills (at about 1–2 ml per minute) the muscular wall (detrusor muscle) expands and the muscular tension increases. In the baby, bladder emptying is purely reflex. Reflex micturition occurs when the stretch receptors in the bladder wall are activated and send impulses to the sacral bladder centre at the base of the spinal cord which then sends impulses back to the bladder muscle making it contract. Eventually, a conscious control over bladder emptying is developed where inhibitory impulses are sent from the cortical bladder centre to block the reflex contracting of the bladder until it is convenient. Once this conscious inhibition of bladder contraction is learnt, continence is achieved.

In old age changes occur which alter the normal patterns of elimination present in younger adults. Brocklehurst (1982) discusses some of the effects of ageing on the anatomy and function of the bladder. Anatomically, the detrusor muscle fibres in many old people show hypertrophy or trabeculation and diverticula are seen. In the urethra, most ageing changes have been seen in females. The closing pressure of the urethra diminishes with age which can lead to problems of urine leakage associated with coughs or movements which suddenly increase pressure inside the bladder. Oestrogen deficiency in some postmenopausal women can lead to non-specific urethritis developing, causing pain and irritation.

The central nervous system changes with age and this has a direct effect on the functioning of the bladder. Cortical neurones change with age and their inhibitory action on the bladder contraction becomes diminished. This means frequency of micturition increases in the elderly, perhaps the most noticeable change being the need to wake up at night to pass urine.

In healthy elderly people normal patterns of elimination differ only slightly from those of younger adults. The bladder will not hold quite so much urine and visits to the toilet will probably have to be more frequent. There may also be residual urine left after voiding. However, the balance between continence and incontinence does become more precarious and a very minor change in health or environment may tip an elderly person into developing incontinence.

THE BOWEL

It is normal to expect the contents of the bowel to be evacuated daily. This is true in the elderly as well. Good bowel management can be achieved by maintaining a high fibre diet, taking plenty of fluids and getting a certain amount of exercise each day.

Again, in the elderly it is very easy to tip the balance between a problem-free existence and the development of difficulties in faecal elimination. The main problem in the elderly is constipation. Unless there are pathological complications, managing bowel problems in the elderly is fairly straightforward.

URINARY PROBLEMS

Incontinence of urine is probably the major problem of urinary elimination in old age. Many surveys have been made to try and estimate the size of the problem. The results of the surveys do depend on the actual population and questions asked but it is well recognized that incidence of incontinence does increase with age. It has also emerged in a postal survey undertaken by Thomas *et al.* (1980) that there are many people who suffer from incontinence but who do not seek medical help. For example in the area they were studying, 2.5 per cent of women over 65 were known to be incontinent by their doctors but a postal survey found 11.6 per cent of women over 65 admitted to having problems with incontinence. The same survey found 6.9 per cent of men over the age of 65 suffered from incontinence.

It is always important to remember that urinary incontinence is a symptom of a particular disorder (or disorders). This is why it is important to diagnose the cause of the incontinence and to treat that. Labelling a person as incontinent is a bit of a blanket term and it is more useful in managing the problem to be more specific about the type of incontinence.

Types of Incontinence

Briefly, causes of incontinence can be classified into the following groups: neurological, pelvic floor damage, urethral disease, outlet obstruction, and urinary infection.

Neurological

This type of incontinence results from damage to the brain or spinal cord. The reaction of the bladder depends on where the damage occurs in the central nervous system. A disease commonly associated with ageing is age-onset diabetes. The posterior nerve roots can be destroyed resulting in loss of bladder-filling sensation. The bladder gradually becomes over-distended and atonic giving retention of urine with overflow incontinence.

Another common neurological problem in old age is damage to the cortical bladder centre in the brain by, for example, cerebrovascular accidents, Parkinson's disease and dementia. Such damage is present to some degree in all elderly people. The ability to inhibit bladder contractions is lost or diminished. The patient suddenly feels an urgent need to empty the bladder, which is followed quickly by a contraction that actually empties it. Some people develop unstable bladders with urge incontinence and have no evidence of neurological disease. The uninhibited contractions are associated with movement, coughing or laughing. Fear or excitement can also start off a contraction and lead to incontinence.

Pelvic floor damage
The pelvic floor muscles support the bladder. If these become weakened – say following childbirth or because of obesity – stress incontinence may occur. Stress incontinence is said to happen after extra pressure is put on the bladder, for example by coughing or movement. Patients with stress incontinence lose smaller amounts of urine than those with unstable bladders.

Urethral disease
Oestrogen deficiency in elderly females can lead to urethritis and leakage of urine through an imperfectly closed urethra.

Outlet obstruction
In men, an enlarged prostate gland can distort the bladder outlet and lead to chronic retention and overflow incontinence. The same can happen to women with ovarian cysts or uterine fibroids. Outlet obstruction is also caused by faecal impaction. This is common in many immobile elderly people.

Urinary infection
Urinary infection leads to urgent and frequent desires to pass urine.

Contributing Factors

In the elderly it is important to remember there are many small things which may contribute to a person developing incontinence. Most elderly people will have a degree of urgency (that is when they feel the need to pass urine they cannot hold off a bladder contraction for very long) and bladder instability (that is a contraction may only be weak and not strong enough to empty the bladder of all the urine). Factors that might lead to incontinence developing include the following: the patient's mobility and dexterity, the environment, clothing, drug regimen, and psychological factors.

Mobility and dexterity

If anything happens to reduce a patient's mobility, such as stiff arthritic joints or even painful corns, it will take longer to get to the toilet. If the patient has any degree of urgency, those extra seconds may lead to an episode of incontinence. Again, if the hands become stiff and arthritic or there is any other reason for loss of dexterity, the extra seconds taken to adjust clothing and pull down pants in order to pass urine could lead to incontinence.

Environment

Finding toilets in a strange environment can be hard for young and able-bodied people, let alone anyone who might be disabled or elderly. Even in homes designed especially for the elderly the toilets are often not well signposted or positioned close enough to the general living areas (Tobin and Riley, 1986).

In many institutions, the actual condition of the toilets is so off-putting it is surprising anyone would want to use them. In some geriatric units, the toilets are at the far end of the ward, often in a cold and draughty corner. There may be no doors to the toilets and the call bell inaccessible or non-existent. In such cases, patients may rather be incontinent than risk frequent trips to such distressing places. Such incontinence is only encouraged if incontinence pads are placed on every bed and chair as Ramsbottom (1982) found in her survey.

Clothing

Tight or restrictive clothing may be hard to manipulate quickly for a person suffering from urgency. Many elderly women wear corsets and these can prove awkward to manage when trying to pass urine in a hurry. Men may have difficulties undoing flies, or the fly opening may not be long enough to allow correct positioning of a urinal bottle. Sloppy slippers may slow a person down.

Drugs

Medical staff can actually provoke urinary incontinence by inappropriate use of drugs. Diuretics are frequently prescribed for elderly people and may exacerbate problems with an unstable bladder and lead to incontinence. Sedatives and tranquillizers can also mask bladder sensations and lead to incontinence, particularly at night.

Psychological factors

The bladder is directly connected to the brain and emotional disturbances are often reflected by a decreased ability to inhibit bladder contractions. Admittance to hospital or to an old people's home is upsetting and is sometimes reflected in an onset of urinary incontinence. Bereavement and other depressing changes in life can lead to people not caring if they are incontinent or even feeling it is right they should be wet, smelly and uncomfortable.

Promotion of Continence

In order to help elderly people remain continent, particularly on admittance to a hospital ward, it is important to anticipate their needs. The position of the toilets should be carefully described, probably more than once. Patients should be encouraged to allow themselves enough time to reach the toilets and to wear non-slippery footwear and easy-to-manage clothes.

From a nursing point of view, a patient should never be labelled as incontinent following just one accident and should certainly never be told off or made to feel dirty. Dignity is all-important in old age.

When urinary incontinence does occur in the elderly positive thinking is essential. It is not an inevitable condition and it is curable. It is important to assess the patient fully to try and find out the cause of the incontinence. Shepherd, Blannin and Feneley (1982) describe the setting up of an incontinence clinic and state that of 109 women with incontinence 26 (nearly 25 per cent) were cured. They also found 18 women who were found to be continent, which shows that in assessing a patient's complaint of incontinence it is important to check they are actually incontinent.

A detailed medical examination allows a diagnosis of the reason for the incontinence to be made. Such an examination will include bladder palpation, vaginal and rectal examinations and a central nervous system examination. Blood is taken for a full blood count and urea and electrolyte estimation. A mid-stream specimen of urine should be taken for laboratory testing regarding urinary infection.

There are special investigations available in some centres which give more detail and help in an accurate diagnosis. Urine flow rate can be measured on a flow rate machine, and this shows up possible problems with urinary tract obstructions. Cystometrograms can be used to study pressure changes in the bladder as it fills and empties and show up abnormalities in the function of the bladder.

Nursing assessments do not aim to make a full diagnosis but to make clear what the patient's problem is. Table 12.1 shows some of the questions that might be asked. It is worth asking what the patient sees as his/her major problem as this often makes a good starting point to managing the problem.

An important and useful step in making an assessment is to get the patient, nurse or carer to record all visits to the toilet and episodes of incontinence on a chart (Figure 12.1). After about a week of using a chart it is often possible to see a pattern to the episodes of incontinence and suggestions can then be made on how to alter toileting patterns to achieve continence.

Nursing Management

Nurses should aim to give active help to their incontinent patients and not just passively mop up after the event. Active nursing management can start once any serious medical causes of the incontinence have been ruled out and/or cured. Initiation of a scheme to promote continence in a ward of elderly, debilitated, incontinent patients requires enthusiastic devotion from a team of dedicated nurses. Copperwheat (1985), a ward sister, describes the success she had in starting a new approach to the promotion of continence on her ward of nineteen females. In a few weeks, nearly all the patients became continent day and night (84 per cent previously incontinent). This did require a great deal of commitment from all the nursing staff and it is easier to start with one or two patients per ward than to try getting all the patients dry at once.

Toileting Schemes

Most elderly people who are incontinent will have small capacity bladders that empty following unstable contractions. They often have symptoms of urgency and frequency accompanied by many episodes of incontinence. The best method of management is to adopt a regime of visiting the toilet at frequent enough intervals to allow the bladder to empty fully and avoid incontinence. There are three types of toileting schemes that can be followed: regular toileting, individualized toileting, and bladder retraining.

Table 12.1 Examples of questions that can be asked to assess a patient's problems with incontinence

History

- When did the problem start?
- What do you think started it?
- Do you have problems during the day or night or both?
- Any other known medical problems?

Type of incontinence

- Any urgency; frequency or pain?
- Does leakage occur:
  - after micturition?
  - with coughing or movement?
  - continuously or are you not aware of it?

How does the patient cope?

- What type of pads and pants are used?
- Any other appliances used?
- Where is the toilet and how does patient get there?
- How mobile and/or dextrous is the patient?

Other

- What medication is the patient on?
- What is the patient's fluid intake?
- Any problems with constipation?
- Any recent emotional upsets?

Regular toileting

This entails fixed regular visits to the toilet at intervals of 2–3 hours. The aim of this is to ensure the bladder is emptied before episodes of incontinence occur due to unstable bladder contractions. Some elderly patients are forgetful and need a reminder to visit the toilet regularly either in the form of a chart to fill in or an alarm clock set at two-hourly intervals, or someone to physically remind or take them to the toilet.

Individualized toileting

The bladder does not fill up at a uniform rate throughout the day and night. For example, some pass most urine in the morning and very little in the afternoon. With careful charting over a week or two it is possible to find the times when a person is most likely to be wet. Once a person's individual pattern of micturition has been found, toileting regimes can be adapted to anticipate bladder-emptying times to avoid episodes of incontinence. For example, a patient may need to visit the toilet every two hours in the morning and four-hourly in the afternoon and evening and perhaps be woken once at night.

Bladder retraining or bladder drill

Bladder retraining is a method of management that can be undertaken when a patient has developed a very low capacity bladder and is visiting the toilet very frequently, at half-hourly or hourly intervals. The intention is to train the bladder to hold more urine and allow the individual to go for 3–4 hours between passing urine; the patient's ability to inhibit the micturition reflex is increased by bladder retraining. It is suggested that bladder retraining schemes are best managed on hospital in-patients (Jarvis, 1981). The programme generally consists of daily charting of micturition and incontinence. Every day the patient is requested to wait an extra fifteen minutes between episodes of micturition; so if they started the programme visiting the toilet hourly on day 1, it would be $1\frac{1}{4}$ hourly on day 2 and so on until day 7 when visits would be $2\frac{1}{2}$ hourly or even three-hourly. During the remaining few days in hospital the patient aims to visit the toilet three-hourly and remain continent between visits as she/he has learnt to inhibit the micturition reflex.

Other Advice

The nurse is in a very good position to suggest changes a patient can make to ease the problems of incontinence. The following two case studies illustrate some methods of managing incontinence in the elderly.

	7	8	9	10	11	12	1	2	3	4	5	6	7	8	9	10	11	12	1	2	3	4	5	6
Mon																								
Tues																								
Wed																								
Thu																								
Fri																								
Sat																								
Sun																								

Please tick in shaded area if you are wet
Please tick in unshaded area if you pass urine normally into the toilet

Figure 12.1 Example of a chart used to record micturition and continence.

Case history

Mrs James is an 81-year-old lady living alone in a small terraced house. She has arthritis and is a bit unsteady on her feet. It seemed to her she was always wanting to go to the toilet but by the time she got there she was wet. She had tried cutting down on her drinks to no effect.

Management

Mrs James was asked to keep a chart recording her visits to the toilet and any episodes of incontinence, and also asked to write down how many drinks she had during the day.

At the end of a week, the chart showed she went to the toilet hourly during the morning and was wet every time. Her visits were not quite so frequent in the afternoon, but she was still often wet. At night, she woke up three or four times to go to the toilet. She took some time to reach the toilet from her front room due to her unsteadiness and when she got there she had obvious difficulty adjusting her clothing and sitting down on the seat.

Arrangements were made for her to have a walking frame and for a raised toilet seat and grab-rails to be fitted in her toilet. She was advised to wear loose-fitting skirts and supplied with Kanga pants and pads which are easy to pull up and down and gave her more confidence as she hated being accidentally wet. She was advised to go regularly to the toilet every two hours whether she felt like it or not. A commode was provided and placed by her bed for use at night.

She only drank three cups of tea during the day, but had another three in the evening. She was advised to try and drink eight cups during the day but to stop drinking after 6 p.m.

Case history

Mr Thompson is an 86-year-old man who had been admitted to a geriatric ward following a fall. He wants to go home to his wife but is worried because he has had a few episodes of incontinence since being in hospital. He has also become constipated since his fall.

Management

In talking to Mr Thompson, it became apparent that he got wet when passing urine into a bottle. He was a little unsteady and shaky and found it difficult to position his bottle.

It was suggested that adjustments should be made to the fly openings of his trousers – the opening should be extended and velcro fasteners attached. He was also provided with a urinal with a non-spill adaptor fitted to the neck. This is a latex rubber valve that allows urine to flow into the bottle but prevents it from spilling out.

His constipation was treated by giving him a high-fibre diet and encouraging him to drink plenty of fluids.

Pelvic Floor Exercises

Simple pelvic floor exercises can be taught to the elderly to help ease the problems of stress incontinence. Patients are taught to recognize where their pelvic floor muscles are by being asked to try and stop their flow of urine whilst micturating. Simple tightening of the pelvic floor muscle around the urethra and anus several times a day is often sufficient to improve the strength of this muscle.

Aids and Equipment

If all else fails, a nurse is able to offer help to an incontinent patient in the form of pads and pants or collection devices. It is important to take time and select a suitable aid for the patient and to explain carefully how the device is to be used.

Pads and Pants

Pads and pants are the incontinence aids used most commonly by women. They need to be chosen to meet certain criteria: the degree of incontinence, mobility, dexterity and size of the patient. If patients are still able to, they should be encouraged to visit the toilet regularly since the pad is only there to prevent embarrassment from accidents. Pads and pants need to be easy to pull up and down.

Selecting Aids by Degree of Incontinence

Stress incontinence or minimal dribbling

Small plastic backed pads with adhesive strips can be fitted into a patient's own knickers. For men, penile drip collectors containing absorbent gel can be held in place with lightweight stretch pants.

Moderate incontinence

Marsupial pants (e.g. Kanga) have a special pouch with a waterproof outer layer which holds a pad. They are easy to manipulate and suitable for mobile patients who can still get to the toilet. They are available in female and male styles and are easy to wash and dry. Alternatively, plastic-backed pads held in place with lightweight stretch knickers (e.g. Molnlycke) can be used.

Heavy incontinence

The more absorbent plastic-backed pads should be used for those likely to void large amounts of urine incontinently (over 100 ml) or who are faecally incontinent. All-in-one disposable diapers are virtually impossible for an elderly person to manipulate on their own and should never be used on mobile patients or those who can use the toilet with help. They may be of some use to bed-fast heavily incontinent patients.

External Collecting Devices

Men are able to use external collecting devices which can be attached to the penis. Urinary sheaths are most commonly used, but they are no good if the penis is retracted or less than 4 cm long. Internal fixing strips with adhesive on both sides are stuck directly on to the penis and the sheath is then rolled into place. Sheaths with external fixing strips are also available, but these do not tend to be so watertight.

There are many other types of male collecting devices available, and expert advice is often needed in fitting them. All these devices drain urine into a bag that can be strapped to the leg.

No satisfactory external collecting devices have yet been designed for women.

Indwelling Urinary Catheters

Urinary catheters are generally used as a final option in helping a patient to cope with intractable incontinence. If they are well managed, they can improve the quality of life for many with uncontrollable incontinence.

Choice of catheter

For long-term use, catheters with an inert coat of silicone should be used, either silicone elastomer or pure silicone. These can be left *in situ* for up to three months. The pure silicone catheters have much thinner walls and larger drainage lumens than coated catheters and are preferable. Latex catheters are only designed for short-term use of a few days.

Catheters with a small diameter or charriere should be used. It has been found that large diametered catheters cause problems such as blocking and bypassing (Kennedy, Brocklehurst and Lye, 1983). A 12 or 14 charriere catheter should be adequate for most patients, and a 16 charriere could be used for patients with very thick urine. The balloon size should also be small; catheters with 10 ml balloons are adequate to retain a catheter *in situ* (if used from the first catheterization). Two lengths of catheter are available, the male length and the shorter female length. The female urethra is much shorter, about 4 cm compared to about 20 cm in males. Use of female-length catheters allows catheterized women to position their drainage bags more discreetly.

Catheter care

The genital area should be cleaned regularly with soap and water. Routine bladder wash-outs or instillations are not necessary and perhaps only helpful when the patient is producing a lot of debris with the urine. Acidic wash-outs or instillations (such as Suby G solution) may then be useful. Routine antibiotic prophylaxis is not a good idea as it encourages the proliferation of resistant bacterial species. Both nurses and patients should always wash their hands before and after touching an individual's catheter or drainage bag to avoid cross-infection.

Drainage Bags

For long-term catheterized patients, some form of body or leg-worn bag should be used, preferably with a night drainage connection so the day bag does not have to be disconnected every night.

BOWEL PROBLEMS

Constipation is a very common bowel problem in old age. The simplest method of management and prevention is to increase the fibre content of the diet by adding bran to breakfast cereals and more fresh fruit and vegetables and wholemeal bread to the diet. An increased fluid intake also helps to bulk up the faecal matter. Exercise and movement stimulate bowel emptying. If a patient has severe constipation and impaction of faeces, then a course of enemas will be required. Enemas may need to be given every day for a week to clear out the bowel.

Faecal Incontinence

Faecal incontinence is often due to constipation. When the bowel becomes full of hard, impacted faecal matter, a lot of mucus may be formed which can seep through the anus and look like faecal soiling. A rectal and abdominal examination should be done to determine whether the patient is impacted, in which case enemas will be required.

Diarrhoea in the elderly can lead to faecal incontinence. Common diseases which cause diarrhoea include diverticular disease, ulcerative colitis, Crohn's disease and carcinoma of the colon or rectum. These all require medical investigation.

Neurological damage in, for example, cerebrovascular disease can lead to faecal incontinence where the patient is unaware of passing a stool. When faecal matter is passed into the rectum, contractions in the rectal muscles are uninhibited by the brain and the anal sphincter becomes relaxed and allows passage of faecal matter. This is quite often a reflex following the first meal or drink of the day. Soiling may be prevented by sitting the patient on the commode when they take their first cup of tea in the morning.

OSTOMIES

Surgical intervention may sometimes be needed in the elderly where there is such severe disease of the bladder or bowel that they have to be removed or bypassed.

If the bladder is resected, one method of treatment is to form an ileal conduit, where the ureters are connected to a section of the ileum. One end of the ileal section is closed and the other end is brought to the surface of the skin as an ileostomy. Urine is collected in a plastic bag which can be fitted directly over the ostomy. Such bags need to be carefully fitted to ensure the correct size is used and no damage done to the stoma.

Faecal matter can also be passed through an ileostomy. The ileum is cut and brought through the abdominal wall to the outer skin. This means faecal matter does not pass into the large intestine but through the opening on the abdominal wall. Again, a special bag has to be carefully fitted to the stoma to collect the liquid faecal matter.

SUPPORT

Many problems with elimination are treatable and patients with incontinence can be cured of their problem, and if not fully cured at least helped to be able to manage the problem in a more socially acceptable way. Nurses are in the best position to educate patients with elimination problems. Specialist nurses called continence advisers are now in post in most health districts in the UK. These nurses are able to educate their fellow nurses and to give advice on how to care for patients with difficult problems. They will also have up-to-date information on the various aids and appliances available and the latest techniques for testing incontinence.

REFERENCES

Brocklehurst, J. C. (1982) The ageing bladder, *Geriatric Medicine,* Vol. 3, pp. 11–15.

Copperwheat, M. (1985) Putting continence into practice, *Geriatric Nursing,* May/June, pp. 4–8.

Jarvis, G. J. (1981) A controlled trial of bladder drill and drug therapy in the management of detrusor instability, *British Journal of Urology,* Vol 53, pp. 565–6.

Kennedy, A. P., Brocklehurst, J. C. and Lye, M. D. W. (1983) Factors related to the problems of long-term catheterisation, *Journal of Advanced Nursing,* Vol. 8, pp. 207–12.

Ramsbottom, F. J. (1982) The use of incontinence underpads in hospital, *Nursing Times,* Vol. 78, pp. 1868–9.

Shepherd, A. M., Blannin, J. P. and Feneley, R. C. L. (1982) Changing attitudes in the management of urinary incontinence – the need for specialist nursing, *British Medical Journal,* Vol. 284, pp. 645–6.

Thomas, M. T., Plymat, K., Blannin, J. and Meade, T. W. (1980) Prevalence of urinary incontinence. *British Medical Journal,* Vol. 281, pp. 1243–5.

Tobin, G. and Riley, M. (1986) The ten-minute hurdle, *Community Care,* 18–19 September.

13. Working and Playing

Steve Goodwin

THE ROLE OF REACTION AND SOCIAL STIMULATION

Sadly, the faces of our elderly in care often show only total boredom, dejection and apathy. Boredom is part of 'institutional neurosis' (Barton, 1966). It 'haunts every institution and does not discriminate between resident and staff. It makes the day dreary, it causes the victim to wish away his life and it takes all interest, initiative and joy out of living' (King's Fund, 1982). The sufferer sinks further into a state of apathy, with declining mobility, wasting muscles and deteriorating mental function at various levels. 'Thus boredom in the extreme can destroy both the brain and the body' (King's Fund, 1982).

Often a state of overwhelming boredom and ritual activity is a permanent feature in hospitals, nursing homes and other institutions (Goffman, 1961; Vladeck, 1980; Martin and Evans, 1984). For many of the elderly, days are long and years short. After a hectic life of hard work, families to raise, long working hours, never a minute to spare for themselves, they suddenly find, through hospitalization or admission to a residential establishment, that they have time to kill. Often, through boredom, time ends up killing them.

Most carers agree that they would like to offer more recreational facilities and sit and talk more, if only they could find the time to do so. However, we dramatically underestimate the damage and abuse caused by not occupying patients' and residents' time in a way that is meaningful, enjoyable and challenging. Recreation can never be viewed as a luxury. It forms the basis of normality and good health and without it sanity declines, behaviour is altered and physical and social illnesses are precipitated (de Beauvoir, 1977). The abuse of elderly people's time in care is absolutely widespread, from the private sector home right through to long-stay geriatric wards. It is not enough to call a lack of recreation or occupational activity unfortunate and blame it on poor resources or being too busy. It is an essential part of care and treatment, and the absence of it amounts to neglect. If on surgical wards nurses could not find time to change dressings or give injections, how would you feel as a patient? If on a coronary care ward you were told your cardiac monitor was not working because there were bits missing, would you want to complain or even sue! And yet on many wards and in many homes, records are scratched or covered in sticky stains, there are jigsaw puzzles with missing pieces, books with pages missing, torn out, stereos with needles missing or held optimistically together by surgical tape, while half sets of dominoes and six-a-side chess games remain on the shelves. These facilities are not considered important or treated with respect and reflects the attitude of nurses and care staff towards recreation. Life itself may not be threatened by this broken or ill-kept equipment, but the quality of many people's lives are threatened. Even where facilities are obtainable and in working order, are they accessible by the elderly, or are they locked away or placed in awkward places? Entertaining patients is a low priority, low status task in the hierarchy of nursing activities (Pearson and Vaughan, 1986).

Quite often pure boredom is misdiagnosed as being 'confused behaviour'. Some of the inappropriate behaviour displayed by elderly people in hospital, especially in 'psychogeriatric'-type settings is too glibly written off as being part of their condition. If we look closely though, perhaps in a doctor's waiting room or airport lounge, we see similar behaviour being shown by younger 'normal' people. We may ourselves whilst waiting read all the notices, magazines we aren't really interested in, gaze endlessly at a spider in a corner, fiddle about in our pockets pulling out any bit of paper or form to read, rummage through a handbag, rub hands together, stamp or tap our feet. If we are kept waiting a long time we may start walking endlessly up and down, keep on asking the time or checking our watch, and we may start to hum or even clap. As soon as someone starts a conversation we are tempted to listen in, even though it may be totally uninteresting, anything that would relieve the boredom and break the monotony. The human animal is such that is needs stimulation; without regular mental exercising and recreation things start to go wrong and health declines (Kastenbaum, 1979).

Of course we all have different levels of needs and wants when it comes to this area of health. There are undoubtedly elderly people who are content with a quiet simple life, but there are also many elderly people who, even at a very late age, have much physical and mental energy and who have a fervent desire and need for action and excitement. We can be misled into thinking that elderly people are grey, uninteresting and insignificant, but let us not forget that may of our elderly in care, especially the very old, have probably seen and done more, and certainly taken more risks, than perhaps any generation before or since them (Elder, 1977). Is this not the generation who criticize their grandchildren because they get bored too easily, especially if the TV is not on? How often have we heard them say they made their own entertainment? The youth of the earlier part of the century were much more involved in the theatre, music-halls, cinemas, sport and family and social gatherings. Even with the limited transport and funds of the time, days out and social events were commonplace. Many of the elderly people in care today have become grey and uninteresting because of the lack of choice, opportunity and motivation to be and act themselves once within the walls of institutional care. Somehow for several decades we have condemned thousands and thousands of elderly people to meaningless miserable and tedious days of mediocrity and yet those responsible for this have done so with extreme kindness and dedicated toil and effort (Wells, 1980). We have failed to realize the essential role in care and cure that recreation and social stimulation should play and the insipid mediocrity that institutional care can be without them.

Firstly, we must recognize that elderly people are generally just young people grown old. Without doubt many miserable old folk were once miserable young folks and many old bores are just young bores with wrinkles and grey hair. Many of the interests and hobbies of elderly people have been with them since their younger days. It is therefore essential to find out what elderly people are interested in and what hobbies and pastimes they have enjoyed (RCN, 1987). Many may have had to give up those things through financial reasons or lack of social contact, immobility, illness or mental frailty. Many of our elderly live alone and when a loss of spouse occurs not only does a marital partner go but also often a best friend, dancing partner, bridge partner, chess or dominoes opponent and the one person who knew you cheated but never seemed to mind. Even though many elderly people may be a little rusty

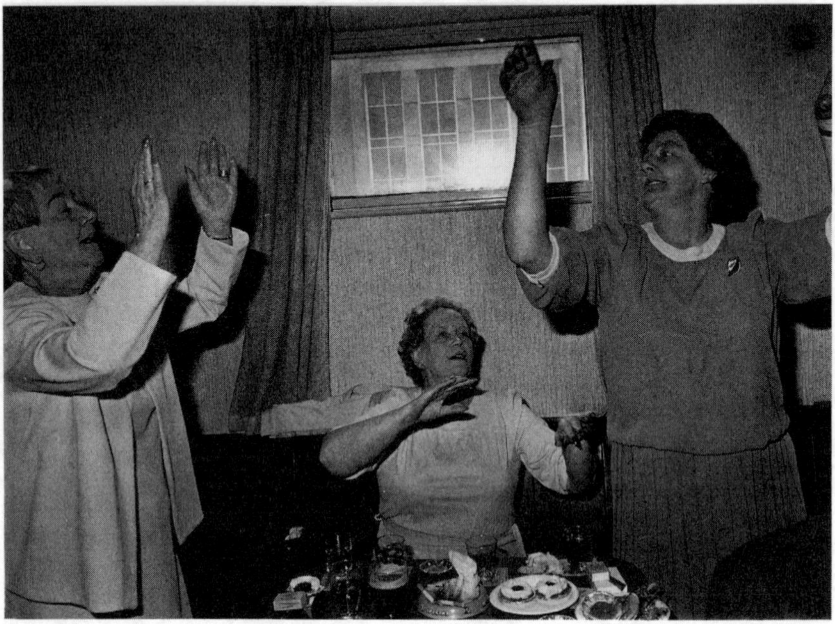

on their previous pastimes, with encouragement and practice the old skilful hand can soon be back to old form.

The interests that can be fostered and redeveloped in elderly people may be purely social, but others can be motivated in other ways. Some elderly people may still have business or political involvements, and they still belong to clubs or other organizations. It is important to encourage elderly people to retain these links and interests even if they are in permanent care. Many of these organizations will provide transport and support if approached or at least keep in contact by means of letters, circulars and news.

PROMOTING LEISURE ACTIVITIES

Nursing in particular has never really identified itself with the role of promoting and carrying out leisure activities. Many still see it as being the role of the occupational therapist and social links perhaps part of a social worker's job or a voluntary organization. Equipment for such activities is often left to charitable groups or hospital friends committees, etc.

What carers really have to do, especially nurses, is to realize how essential these social activities are and how closely and relevantly linked to health they are. They must be included in individual programmes whether elderly people are in hospital or care for a short or long stay. Just by making therapies more interesting and enjoyable the two things can be achieved at once with great benefit. For instance, if an elderly man on a ward or in a home needs mobility practice, that practice is likely to be more productive and beneficial if, instead of just walking down a corridor or in a physiotherapy department, the walk is round the corner to a pub or takes place in the hospital garden, or is out to a car or even with the home's dog trotting alongside. This is the kind of invisible mending that seems often to reap the best results. Therapy should be enjoyed and is more likely to be if people do not recognize it as therapy at all. I could name one or two old men with arthritis who won't lift their arms above shoulder height to wash their faces for the nurses or the occupational therapist. However, when a pint glass is put in the hand they can suddenly manage to lift their arm up all the way to their mouths!

Close observation of elderly people with mobility problems reveals how much they can achieve away from the ward or residential setting. Even people with major problems and disabilities can achieve much more than they expect in a social setting, often forgetting their aches and pains when the environment around them is geared towards ability and normality.

Linking physiotherapy and occupational therapy to social activities may seem obvious but in fact the benefit to health and nursing is not always realized. Where social acitivities and recreation are restricted on a ward or in a home the level of dependency and the level of physical and mental ill-health will probably rise and create the conditions so many nurses find themselves in. Where it is thought that such activities should not take precedence over other nursing practices like dressings, bathing and toileting and feeding then there is little hope of escaping the snare that has caught generations of conscientious carers. 'Cosmic nursing' is a philosophy of care that demands attention to be paid to what is right with elderly people in care, and what they can achieve even with highly infirm and disabled people (Goodwin and Mangan, 1985).

At ward level working with elderly mentally frail people in particular it has been shown that if social and recreational activities are increased, especially those away from the hospital, then physical and mental ability increases. As mobility improves through regular walking, gentle sport and regular outings to public facilities like pubs, cinemas and relatives' or friends' houses, then continence improves, even more so where particular attention is drawn to an elderly person's smart appearance. Even with chair-fast and highly infirm elderly people mental capability and incontinence can be improved. This saves nursing time dramatically because less incontinence and improved mobility reduce nursing time spent changing and bathing, and pressure area care can be decreased. The time saved each day from being tied to these duties is reinvested into social and psychological activities. Even bathing can be transformed from a beat the clock sheep-dip-style activity to a leisurely soak that an elderly person can enjoy rather than endure.

A bath is a nursing task but can also be a social event. By spending a little more time and asking how people want the bath, either full to the brim and hot or a few inches of lukewarm water. A bath may mean for some a soak with a newspaper, cigarette and cup of tea. Wherever the elderly bath with minimum supervision then they should be encouraged to do so, rather than having a nurse hovering around like an anxious life-guard.

Although nursing is not taught along these lines it does not mean to say that nursing is a single track even though many have one-track minds - cure, and of course safety first.

RISK AND EXCITEMENT

Risk does have to enter into nursing somewhere along the line. Unfortunately where elderly people are concerned the cushion of safety is so huge and undefined that it ends up smothering every last breath of inspiration from them and suffocates their very life-styles. Yet this is a generation of people who have lived through at least one world war and maybe a blitz. Many of them spent months or years in the front line, perhaps even in the trenches of the Great War. They have lived and worked without Health and Safety Acts. Wasn't this the generation who never wore crash helmets but just turned their caps back to front? Rightly or wrongly, they have on many occasions had to face great risk.

Excitement may seem an extreme word to use with elderly people living in care but it should not have to be excluded. Often excitement and risk go hand in hand, for instance with many circus and theatrical acts, sport, fun-fairs, gambling, and of course good cinema and television. Risk, dare and excitement should not be withheld from all elderly people just because they are in care. On admission to a residential home elderly people are generally told they've got 'nothing to worry about now'. Unfortunately some people need something to worry over, something to get concerned about. What usually happens is they end up becoming totally neurotic about their shawl not being straight or that their Zimmer frame is too far away or that someone else is in their place at dinner. A lack of constructive risk and anticipation in their lives turns many elderly people into grey, uninteresting, insignificant beings who fade into apathetic irrelevance, slowly being bored to death.

Cosmic nursing's motto is quite simply 'Come out death and fight'. It has helped many elderly people to more interesting and fulfilling lives and given many individuals the opportunity of continuing with old interests and achieving new objectives. It has added life to their final years and moments of excitement and thrills. This has been done by involving nursing and other staff in setting up special days for different individuals, like Fred, a 92-year-old Great War veteran, a bugler and drummer in his days at the Somme. Seventy years later, finding himself in a social services' home, he went back with care staff to be guest of honour with his old regiment and out for a ride in a tank, played out in style to bugles and drums. Weeks before that he and two other war veterans in similar homes had been down on army rifle ranges trying out the modern army's firepower and enquiring, 'Do they still put that funny stuff in your tea?'

Case study

Sister Burke's 'long stay' ward had a large number of patients of limited mental abilities, while the ward itself was old with poor facilities. With her colleagues, however, she had successfully put into action a range of activities - some for groups, some individually planned - to minimize the potential institutionalizing effect on the patients. There was little time for boredom on this ward.

The organization of the ward kept routines to the minimum. She had some years ago cut down on the obsessive weekly bath days and the rigid toilet rounds. She had also made a concerted effort to minimize the use of safety rails and chairs with tables fastened in place. 'Getting up' and 'going to bed' times were more attuned to the patient's choice. The day-room not only had TV and games, but also a bar stocked and funded by donations from relatives, local pubs and the occasional staff fund-raising effort. Patients would use their own money to buy drinks (at very modest cost). The bar was open at usual pub hours. Liaison was maintained with the medical staff and drugs which might adversely effect them socializing were minimized.

There was open visiting on the ward, but there was a tendency for visitors to arrive at pub times - the day-room becoming a social centre for the whole ward.

In addition, the staff organized regular outings to clubs, shops, pubs and places of interest. Group games on the ward were a common feature, with outdoor games – such as bowls in the summer, or simply sitting in the garden and enjoying the sunshine. One nurse took a special interest in reminiscence therapy, another in relaxation therapy. Both taught the skills to their colleagues and organized sessions for individuals and groups on the ward. Voluntary helpers, friends and neighbours were encouraged to call in for a chat, write a letter or read to someone. These patients who had no relatives were taken under an 'adoption' enabling them to take trips out at weekends and holiday times.

The nurses worked hard, but the work had been changed in a few years, with a little imagination, from the hard 'slog' of the institutionalized regime, to a more open and stimulating environment – less of a ward, more of a social centre.

There have been special outings for many elderly individuals away from institutional care, from a couple of hours in a window cleaner's hoist up the side of a tower block to a couple of old ladies having rides out in a fire engine and going up eighty feet on the hydraulic lift to put a new perspective on their lives. An hour or two like this for the elderly person who enjoys risk and a dare and something a little more than just the weather to talk about is important.

Although we may think by looking at an elderly person that they will want to do very much, or anything at all daring or unusual, we must not judge them by our own biased opinions. Sometimes it might be better if the staff took the tranquillizers and let the elderly people get on with their own lives, as it is often our own limited imaginations and conceptions of old age and disability that prevents many old folk from achieving more! Many nurses and carers following the cosmic nursing philosophy have been surprised, even shocked, by what many elderly people have asked to do, and, in fact, on some occasions it has been difficult to find a staff member willing to accompany an elderly patient because of their own anxiety about the situation. Witnessing elderly people who are infirm or disabled, confused or highly impaired achieving and succeeding and disproving the myths and biases about old age can have major consequences. Certainly it does alter the opinions and attitudes about old age not only of the staff, especially learners, but of the elderly people themselves.

WHAT NURSES CAN DO

Whether we jump in at the deep end or start to paddle out from the shallow end with recreational activities, we cannot avoid getting our feet wet. We need to plan activities, discuss and record what people enjoy doing and what they have interests in, and ask their permission where possible to set things up for them. If there is a lack of interest or motivation then it may be necessary to cheat a little, perhaps by asking a reluctant or shy person to participate as a favour to Mrs Jones, who would love a game but was no one to play with, and that half hour of dominoes would help her no end. Nursing staff don't always need to be actively involved but where possible it may help. Often if the facilities are readily available it only takes a suggestion and a little persuasion from staff to instigate activity. Here it is important that we don't become too presumptuous or careless in what we provide. For instance, though books may be available on a ward there need to be some large print, which are easily available from libraries, and none should have pages missing. There should also be a wide selection of subjects both fiction and non-ficton and geared towards both sexes and for the elderly who are broad-minded.

Magazines and newspapers too are often geared towards middle of the road readers or what the staff prefer. Elderly people who can afford it should have access to their own weekly or monthly journal, especially those who have particular interests. Often elderly people who have been displaced from their own locality to move nearer family find themselves in care and alienated miles from their real home. Here a local paper ordered could keep them in touch with their old homestead especially those from overseas. The last thing a Yorkshireman may want is to read *Lancashire Life*.

Reading material is important but without proper spectacles it is useless. Some may need a magnifying glass; the blind may perhaps benefit from talking books and newspapers. For some a nurse, volunteer or relative sitting down reading out bits of news from the press can be rewarding. Done in a small group this often leads to regular discussion groups. Again we may feel the elderly shouldn't have access to the bad news, but old folk are people and people love to hear about a good gruesome murder or terrible accident.

Reminiscence therapy groups can be used as social occasions. Here elderly people can recall and comment on past events and memories from their often colourful histories. These reflections are prompted by tapes/slides or by articles brought in specially, like old gas masks, scrubbing boards, cigar tins and the like. These are often lent out by local organizations or museums at little or no cost. The best results of therapy of this kind come when it is done in very small groups or even one to one, outside the ward or home. This may be a bus or taxi ride down the local streets or to a local museum or permanent exhibition that reflects days gone. Children from local schools may get involved by coming to inquire from the elderly people in care what school was like when they were young, what games they played or what used to be where the new housing estate is now sited. Elderly people in care can be a great resource of knowledge and entertainment for other generations of all ages.

Music can be a great asset and source of comfort for many elderly people but it can also be greatly abused. Too many elderly people in care have to suffer hours upon hours of piped pop and rock music. Loud music like this can vastly alter people's behaviour, creating agitation and aggravating confusion and wandersome behaviour. The television is as guilty as radio for this. Television in hospitals and homes for the elderly is the most common form of entertainment and yet is widely abused and misused. Apart from constant noise, often intolerable to those who are hard of hearing, it is also misused and poorly planned. Television can be used successfully if staff prepare the elderly people's programmes. It is not good enough to just switch on a TV and expect instant involvement and interest halfway through a film or series. Most television that elderly people in care get to watch children's TV and hardly appropriate. Often when adult and peak-time viewing is on they are either in bed or at a meal. Here a video can be a great resource, especially recording sport, old black and white films, documentaries, cup finals or that episode of Coronation Street someone was eager to watch but had to have those miserable visitors instead!

By planning what people can watch enthusiasm can be drummed up, old actors and film stars can be discussed and the whole programme can be enjoyed. Music played on record can be very entertaining but nothing beats a good sing-along round a piano. Here volunteers can come in handy, and there may even be elderly patients who can still play an instrument, be it only a comb and tissue paper. If one person alone wants to listen to music while others are perhaps watching TV or are with visitors, then personal stereos with headphones are very reasonably priced and can easily fit inside a handbag or jacket pocket. Why should teenagers have a monopoly on fun?

Trips to a concert are of course much more enjoyable for many, not just for the music but for the preparation and anticipation of the occasion: the getting ready with the glad-rags and finery. Occasions like these start the adrenaline flowing again. For elderly men too getting out into a crowd at a soccer match can be a thrill regained, especially now as more grounds are increasing seating facilities. A meat pie and a pint of bitter beforehand and pretend the referee is matron or the ward sister and let the abuse fly, that's what Saturday afternoon can be like even if home is for some a hospital.

Sundays too may be special for many elderly people in care. Many have been regular church attenders. Churches offer wide varieties of activities and organizations that can still be enjoyed by a large proportion of people in care. Spiritual needs as well as the social needs often met by the church are often neglected or biased by staff failing to encourage people to remain spiritually active whatever their creed or culture, especially in some highly ethnic communities.

An increasingly popular interest is being shown by staff and charities in introducing pets and animals on to wards and homes for elderly people. Charities like the PAT dogs (Pro-Dogs Active Therapy) bring dogs into the ward with a volunteer handler to give elderly people an opportunity to have contact with animals. This contact has recently been shown to be very important and beneficial to people who have or are recovering from illness (see Chapter 5). Pets do lower stress levels and help some people fare better and recover more successfully. The roles that pets play in the lives of many elderly people should not be underestimated. How many old folk won't go into hospital for a minor operation or attend day care or have a rest break in a home because they have no one to look after their pets? Many old folks worry about their pet more than they worry about themselves; some pay out a large proportion of their pension on pet foods and accessories and neglect themselves. A cat, dog or budgie can be the best friend of many a lonely and isolated elderly person at home.

More and more homes and wards have their own permanent pets now and the results of this are very encouraging. Some establishments for the elderly have animals like doves, hens, ducks and farm animals like goats, donkeys and ponies. How much nicer it is to be awakened by a rooster than the rattling of a linen trolley. Even if no land is available as is commonly the case, then cats, dogs, cage birds and aquariums can be beneficial and easy to manage. It is surprising how many elderly people kept livestock like bantams during the war or just for a hobby. Much fun can be gained from keeping pets and many a ward dog or cat has won a prize at a show thanks to the skill and interest shown by elderly patients.

Gardens too are easy to set up, from window-boxes in a multistorey hospital to allotments in the back garden. Most establishments for the elderly are generally kept very warm and well lit and this is often an ideal situation for many plants, even exotic ones, and for indoor tomatoes. Some wards and one-day hospitals have grown grapes from vines and some make a healthy cash turnover in plants and salads which subsidizes holidays and outings on the ward.

One conscientious old soldier makes cigarette money through selling manure from the pony at the hospital. Flower shows and competitions of blooms between wards and different hospitals can produce very aggressive competition among green-fingered patients.

In poor weather, when it is difficult to take elderly patients out regularly, more needs to be found to do inside, though trips and excursions out in winter and autumn should still be encouraged. Indoor sport and leisure activities are often limited by the ability and interest of the elderly person. Confused elderly people and those with a dementia or forgetfulness may have poor or short span concentration. Even highly confused elderly people though can surprise staff with their ability to play games like dominoes or bowls, since some skills hardly diminish. Often table-top games, like table skittles as played in pubs, are ideal for those confined to a wheel-chair or chair-fast. There are numerous hobbies and pastimes that can easily be encouraged on a ward like potting plants, baking, knitting, crocheting, painting, in fact all the things that many of the nursing or care staff may have an interest in. Of course no one should ever be forced or bullied into any activity and for most of the day most of the elderly people may choose to do little or nothing, which is fine. However there should always be access to some activity as few elderly people will ask because they believe staff are too busy, or they may not think it part of the nurses' role.

Cooking and perhaps other activities like knitting and sewing can be made more interesting where there is a purposeful outcome for the fruit of people's labours. This may mean knitting or making clothes for an expected baby or for charity purposes or making cakes for thier own tea, or, even better, trying out recipes old and new for their own meals. This is especially so on special occasions like Pancake Day and Bonfire Night. Few hospitals or homes seem to get involved in Bonfire Night but it is a great opportunity for elderly people in care to carry out their role as grandparents or even great-grandparents. Sadly, this is a role that is denied to too many old folk in care. But maybe all it needs is Gran's special treacle toffee, inviting in children and getting together round a bonfire somewhere in the grounds, toffee apples and all.

There are many special occasions in the calender for a celebration, especially Christmas. There can be a good social build-up to Christmas, with patients, staff and helpers, perhaps even a local school or nursery creating decorations and fancy goods for the big occasion. We may think that a ward is too busy to halt or slow down during Christmas but let us bear in mind that in 1914 the Great War actually had to halt for the worst of enemies to celebrate Christmas. This is a perfect time to reassure our elderly in care that we are not on opposite sides.

Day excursions and trips out succeed best in small groups, and families and volunteers are becoming more an essential ingredient as staffing levels are limited. Sometimes staff are reluctant to run trips and outings for confused or forgetful elderly people because after all the effort and expense they can't even on the way back remember where they've been. Dare we admit that there have been nights out when we can't remember where we have been or what we did, but this doesn't seem to deter us from ever going out again.

If we do not treat our elderly with the respect their often colourful and eventful histories deserve, or plan meaningful futures for them, then surely they can at least have the pleasure of living for today. Not every day in hospital or an elderly persons' home can be a holiday camp and nor can nursing staff or care staff become 'redcoats'. What can, and indeed has been shown, is that elderly people can sometimes enjoy therapy, expect happiness and have a basic right to social recreation, something not even denied to prisoners.

We must not sentence elderly people in care to be bored to death. We must remember that he who laughs ... lasts.

REFERENCES

Barton, R. (1966) *Institutional Neurosis*, Wright, Bristol.
de Beauvoir, S. (1977) *Old Age,* Penguin, Harmondsworth.
Elder, G. (1977) *The Alienated: Growing Old Today*, Writers and Readers Publishing Co-operative, London.
Goffman, I. (1961) *Asylums*, Penguin, Harmondsworth.
Goodwin S. and Mangan P. (1985) Cosmic nursing, *Nursing Times,* series of monthly articles, May to December.
Kastenbaum, R. (1979) *Growing Old: The Years of Fulfilment*, Harper & Row, London.
King's Fund (1982) *Living in Hospital*, Kings Fund, London.
Martin, J. P. and Evans, D. (1984) *Hospitals in Trouble*, Blackwell, Oxford.
Pearson A. and Vaughan, B. (1986) *Nursing Models for Practice*, Heinemann, London.
Royal College of Nursing (1987) *Improving the Care of Elderly People in Hospital*, London.
Vladeck, B. C. (1980) *Unloving Care: The Nursing Home Tragedy*, Basic Books, New York.
Wells, T. (1980) *Problems in Geriatric Nursing*, Churchill Livingstone, Edinburgh.

14. Resting and Sleeping

Rosemary Webster and David Thompson

INTRODUCTION

Effective nursing seeks to provide care for patients over a 24-hour period. As most people, including the elderly, spend about one-third of their time asleep the promotion and maintenance of sleeping patterns would seem sensible. The accomplishment of this requires a knowledge and understanding of the nature of sleep with particular reference to the norms and problems of sleep in the elderly.

NORMAL SLEEP

All humans sleep although each individual has differing behavioural patterns pertaining to it. Many definitions of sleep exist depending on the context in which it is being studied. From a neurobiological perspective, McGinty and Beahm (1984) define sleep as 'Recurrent spontaneous episodes of motor quiescence accompanied by raised thresholds of sensory response. Greatly diminished recall or continuity of mental activity, that is, unconsciousness, accompanies human sleep.'

Loomis, Harvey and Hobart (1937) first described separate and distinct electroencephalographic (EEG) stages within sleep, and thus established the fact that sleep is not a steady state. In 1953, Aserinsky and Kleitman reported that periods of rapid eye movement occur during sleep. A few years later, Dement and Kleitman (1957) linked these periods of rapid eye movement (REM) to dreaming. However, it is evident that dreaming does occur outside of REM sleep (Foulkes, 1962).

Sleep is conveniently divided into two distinct types: REM (paradoxical) sleep and non-REM (orthodox) sleep. Human non-REM (NREM) sleep is divided into four stages (Rechtschaffen and Kales, 1968) on the basis of specific EEG patterns. Individuals become more deeply asleep as they pass from stage 1 to stage 4. The stages and their most prominent features are summarized in Table 14.1.

The sleep stages described follow a fairly orderly cyclic pattern. In normal human adults, REM sleep begins about ninety minutes after sleep onset and recurs again at 90–100 minute intervals. On average, the individual progresses through 4–5 cycles of sleep per night. Stage 4 sleep decreases and REM sleep increases in proportion progressively with each cycle so that most stage 4 sleep occurs early in the night and most REM sleep occurs during the last few hours before arising.

Table 14.1 Sleep stages and the most prominent features of the EEG

Stage	*EEG activity*
W (wakefulness)	Alpha activity and/or low voltage, mixed frequency activity.
1	Relatively low voltage, mixed frequency EEG without REMs.
2	12–14 cycles per second sleep spindles and K complexes on a background of relatively low voltage, mixed frequency EEG activity.
3	Moderate amounts of high amplitude, slow wave activity.
4	Large amounts of high amplitude, slow wave activity.
NREM	Stages 1,2,3 and 4 combined.
REM	A relatively low voltage, mixed frequency EEG in conjunction with episodic REMs and low amplitude EMG.

Source: Rechtschaffen and Kales, 1968.

Function of Sleep

The various functional theories concerning sleep may be roughly divided into two categories: behavioural and restorative-synthetic.

Traditionally sleep is looked upon as a time of restoration and preparation for the next period of wakefulness. It has been suggested that sleep is a period of bodily and brain restitution (Oswald, 1974; Adam and Oswald, 1983). However, the idea that sleep is a restorative process has been challenged by Horne (1983) who postulates that for the majority of tissues, excluding the brain, sleep is probably a state of tissue degradation caused by lack of food intake during the night.

Meddis (1977) challenges the idea that sleep is necessary at all, believing that sleep is an instinct which has the function of merely segregating periods of inactivity and activity in animals. He suggests that, in principle, man is quite capable of living without it.

Much of the evidence for the various functional theories of sleep has been derived from examining the effect of sleep deprivation. If sleep does have a biological or behavioural function then elimination of sleep should theoretically produce alteration in this function. However, total sleep deprivation does not appear to result in any specific bodily dysfunction but there does appear to be related biological and behavioural changes (Vogel, 1975; Horne, 1978) such as alterations in proportion of sleep stages, and performance and mood changes. The type of sleep lost appears to be relevant: for example, Williams, Agnew and Webb (1967) showed that loss of stage 3 and 4 sleep caused subjects to feel withdrawn and physically uncomfortable; loss of REM sleep resulted in feelings of confusion and suspicion. When recovering from a lack of sleep people rarely sleep for more than twenty hours at a stretch regardless of the amount of sleep lost, and the composition of this recovery sleep differs from normal sleep.

Sleep research tends to be carried out in controlled laboratory conditions over relatively short periods of time: little is known about the long-term effect of sleep loss or its effect on life-long health. For many, sleep has important psychological and social purposes; people expect to sleep for certain periods of time at different stages and times in their lives and the implications of lack of sleep will be dependent on such expectations.

Circadian Rhythms

Sleep, in common with many other bodily functions, follows an approximate 24-hour pattern referred to as a circadian rhythm (derived from the Latin *circa* meaning about, and *dies* meaning day) (Halberg, 1953).

Factors such as social and work commitments influence normal sleep patterns but there is evidence that an innate circadian rhythm will continue to operate in the absence of these external mediators. The free-running sleep–wake cycle is though to be about twenty-five hours, although there is much individual variation (Moore-Ede, Czeisler and Richardson, 1983).

It appears that people also differ in the time of day at which they function at their best and choose to sleep. Horne and Ostberg (1976) categorized two distinct groups of sleepers: 'morning' types, who preferred to go to bed early, get up early, and who functioned best early in the day; and 'evening' types, who chose to go to bed late, get up late, and performed best in the evenings.

The maintenance of the sleep–wake cycle is an important factor in the synchronization of other physiological cycles and as such is an important component in the maintenance of health. Unfortunately, circadian rhythms in hospital patients are likely to become desynchronized or 'phase shifted' resulting in poorer quality of sleep (Taub and Berger, 1976).

CHANGES IN SLEEP ASSOCIATED WITH OLD AGE

Age is regarded as the most powerful determinant of a person's sleep behaviour (Williams, Karacan and Hursch, 1974). Most sleep research has been carried out on healthy young volunteers and there is a paucity of information about the specific nature of sleep changes with ageing from which to derive norms for the elderly. The plausibility of research findings depends very much on the accuracy and appropriateness of the research method, and a certain amount of variability in research findings may be attributable to this.

Objective studies of sleep which derive patterns from all-night polygraphic recordings, demonstrate certain well-established attributes (Dement, Miles and Carskadon, 1982), including:

- Time in bed is increased: elderly people seem to spend more time in bed either (a) without trying to sleep, (b) unsuccessfully trying to sleep, or (c) resting or napping during the day.
- Total sleep time is generally reduced or unchanged in comparison with younger age groups.
- Awakenings after sleep onset are generally increased. There may be either relatively short arousals or several long periods of wakefulness.
- Sleep efficiency is usually reduced in the elderly.

Amount of Sleep in the Elderly

Bahr (1983) reports that researchers have found that neither the amount of sleep per twenty-four hours or the need for sleep decreases with age. The total sleep time for any 24-hour period may not change by more than one hour over adult lifetime, but the timing and quality of the sleep are altered considerably. Total sleep time has been found to be between 6.0 and 6.5 hours in the elderly (Feinberg, Koresko and Heller, 1967; Williams, Karacan and Hursch, 1974), although the elderly seem to spend much more time than this actually in bed. Webb and Swinbourne (1971) found the average time in bed for the elderly to be 12.1 hours in males and 11.7 hours per day in women. Sleep efficiency thus declines in the elderly, falling to between 75–85 per cent of middle life norms (Williams, Karacan and Hursch, 1974; Prinz, 1977).

The decline in sleep efficiency may be as a result of lengthier and more numerous arousals (Feinberg, Koresko and Heller, 1967; Kahn and Fisher, 1969: Webb, 1982). McGhie and Russell (1962) found that between one-quarter to one-third of a sample of people aged over 65 years reported frequent night-time awakenings. Dement, Miles and Carskadon (1982) and Webb (1982) report that elderly men have more disturbed sleep than elderly women. Hayter (1983), in a study of healthy subjects aged between 65 and 95 years, found a significant increase in time spent in bed, total sleep time, number and length of naps, and number and length of periods awake after sleep onset after the age of 75 years, and a significant increase in day-time sleepiness and total sleep time after 85 years.

Webb and Campbell (1980) found that it could take up to four times as long for the elderly to get back to sleep once awakened than a younger age group. Early morning awakening has been found to be a feature of ageing. McGhie and Russell (1962) found that 15 per cent of their sample of over 65-year-olds awoke before 0500 hours.

Sleep Stages

Characteristics of the sleep EEG in the elderly show considerable variation to those observed in the younger adult. Sleep stages differ in both nature and amount and are less clearly defined (Kales *et al.*, 1967) making them difficult to quantify.

Evidence suggests that the elderly have longer periods of stage 1 sleep and significantly reduced amounts of slow-wave (stage 3 and 4) sleep. In fact, the amounts of stages 3 and 4 sleep can fall to almost negligible amounts in the elderly (Agnew, Webb and Williams, 1967; Feinberg, 1968; Williams, Karacan and Hursch, 1974).

The distribution of REM sleep throughout the night becomes increasingly more uniform in the elderly as there is an increase in the amount of REM sleep earlier in the night. In general, absolute amounts of REM sleep decline slightly but relative amounts are well maintained until extreme ageing at which time they decline rapidly (Williams, Karacan and Hursch, 1974).

Circadian Rhythms

The elderly demonstrate a tendency towards dissociation and asynchrony of certain circadian rhythms (Cahn, Folk and Huston, 1968). This may be a consequence of normal ageing caused by deterioration of regulatory mechanisms (Shock, 1977). Colling (1983) reports that it is thought that a progressive decrease in cerebral blood flow or a loss of specific neurones involved in sleep regulation may account for the apparent decline in maintenance of the sleep–wake cycle in the elderly. Some researchers have concluded that the elderly return to a child-like pattern of sleeping on multiple occasions in a 24-hour period (Webb, 1982), or that the sleep pattern of the elderly becomes a reversal of previous day and night patterns (Armstrong-Esther and Hawkins, 1982).

Sensory impairment often associated with ageing may inhibit perception of external time cues necessary to maintain regulatory processes. Diminished eyesight limits light-dark stimulation and restricts the capacity for gaining information from clocks and watches or carrying out activities which could give some framework and concept of time to the day. Difficulty in hearing reduces the likelihood of the elderly picking up time-cues from noises around them, including television and radio.

The time chosen or made available for sleeping is dependent on what occupies the waking hours and the priority placed on sleep. The elderly, who have often retired and live alone, lack the commitments of work and family on a daily basis. They may also have a limited social life due to disability, disinclination or financial disincentives. Thus, for many, sleep time is of their own making. Some may choose to continue with regimes followed throughout their working lives to give some structure to the day, whereas others may try to sleep for longer periods through boredom, to keep warm, or perhaps because they feel they need more sleep now they are older.

Napping

Many elderly people nap during the day, possibly in an attempt to increase their total sleep time. Evidence suggests that the total sleep time for the elderly over 60 years is the same as at 40 years of age if naps are included (Zepelin, 1973). Sleeping during the day modifies the sleep–wake rhythm from a biphasic to a polyphasic one. Day-time naps do not consist of the same sleep stage components as night-time sleep. REM sleep is more prominent in morning napping whereas slow wave sleep occurs most in afternoon naps.

People may attempt to sleep during the day because they have nothing else to do or because they feel that it is the norm for their age group. Those who feel that they do not sleep very well at night may attempt to sleep during the day to compensate for their perceived sleep deficit. Johns (1975) found that episodes of wakefulness during the night coincided with increasing amounts of sleep taken during the day.

Effects of Change in Sleep Pattern with Ageing

Dement, Miles and Carskadon (1982) conclude that in general the elderly are dissatisfied with their sleep. There is no evidence of cause and effect to link this dissatisfaction with actual sleep changes occurring with ageing, but the nature and type of sleep had will influence how the person feels and behaves the following day. The image of the elderly dozing in a chair during the day is a stereotype of ageing. Carskadon, van den Hoed and Dement (1982) found that a substantial number of the elderly persons they studied were pathologically sleepy during the daytime.

Prinz (1977) reported a correlation between declining intellectual function and reduced REM sleep in the elderly. Feinberg (1968) described a relationship between chronic brain syndrome and loss of REM sleep in the elderly. Bahr (1983) reports that if the sleep pattern allows less complete rest than is required psychologically or physiologically then the elderly person may exhibit symptoms of fatigue, headaches, visual disturbances, poor concentration, apathy, depression, and problems with musculoskeletal co-ordination. Dement, Miles and Carskadon (1982) report that there is some evidence that the elderly may be less tolerant to phase shifts in the sleep-wake cycle than a younger age group. As a result of a pre-existing increase in awakenings throughout the night they are likely to be particularly sensitive to any additional sleep loss.

SLEEP PROBLEMS IN THE ELDERLY

A detailed review of sleep disorders in the elderly is beyond the scope of this chapter. Nevertheless, a basic knowledge of such disorders is important for those caring for the elderly as recent evidence accumulates to suggest that they are more prevalent than was first realized. They often present in the absence of specific complaints, and the initial identification of sleep problems will be dependent on the subjective assessment of the sleeper and the differentiation between normal and abnormal.

Dement, Miles and Carskadon (1982) report that complaints about difficulty sleeping tend to be more frequent than in other age groups. Common complaints involve various aspects of insomnia, but respiratory impairment during sleep is likely to be the most prevalent sleep disorder in the elderly.

Respiratory-Related Sleep Problems

Sleep-related respiratory disturbances are thought to increase substantially in mid-life and rise markedly during the eighth decade (Bliwise *et al.*, 1984).

Snoring

The prevalence of snoring increases with age, partly as a result of tissue relaxation. Approximately 60 per cent of men in their 60s and 45 per cent of women in their 60s are habitual snorers (Lugaresi, Coccoagna and Cirignotta, 1978). Guilleminault, van den Hoed and Mitler (1978) have emphasized that heavy snoring almost always precedes development of an apnoea syndrome. Snoring can also cause embarrassment on behalf of the sleeper and irritability and disturbance for those in close proximity.

Sleep Apnoea

Sleep apnoea is defined as apnoea lasting at least ten seconds and occurring thirty or more times per night. Dement, Miles and Carskadon (1982) cite a study of non-institutionalized elderly subjects (aged 62–86 years) revealing mean apnoeic episodes of fifty but reaching as high as 216 per night. Based on such findings it has been estimated that sleep apnoeas may affect over one-third of all elderly persons judged to be in good health (Dement, Miles and Carskadon, 1982). Carskadon, van den Hoed and Dement (1982) found that respiration during sleep was significantly disturbed in nine of twenty-four elderly subjects and that virtually all the disturbances during sleep resulted in at least a brief arousal. They concluded that sleep apnoeas could account for much of the sleep fragmentation in the elderly. Many sufferers are unaware of the reason why they have had disturbed sleep but complain of headaches and disorientation on waking and excessive day-time tiredness. It is possible that sleep apnoeas can trigger lethal cardiac arrhythmias although the possibility that they have developed to serve a physiological function, such as to initiate awakenings to improve the ventilatory response to hypoxia, or to prevent upper airway obstruction by encouraging coughing and swallowing (Orr, 1980), must not be overlooked. Most apnoea sufferers have no apparent anatomical defect although weight loss, drug therapy and surgery (tonsillectomy and tracheotomy) have been used as treatment measures.

Insomnia

Insomnia tends to be concerned with poor sleep associated with day-time tiredness. Symptoms include difficulty falling asleep, frequent awakenings, inability to go back to sleep once awakened and awakening early in the morning. Complaints of excessive sleep and persistent day-time tiredness are symptoms of hypersomnia and tend to be associated with inappropriate sleep, weakness and learning and memory problems.

Unusual Nocturnal Behaviour

The elderly may be prone to nocturnal disorientation and wandering which may be aggravated by illness, medication, or a change in environment. Abnormal night-time behaviour can include screaming, talking, moaning, scratching and tooth grinding.

Night-Time Leg Movements (Restless Leg Syndrome)

Restless leg syndrome is characterized by recurrent rhythmic movements of the legs and feet causing difficulty in keeping the lower extremities still enough to permit falling asleep. This behaviour tends to occur during the waking stage of the sleep cycle. The cause is unknown but it is thought that circulatory inefficiency or motor neurone problems may play a part. This syndrome seems to increase with age and is exacerbated by a lack of sleep. Sleep-related leg movements or leg jerks are also found in the elderly. These tend to occur every 30–40 seconds resulting in a period of arousal or awakening. The leg movements themselves are not perceived by the sleeper and are invisible to the naked eye but the sleeper tends to complain of frequent awakenings and poor quality sleep.

Nocturia

This is a common problem in the elderly, causing disruptions in the sleep cycle. An inability to get out of bed, diuretic therapy, anxiety and a change in environment and/or routine can exacerbate the problem.

Emotional Factors

Studies have shown that poor sleepers tend to have higher anxiety levels (Monroe, 1967). Hicks and Pellegrini (1977) demonstrated that short sleepers had significantly higher levels of anxiety than long sleepers. People who consider themselves to be nervous tend to have greater difficulty getting off to sleep and have more disturbed sleep (McGhie and Russell, 1962).

Colling (1983) reports that the intensity and duration of emotions may increase with age. Ageing brings an exposure to a variety of potentially anxiety-provoking events. These may include physical decline, loss of spouse and peer group members, decrease in material wealth, and a possible decline in status, sense of worth, and ability to control events. Depression and anxiety are not uncommon in the elderly and the symptoms tend to highlight those associated with normal ageing, including increased time before sleep onset, frequent arousals, longer time in bed, early morning awakenings, and expectations of poor sleep. Anxious persons may feel exhausted during the day but unable to nap. Highly anxious or depressed people may lack the inclination to do anything else but try to sleep and return to bed to sleep during the day. Others find it difficult to remain awake during the day. Some become fully alert through trying too hard to fall asleep resulting in arousal of the central nervous system. The latter may find that they fall asleep at inappropriate times such as when they are reading or watching television.

Bliwise *et al.* (1986) report that clinical observations suggest that sleep-related respiratory disturbances are associated with higher levels of depression in the elderly.

FACTORS INFLUENCING REST AND SLEEP FOR THE ELDERLY IN HOSPITAL

Various aspects of hospitalization can adversely influence rest and sleep behaviour of the elderly patient. Exisiting disorders may be aggravated by illness and people who have previously had no sleep complaints may find that they do have once they feel unwell and become a patient. Pacini and Fitzpatrick (1986), in a study of hospitalized and non-hospitalized elderly, found significant differences in the timing and duration of sleep. The hospitalized elderly reported less nocturnal sleep time, more 'other' sleep time and went to bed and awakened earlier.

Many potential sleep disturbances result from inappropriate environmental factors. The elderly person may be less ready to adapt to different situations and may become worried about the prospect of being unable to sleep in a strange setting. Those who through illness, impaired mobility or cognitive dysfunction, are unable to initiate appropriate changes in their environment will depend on others to do so. The mere fact of becoming a patient, especially an elderly patient, may be perceived by nurse and patient alike as justifying passivity and delegation of control over environment and routine to others. Certainly most environmental factors are capable of being effectively controlled by nurses provided they have the knowledge and motivation, and collaborate with the patient.

Alteration in Routine

Hospital patients may suddenly find themselves becoming a relatively minor part of the social system of ward environment with its own predetermined sleep–wake pattern which may or may not consider or accommodate individual preferences. Social and environmental cues which to some extent govern sleep rhythms will be different in hospital and sleep cycles and circadian rhythms are likely to become 'phase-shifted' or desynchronized resulting in poorer quality of sleep (Taub and Berger, 1976). Hayter (1986) reports that various studies show that sleep will be maximized by adherence to habitual sleep timings and routines. People who are in hospital for a short while will not have time to adjust to new regimes and those in long-term care find that their sleep requirements change as a result of restructuring of day-time activities.

The sleep patterns of the elderly in long-term institutions may, as a group, become more homogeneous and synchronized (Wessler, Rubin and Sollberger, 1976). This may not necessarily be beneficial for the individual and may in fact occur for the benefit of staff who organize care around their own priorities and shift patterns. Clapin-French (1986), looking at sleep patterns of 102 elderly patients in long-term care, found that there were significant shifts in sleep patterns following admission. If patients' nocturnal schedules do not coincide with those of the institution then they may be awakened at endogenously inappropriate times for meals, treatments and other interventions. Bearing in mind that an average sleep cycle lasts ninety minutes, someone who is disturbed hourly will not complete one full sleep cycle throughout the night.

The day-time atmosphere of many hospital wards is one of hustle and bustle with patients never being quite sure of when they will next be approached for some intervention. This is hardly conducive to rest since patients anticipating being disturbed at any moment will find it difficult to relax. Constant stimulation from surrounding activities will also limit relaxation.

Activity

Elderly patients in hospital may be less active as a result of ageing and/or illness. A lack of new interests and stimulation within the hospital confines may lead to patients sleeping through boredom or because of difficulty sleeping at night due to day-time inactivity. However, some patients may be more active in hospital than at home, and physiotherapy and occupational therapy sessions may leave them exhausted. Hayter (1980) notes that physical exercise promotes stage 4 sleep in the well person, but that it needs to be taken more than two hours before the person's bed-time in order to be effective. Excessive activity immediately before going to bed leads to increased arousal and stress (Hobson, 1968).

Patients will have developed their own routines prior to settling down for the night such as an evening stroll, watching television or quietly reading. Long-term illness resulting in the elderly becoming bedridden will influence activity levels and sleep needs. Ryback *et al.* (1971) found that people who had been confined to bed for over five weeks had increased amounts of stage 3 and stage 4 sleep. Dement, Miles and Carskadon (1982) comment on studies that illustrate that prolonged bed rest leads to alterations in circadian rhythms, the cause of which is thought possibly to be postural.

Noise

Hospital nurses may become habituated to noises that can be very disturbing for patients. It is well established that the auditory awakening threshold decreases with age (Lukas, 1972; Roth, Kramer and Trinder, 1972). Sound may also appear to be amplified at night (Gress, Bahr and Hassanein, 1981). There is evidence that noise, especially noise stimuli occurring during sleep, results in marked physiological changes in endocrine and cardiovascular systems such as peripheral vascular constriction and electrocardiographic changes (Falk and Woods, 1973). The auditory awakening threshold seems to depend on the stage of sleep, stage 1 sleep being the lightest and stages 3 and 4 the deepest. Rechtschaffen, Hauri and Zeitlin (1966) found that the awakening threshold depended on how much sleep had already been had. Ogilvie (1980), looking at noise levels on wards at night, found that noise levels were greater than those recommended for a bedroom at night and equated to noise levels similar to a living-room during the day. The loudest sources of noise were telephones, metal bins and doors banging, and the most frequent from staff talking and using equipment. Close proximity of other people, noise from confused and very ill patients, and the disturbances caused by emergencies and admissions during the night add to the problem.

Temperature

Hospital wards may be kept at temperatures higher than the elderly are used to. Many elderly, in an attempt to keep heating bills at a minimum, live in cold conditions, especially during the winter. Temperature regulatory mechanisms are also less efficient in the elderly. Sleeping at temperatures greater than 24°C is likely to cause less efficient sleep (Schmidt-Kessen and Kendel, 1973), and too much or too little fresh air from air conditioners or open windows will affect comfort and influence rest and sleep. Feelings of being too hot may be aggravated by pyrexia and restlessness.

The cooling effect of sweating or being left in a wet bed when incontinent will also adversely affect sleep. Horne and Reid (1985) have shown that heating the body in a hot bath (41°C) during the afternoon produces a significant increase in sleepiness at bed-time, more slow wave sleep, and a reduction in REM sleep.

Lighting

The elderly will have become accustomed to certain levels of lighting when sleeping or resting. It may be difficult for them to nap during the day with bright lights on. At night they may have been used to leaving a landing or bed-side light on and feel insecure in hospital in darkness. Many elderly people have failing eyesight and need extra light to help them find their way to the toilet at night especially in the unfamiliar environment of the hospital.

Bed Positioning

The different positioning of the hospital bed and lack of familiar objects may cause disorientation upon awakening. Patients used to sleeping next to a wall may feel vulnerable in their hospital bed. Close proximity to other people and the communal atmosphere of the ward may also inhibit sleep. People normally move away from their day-time area to sleep at night, and the fact that the hospital bed serves as a focal point for eating, receiving visitors, treatment and spending time awake may detract from its intended purpose of a place for rest and sleep. Some patients may be used to sleeping in a chair at home and may wish to continue with this practice in hospital.

Diet and Nutrition

It seems that a continuation of an individual's normal eating habits is more crucial to effective sleeping than any particular food or drink (Adam, 1980). Many people have a hot milky drink before going to bed and it is thought that the amino acid tryptophan found in milk may help towards inducing and maintaining sleep. Ovaltine and Horlicks have been shown to significantly improve sleep when taken before bed-time (Brezinova and Oswald, 1972). Coffee apparently disturbs sleep even in those who feel unaffected by it (Karacan *et al.*, 1976a) and the sleep-disrupting effect of caffeine has been shown to increase greatly with age (Karacan *et al.*, 1976b), two cups of evening coffee causing very disturbed sleep in the elderly (Adam, 1980). Alcohol before bed-time can produce more awakenings and changes in sleep stage duration (Williams, McLean and Cairns, 1983).

Adam (1980) reports that body weight and changes in body weight are reflected in the sleep pattern. It has been found that as obese persons lose weight they sleep less, and as underweight persons regain weight they sleep longer. In general, fat people sleep longer than thin people. A report by Beecham Foods Nutrition Information Centre (1978) cites a study which revealed that a four-day period of starvation resulted in a slight fall in the amount of REM sleep with an increase in NREM sleep.

Comfort

The elderly may find hospital beds harder than those they are accustomed to at home. Hard surfaces cause more bodily movements, which may affect sleep, and plastic protective covers which are a feature of most hospital beds can lead to patients becoming uncomfortable, hot and sweaty. Patients used to sleeping in a double bed may feel restricted or indeed fearful of falling out of a hospital bed and they miss the comfort and security of sleeping with their partner. Hospital beds are likely to be of different dimensions to those which the elderly are used to and some elderly may have difficulty getting in and out of bed unaided. Patients used to continental quilts find the differing weight and feel of blankets difficult to get used to.

The nature of the illness itself may mean that normal sleeping positions become impossible; for instance, the patient who is unable to lie flat because of shortness of breath or who has to attempt to sleep in an awkward position on traction. Elderly patients used to an afternoon fireside nap in their favourite easy chair may find hospital furniture clinical and uncomfortable and the environment not conducive to day-time sleeping. Invasive procedures such as catheterization, the discomfort and embarrassment caused by incontinence, and the disturbance for the recording of observations, may also limit the comfort of patients.

Pain

With the increased likelihood of chronic disease it is apparent that the elderly may suffer pain during the night. This is particularly so if the effect of medication taken prior to bed-time has worn off or if routine analgesia is stopped on admission to hospital. Acute illness episodes will also produce pain in some which will be reported to variable extents by patients.

Anxiety

The ease of going to sleep will be greatly affected by whether the patient is anxious or depressed (Kleitman, 1963). Hospitalization plays an important role in the production of anxiety. Pacini and Fitzpatrick (1986) consider that higher anxiety levels during hospitalization attributed to the significant differences found in sleep between hospitalized and non-hospitalized elderly patients. The elderly may be worried about leaving the security and familiarity of their home environment for the unknown. They may be used to being on their own and feel uncomfortable in the presence of so many other people. They may feel embarrassed by their disabilities and be uncertain of what is expected of them as patients. Fear and worry over their illness and outcome may be paramount, and understandable, in a population group who have experienced the loss of many of their peers – many of them in hospital. Possible investigations and surgery are a further source of anxiety. Patients may worry about their personal sleep characteristics such as snoring, and feel embarrassed about preparing for sleep – removing dentures, getting undressed, etc – in the presence of strangers. They may worry about the possible need to go to the toilet in the night, about wetting the bed, or just 'bothering the nurses', all inhibiting sleep. It is possible that certain aspect of anxiety will be reduced in hospital as patients no longer feel they are struggling on without help but feel that something positive is being done to help them overcome their problems.

Illness

Colling (1983) reports that physical illness is a major factor implicated in sleep disturbances in the elderly and sleep will improve only when the underlying problem is alleviated.

It is well recognized that sleep is associated with a fall in blood pressure, heart and respiratory rates and temperature. Karacan *et al.* (1976a) point out that cardiovascular crises often occur with a high frequency during sleep. Hayter (1980) notes that the pulse is irregular during REM sleep and that cardiac arrhythmias are more likely to occur at this time.

Duodenal ulcers producing increased gastric acid secretion at night can lead to nocturnal epigastric pain. Gastric secretions appear to increase during REM sleep. For patients with arthritis, there may be a build-up of pain during the night as the joints stiffen through inactivity. Patients with heart failure may experience asthma-like symptoms during the night as a result of fluid build up around the lungs and sleeping supine may cause breathing difficulties for patients with chronic obstructive airways disease. Conditions affecting the central nervous system are likely to interfere with the quantity and quality of sleep, although it is not known to what extent degenerative changes in the central nervous system are responsible for changes in the sleep pattern in normal ageing. Raised intracranial pressure from any cause and many toxic infective conditions are likely to cause increased sleepiness. Patients with Parkinson's disease experience alteration in sleep patterns and an increase in the time spent awake. They can awaken during the night with recurrence of rigidity making change of position in bed impossible. Many endocrine and metabolic disorders will adversely affect sleep. For instance, renal failure and uraemia will both produce excessive sleepiness. Liver failure seems to cause day–night reversal of sleep patterns, and hypothyroidism is associated with a decrease in stage 4 sleep.

Psychiatric problems such as obsessive, compulsive and phobic disorders may influence sleep patterns. Patients with psychotic depression tend to wake frequently and early in the morning; schizophrenia can result in inversion of the night–day pattern; and mania or hypomania produces difficulty in falling asleep or shortened sleep time.

Episodes of illness, particularly acute, are likely to be accompanied by a perceived need, if not an actual need, for more sleep. People tend to take to their beds when ill in accordance with cultural or social norms, presumably supposing that time spent asleep or resting is a bonus to the healing process. The feeling of being unwell seems to be diminished by reduced activity and opting out of responsibilities and day-to-day commitments until feeling better. Although individual responses to illness vary, it would seem appropriate to facilitate adequate rest and sleep in hospital.

Drug Therapy

The elderly are often prescribed medication which results in a change in their sleep pattern. Such an effect may be intentional when drugs are given to promote sleep, or the effect may be a secondary consequence. The elderly are often prescribed multiple drugs and are therefore at increased risk of drug interaction and iatrogenic problems. Drug efficacy may differ in the elderly population as body composition changes influencing distribution of the drug, and reduced renal function limits elimination. Those drugs affecting the central nervous system tend to have a heightened effect in the elderly and so are more disrupting to their sleep architecture. Drugs that stimulate the central nervous system, include amphetamines and sympathomimetic agents and these decrease total sleep time and delay sleep onset. They may also produce episodes of day-time sleepiness and feelings of anxiety and irritability. Drugs which suppress the central nervous system include hypnotics, sedatives, tranquillizers, anticonvulsants, antihistamines, beta-adrenergic blocking agents and antidepressants. These are likely to produce increased day-time sleepiness and may result in feelings of depression, episodes of amnesia, or alveolar hypoventilation if used over long periods of time in the elderly.

The elderly population is a frequent user of both prescriptions and over-the-counter medications designed to improve sleep (Basen, 1977). The incidence of elderly persons taking sleeping tablets in hospital or institutions is possibly higher than in the community. Clapin-French (1986), looking at institutionalized elderly, found that 71 per cent of patients were receiving sleeping tablets on a regular basis.

Ideally, a sleeping tablet should not modify the normal sleep architecture and should not continue to exert the sedative effect for longer than the normal sleep period. As Dement, Miles and Carskadon (1982) point out, the general body of knowledge about sedatives and hypnotics has been largely derived from studies of younger adults and does not necessarily apply to the elderly. Thus, sleeping tablets should not be liberally prescribed to elderly patients as a matter of routine.

There are various types of medication taken to improve sleep. Anxiolytics such as benzodiazepines are prescribed to reduce anxiety, and depression is often treated with antidepressant drugs such as amitriptyline. Barbiturates, once the most preferred sleeping agents, are now avoided, particularly in the elderly, because of marked hangover effects during the day-time. Benzodiazepines are increasingly being used as hypnotics, the most common being nitrazepam, flurazepam, temazepam, and diazepam. These are advantageous in that they have less side-effects and dependence is less likely to occur although they can produce morning drowsiness. Chlormethiazole is often used with the elderly as it is free from hangover effects.

If people continue to take hypnotics and sedatives over a long period the dosage required to produce sleep gradually increases until natural sleep becomes impossible (Kales and Kales, 1974). Most, if not all, hypnotics and sedatives interfere with REM sleep. The elderly may experience more of a hangover effect with sleeping tablets as slower drug metabolism increases the half-life of the drug and the drug is therefore still effective the following day.

Problems arise when people who have been taking sleeping tablets regularly try to stop them. REM sleep increases without the tablets and there may be complaints of increased dreaming, nightmares, and feelings of nausea, muscle tension and of not having slept well. This may be a problem for the elderly who suddenly have their sleeping tablets omitted on coming into hospital. Gradual withdrawal from sleeping tablets will eventually result in an improvement of sleep for most.

Clapin-French (1986), in her study of institutionalized elderly, concluded that patients were possibly receiving inappropriately large amounts of sleeping medication without much inquiry into the factors promoting their insomnia. It is possible that nursing intervention aimed at increasing relaxation and comfort would be more effective. It is the quality rather than the quantity of sleep which is important. Gerard *et al.* (1978), in a study of the elderly, reported that quality of sleep was worse for those taking hypnotics. Hindmarch (1980) concluded that the improved ease of getting to sleep and reported sleep quality experienced when taking sleeping tablets was at the expense of a 'hangover' effect the next day. It is possible that changes that occur in sleep with ageing are adaptive and sleeping tablets counterproductive. Restless sleep may in fact be desirable in strange situations where the increased REM sleep helps restore the body mentally after stressful experiences (Muncy, 1986).

Patients who are heavily sedated at night may suffer from the consequences of reduced body movements during sleep and may also have an increased incidence of night-time incontinence. Muncy (1986) reports that hypnotics have been shown to increase the amount of noise necessary to awaken people, but that medication has never been shown to be of benefit in sleeping problems and is in fact the cause of the most common sleeping disorders. Studies reported by Barnes (1968) concluded that sleeping tablets were often given to relieve the nurse's frustration over a wakeful patient rather than to benefit the patient.

Sleeping tablets have psychological effects which may be as important as the actual pharmacological composition of the drug. Patients used to taking sleeping tablets at home may worry that they may be omitted in hospital or that they will be given different ones that they expect to be less effective.

The elderly who smoke may adversely influence their sleep patterns. Palmer, Harrison and Hiorns (1980) found that cigarette smokers had significantly shorter sleep duration than non-smokers.

SLEEP ASSESSMENT

Accurate sleep assessment will be necessary before planning and evaluating nursing intervention designed at promoting sleep. A review of the most commonly used methods for assessing sleep has been provided by Johns (1971). Objective measures such as polygraphic recordings are generally inappropriate for the elderly in hospital. It is subjective evidence that is most useful in this setting.

Elderly people will judge their sleep by how it compares to habitual patterns, including how they feel the following day, and how much sleep they expect. This will depend on perception, memory and recall. The elderly tend not to complain about sleep problems (Carskadon, van de Hoed and Dement, 1982) and may expect poorer sleep in hospital making accurate evaluation of subjective reports difficult.

Nursing assessment will be a reflection of expectations held by nurses and if the elderly are judged by middle age adult norms, inaccuracies will occur. Day-time symptoms of apathy and sleepiness may be considered normal for the elderly in hospital and thus sleep problems may be missed. Often patients who spend some time in bed are assumed, often wrongly, to be asleep. Cohen *et al.* (1983), comparing patients' and nurses' ratings of sleep quality for elderly persons with disturbed and undisturbed sleep, found that patients with sleep disturbances rated their quality of sleep significantly lower than their peers with undisturbed sleep. Nurses' ratings did not discriminate between either group of patients' sleep and were poorly correlated with patients' ratings, suggesting that nurses are not skilled at assessing patients' sleep quality.

Methods of recording subjective reports include sleep diaries and questionnaires. Researchers have demonstrated that these can provide information which correlates significantly with objective assessments of sleep (Johns, 1977).

Assessment needs to be a continuous process, with nursing goals being regularly defined. Nursing considerations for patients' sleep are listed in Table 14.2.

Table 14.2 Nursing considerations in sleep assessment

From the patient

- Amount of sleep patient feels he/she needs.
- Patient's level of satisfaction with sleep.
- Factors influencing sleep as identified by patient.
- Patient's suggestions for improving sleep.

From the nurse

- Evaluation of sleep time and duration.
- Observation of number and cause of awakenings.
- Observation of rest and sleep periods during the day.
- Observation of patient's behaviour during the day – alertness, apathy, etc.
- Awareness of possible contributory factors – underlying illness, emotional factors, nutritional status, etc.
- Awareness of relevant drug therapy.

The use of a sleep questionnaire might be a useful instrument in some instances, although not all elderly persons may be able to complete them. We recommend the St Mary's Hospital Sleep Questionnaire (Ellis *et al.*, 1981). However, many researchers and clinicians develop their own sleep questionnaires and this may be more appropriate in certain circumstances.

Case history

Since her admission to the home, Miss Priestly had difficulty sleeping in the strange environment. To help her get a normal night's sleep, the nurse considered the following points:

- Provide peaceful/quiet environment and ensure general comfort in bed.
- Help to take rest periods on bed during the afternoon – she usually takes an hour's 'nap' at home mid-afternoon.
- Help with general comfort in bed.
- Talk with patient to discover anxieties, listen and problem-solve.
- Offer help if awake/restless, for example assistance to the toilet.
- Provide adequate bedding/pillows as preferred (likes two).
- Offer drink/snack of choice to help settle if disturbed.
- Review with patient if problem persists to see if sedation may help.
- Give time to sleep/rest according to normal pattern. She likes to remain in bed until about 7 a.m. and goes to bed usually about 10.30 p.m.
- Ensure curtains are drawn together at night and keep lamp within reach at bedside to use if needed.
- Provide bell to summon help if required.

PROMOTION OF REST AND SLEEP

Effective promotion of rest and sleep for the elderly in hospital depends on a variety of factors including:

- Knowledge of the normal ageing process in relation to sleep.
- Knowledge of how illness and sleep disorders affect sleep in the elderly.
- Knowledge of factors likely to inhibit or promote sleep in hospital.
- Knowledge of patients' normal sleep and rest patterns, e.g.:

  Time and duration of rest and sleep.
  Satisfaction with rest and sleep.

Table 14.3 Nursing intervention to promote rest and sleep

Maintenance of sleep routines

- Continuing habitual timing and duration of sleep.
- Continuing habitual bed-time routines.

Promotion of a restful environment

- Controlling environmental factors, e.g. noise, temperature, etc.
- Limiting and co-ordinating interventions.
- Minimizing anxiety.

Provision of comfort

- Ensuring comfortable positioning for rest and sleep.
- Using aids for comfort, e.g. bed cradle, adequate pillows, etc.
- Minimizing sweating and incontinence.
- Preventing harmful effects of immobility.
- Relieving pain.

Promotion of optimum sleep

- Providing stimulation and activity to relieve day-time boredom.
- Avoiding vigorous activity nearing bed-time.
- Encouraging relaxation.
- Adopting habitual sleep routines, where appropriate, whilst ill.
- Ensuring the environment is made familiar and personal to the individual by encouraging personal items, e.g. photographs, pillows, clocks, windows for orientation.
- Encouraging the involvement of relatives and friends.
- Using sleep-promoting agents if appropriate.

Position and place of rest and sleep.
Pre-sleep routines.
Reliance on sleeping tablets.

Some information may need to be obtained from the patient, relative or other reliable source. Care plans to promote rest and sleep need to be devised in collaboration with the patient. Plans will involve the elimination or reduction of unnecessary interruptions to wake or disturb patients. Patients need to be provided with the information and sources necessary to promote and improve rest and sleep and to expect changes in these occurring with ageing.

Nurses are ideally placed at assessing and meeting these needs by virtue of their being available twenty-four hours a day. Bahr (1983) considers that professional nurses are the key to ensuring that institutionalized elderly enjoy a higher quality of life in the area of sleep. Lerner (1982), discussing sleep loss in the aged, provides an eight-point check-list for nurses to use in planning care in the realm of sleep. It is vital that the patient has input into his or her care plan promoting sleep (Schirmer, 1983). Although care has to be provided within the constraints of staffing levels and patient dependency etc., an understanding of the importance of sleep should place its promotion as a high priority. Nurses need to make themselves aware of existing research in this area and base their care on scientific foundations. Protocol and established ward routines often form barriers to change and innovation based on sound rationale and research findings (Webster and Thompson, 1986). There is certainly a need for further nursing research based specifically on the sleep of the elderly in hospital.

REFERENCES

Adam, K. (1980) Dietary habits after bedtime food drinks, *Sleep,* Vol. 3, pp. 47–58.

Adam, K. and Oswald, I. (1983) Protein synthesis, bodily renewal and the sleep-wake cycle, *Clinical Science,* Vol. 65, pp. 561–67.

Agnew, H. W., Webb, W. B. and Williams R. L. (1967) Sleep patterns in late middle aged males: an EEG study, *Electroencephalography and Clinical Neurophysiology,* Vol. 23, pp. 168–71.

Armstrong-Esther, C. A. and Hawkins, L. H. (1982) Day for night. Circadian rhythms in the elderly, *Nursing Times,* Vol. 78, pp. 1263–66.

Aserinsky, E. and Kleitman, N. (1953) Regularly occurring periods of eye motility and concomitant phenomena during sleep, *Science,* Vol. 118, pp. 273–4.

Bahr, R. T.(1983) Sleep–wake patterns in the aged, *Journal of Gerontological Nursing,* Vol. 9, pp. 534–40.

Barnes, E. (1968) *Psychosocial Nursing: Studies from the Cassel Hospital, London,* Tavistock, London.

Basen, M. (1977) The elderly and drugs: problems, overview and program strategy, *Public Health Reports,* Vol. 93, pp. 38–43.

Beecham Foods Nutrition Information Centre (1978) How diet affects your sleep, *Nursing Mirror,* Vol, 147, no. 20, pp. 32–5.

Bliwise, D., Carskadon, M., Carey, E. and Dement, W. (1984) Longitudinal development of sleep-related respiratory disturbance in adult humans, *Journal of Gerontology,* Vol. 39, pp. 290–3.

Bliwise, D. L., Yesavage, J. A., Sink, J., Widrow, L. and Dement, W. C. (1986) Depressive symptoms and impaired respiration in sleep, *Journal of Consulting and Clinical Psychology,* Vol. 54, pp. 734–5.

Brezinova, V. and Oswald, I. (1972) Sleep after a bedtime beverage, *British Medical Journal,* Vol. 2, pp. 431–3.

Cahn, H. A., Folk, G. E. and Huston, P. E. (1968) Age comparison of human day–night physiological differences, *Aerospace Medicine,* Vol. 39, pp. 608–10.

Carskadon, M. A., van den Hoed, J. and Dement, W. C. (1982) Insomnia and sleep disturbances in the aged. Sleep and daytime sleepiness in the elderly, *Journal of Geriatric Psychiatry,* Vol. 13, pp. 135–51.

Clapin-French, E. (1986) Sleep patterns of aged persons in long-term care facilities, *Journal of Advanced Nursing,* Vol. 11, pp. 57–64.

Cohen, D., Eisdorfer, C., Prinz, P., Breen, A., Davis, M. and Gadsby, A. (1983) Sleep disturbances in the institutionalized aged, *Journal of the American Geriatrics Society,* Vol. 31, pp. 79–83.

Coleman, R. M., Miles, L. E., Guilleminault, C. C., Zarcone, V. P., van den Hoed, J. and Dement, W. C. (1981) Sleep–wake disorders in the elderly: a polysomnographic analysis, *Journal of the American Geriatrics Society,* Vol. 29, pp. 289–96.

Colling, J. (1983) Sleep disturbances in aging: a theoretic and empiric analysis, *Advances in Nursing Science,* Vol. 6, pp. 36–44.

Dement, W. C., Miles, L. E. and Carskadon, M. A. (1982) 'White paper' on sleep and aging, *Journal of the American Geriatrics Society,* Vol. 30, pp. 25–50.

Dement, W. and Kleitman, N. (1957) Cyclic variations in EEG during sleep and their relation to eye movements, body motility, and dreaming, *Electroencephalography and Clinical Neurophysiology,* Vol. 9, pp. 673–90.

Ellis, B. W., Johns, M. W., Lancaster, R., Raptopoulos, P., Angelopoulos, N. and Priest, R. G. (1981) The St Mary's Hospital Sleep Questionnaire: a study of reliability, *Sleep,* Vol. 4, pp. 93–7.

Falk, S. A. and Woods, N. F. (1973) Hospital noise levels and potential health hazards, *New England Journal of Medicine,* Vol. 289, pp. 774–81.

Feinberg, I. (1968) The ontogenesis of human sleep and the relationship of sleep variables to intellectual function in the aged, *Comprehensive Psychiatry,* Vol. 9, pp. 138–47.

Feinberg, I., Koresko, R. and Heller, N. (1967) EEG sleep patterns as a function of normal and pathological aging in man, *Journal of Psychiatric Research,* Vol. 1, pp. 107–44.
Foulkes, W. D. (1962) Dream reports from different stages of sleep, *Journal of Abnormal and Social Psychology,* Vol. 65, pp. 14–25.
Gerard, P., Collins, K. J., Dore, C. and Exton-Smith, A. N. (1978) Subjective characteristics of sleep in the elderly, *Age and Ageing,* Vol. 7, pp. 55–9.
Gress, L. D., Bahr, R. T. and Hassanein, R. S. (1981) Nocturnal behaviour of selected institutionalized adults, *Journal of Gerontological Nursing,* Vol. 7, pp. 86–92.
Guilleminault, C., van den Hoed, J. and Mitler, M. (1978) Clinical overview of the sleep apnea syndromes, in C. Guilleminault and W. Dement (eds) *Sleep Apnea Syndromes,* Alan Liss, New York.
Halberg, F. (1953) Some physiological and clinical aspects of 24 hr periodicity, *Lancet,* Vol. 73, pp. 20–32.
Hayter, J. (1980) The rhythm of sleep, *American Journal of Nursing,* Vol. 80, pp. 457–61.
Hayter, J. (1983) Sleep behaviours of older persons, *Nursing Research,* Vol. 32, pp. 242–6.
Hayter, J. (1986) Advances in sleep research: implications for nursing practice, in A. J. Tierney (ed.) *Clinical Nursing Practice,* Churchill Livingstone, Edinburgh.
Hicks, R. A. and Pellegrini, R. J. (1977) Anxiety levels of short and long sleepers, *Psychological Reports,* Vol. 41, pp. 569–70.
Hindmarch, I. (1980) Calling time on hypnotic drugs, *Nursing Mirror,* Vol. 150, no. 11, pp. 37–8.
Hobson, J. A. (1968) Sleep after exercise, *Science,* Vol. 162, pp. 1503–5.
Horne, J. A. (1978) A review of the biological effects of total sleep deprivation in man, *Biological Psychology,* Vol. 7, pp. 55–102.
Horne, J. A. (1983) Human sleep and tissue restitution: some qualifications and doubts, *Clinical Science,* Vol. 65, pp. 569–78.
Horne, J. A. and Ostberg, O. (1976) A self-assessment questionnaire to determine morningness–eveningness in human circadian rhythms, *International Journal of Chronobiology,* Vol. 4, pp. 97–110.
Horne, J. A. and Reid, A. J. (1985) Night-time sleep EEG changes following body heating in a warm bath, *Electroencephalography and Clinical Neurophysiology,* Vol. 60, pp. 154–7.
Johns, M. W. (1971) Methods for assessing human sleep, *Archives of Internal Medicine,* Vol. 127, pp. 484–92.
Johns, M. W. (1975) Factor analysis of subjectively reported sleep habits and the nature of insomnia, *Psychological Medicine,* Vol. 5, pp. 83–8.
Johns, M. W. (1977) Validity of subjective reports of sleep latency in normal subjects, *Ergonomics,* Vol. 20, pp. 683–90.
Kahn, E. and Fisher, C. (1969) The sleep characteristics of the normal aged male, *Journal of Nervous and Mental Disease,* Vol. 148, pp. 477–94.
Kales, A., Wilson, T., Kales, J. D., Jacobson, A., Paulson, M. J., Kollar, E. and Walter, R. D. (1967) Measurements of all-night sleep in normal elderly persons: effects of aging. *Journal of the American Geriatrics Society,* Vol. 15, pp. 405–14.

Kales, A. and Kales, J. D. (1974) Sleep disorders: recent findings in the diagnosis and treatment of disturbed sleep, *New England Journal of Medicine,* Vol. 290, pp. 487–99.

Karacan, I., Thornby, J. I., Anch, M., Booth, G. H., Williams, R. L. and Salis, P. J. (1976a) Dose-related sleep disturbances induced by coffee and caffeine, *Clinical Pharmacology and Therapeutics,* Vol. 20, pp. 682–9.

Karacan, I., Thornby, J. I., Anch, M., Booth, G. H., Williams, R. L. and Salis, P. J. (1976b) Dose response effects of coffee on the sleep of normal middle aged men, *Sleep Research,* Vol. 5, pp. 71.

Kleitman, N. (1963) *Sleep and Wakefulness,* University of Chicago Press, Chicago.

Lerner, R. (1982) Sleep loss in the aged: implications for nursing practice, *Journal of Gerontological Nursing,* Vol. 8, pp. 323–6.

Loomis, A. L., Harvey, E. N. and Hobart, G. A. (1937) Cerebral states during sleep as studied by human brain potentials, *Journal of Experimental Psychology,* Vol. 21, pp. 127–44.

Lugaresi, E., Coccoagna, G. and Cirignotta, F. (1978) Snoring and its clinical implications, in C. Guilleminault and W. Dement (eds) *Sleep Apnoea Syndromes,* Alan Liss, New York.

Lukas, J. S. (1972) Awakening effects of simulated sonic booms and aircraft noise on men and women, *Journal of Sound and Vibration,* Vol. 20, pp. 457–66.

McGhie, A. and Russell, S. M. (1962) The subjective assessment of normal sleep patterns, *Journal of Mental Science,* Vol. 108, pp. 642–54.

McGinty, D. J. and Beahm, E. K. (1984) Neurobiology of sleep, in N. A. Saunders and C. E. Sullivan (eds) *Sleep and Breathing,* Marcel Dekker, New York.

Meddis, R. (1977) *The Sleep Instinct,* Routledge & Kegan Paul, London.

Monroe, L. J. (1967) Psychological and physiological differences between good and poor sleepers, *Journal of Abnormal Psychology,* Vol. 72, pp. 255–64.

Moore-Ede, M. C., Czeisler, C. A. and Richardson, G. S. (1983) Circadian time keeping in health and disease: Part 1, Basic properties of circadian pacemakers, *New England Journal of Medicine,* Vol. 309, pp. 469–76.

Muncy, J. H. (1986) Measures to rid sleeplessness, *Journal of Gerontological Nursing,* Vol. 12, pp. 6–11.

Ogilvie, A. J. (1980) Sources and levels of noise on the ward at night, *Nursing Times,* Vol. 76, pp. 1363–6.

Orr, W. C. (1980) Arousals from sleep: is a good night's sleep really good?, *International Journal of Neuroscience,* Vol. 11, pp. 143–4.

Oswald, I. (1974) *Sleep,* Penguin, Harmondsworth.

Pacini, C. M. and Fitzpatrick, J. J. (1986) Sleep patterns of hospitalized and nonhospitalized aged individuals, *Journal of Gerontological Nursing,* Vol. 8, pp. 327–32.

Palmer, C. D., Harrison, G. A. and Hiorns, R. W. (1980) Association between smoking and drinking and sleep duration, *Annals of Human Biology,* Vol. 7, pp. 103–7.

Prinz, P. (1977) Sleep patterns in the healthy aged: relationship with intellectual function, *Journal of Gerontology,* Vol. 32, pp. 179–86.

Rechtschaffen, A., Hauri, P. and Zeitlin, M. (1966) Auditory awakening thresholds in REM and NREM sleep stages, *Perceptual and Motor Skills,* Vol. 22, pp. 927–42.

Rechtschaffen, A. and Kales, A. (1968) *A Manual of Standardized Terminology, Techniques and Scoring System for Sleep Stages of Human Subjects,* US Department of Health, Education and Welfare, Bethesda.

Roth, T., Kramer, M. and Trinder, J. (1972) The effect of noise during sleep on the sleep patterns of different age groups, *Canadian Psychiatric Association Journal,* Vol. 17, pp. 197–201.

Ryback, R. S., Trimble, R. W., Lewis, O. F. and Jennings, C. L. (1971) Psychobiologic effects of prolonged weightlessness (bed rest) in young healthy volunteers, *Aerospace Medicine,* Vol. 42, pp. 408–15.

Schmidt-Kessen, W. and Kendel, K. (1973) Einfluss der Raumtemperatur auf den Nachtschlaf, *Research in Experimental Medicine,* Vol. 160, pp. 220–33.

Schirmer, M. S. (1983) When sleep won't come, *Journal of Gerontological Nursing,* Vol. 9, pp. 16–21.

Shock, N. (1977) Biological theories of ageing, in J. Birren and K. Schaie (eds) *Handbook of the Physiology of Ageing,* Van Nostrand Reinhold, New York.

Snyder, F. (1965) Progress in the new biology of dreaming, *American Journal of Psychiatry,* Vol. 122, pp. 377–90.

Taub, J. M. and Berger, R. J. (1976) The effects of changing the phase and duration of sleep, *Journal of Experimental Psychology: Human Perception and Performance,* Vol. 2, pp. 30–41.

Vogel, G. W. (1975) A review of REM sleep deprivation, *Archives of General Psychiatry,* Vol. 32, pp. 749–61.

Webb, W. B. (1982) Sleep in older persons: sleep structures of 50 to 60-year-old men and women, *Journal of Gerontology,* Vol. 37, pp. 581–6.

Webb, W. B. and Campbell, S. S. (1980) Awakenings and the return to sleep in an older population, *Sleep,* Vol. 3, pp. 41–6.

Webb, W. B. and Swinbourne, H, (1971) An observational study of sleep in the aged, *Perceptual and Motor Skills,* Vol. 32, pp. 895–8.

Webster, R. A. and Thompson, D. R. (1986) Sleep in hospital, *Journal of Advanced Nursing,* Vol. 11, pp. 447–57.

Wessler, R., Rubin, M. and Sollberger, A. (1976) Circadian rhythm of activity and sleep-wakefulness in elderly institutionalized patients, *Journal of Interdisciplinary Cycle Research,* Vol. 7, pp. 333.

Williams, R. L., Agnew, H. W. and Webb W. B. (1967) *Effects of Prolonged Stage Four and 1-REM Sleep Deprivation. EEG, Task Performance and Psychologic Responses,* SAM-TR-67-59, United States Airforce School of Aerospace Medicine, Florida University, Gainesville.

Williams, R. L., Karacan, I. and Hursch, C. J. (1974) *Electroencephalography (EEG) of Human Sleep: Clinical Applications,* Wiley, New York.

Williams, R. L., McLean, A. W. and Cairns, J. (1983) Dose-response effects of ethanol on the sleep of young women, *Journal of Studies on Alcohol,* Vol. 44, pp. 515–23.

Zepelin, H. A. (1973) A survey of age difference in sleep patterns and dream recall among well-educated men and women, *Sleep Research,* Vol. 2, pp. 81.

15. Sexuality and the Older Person

June Andrews

INTRODUCTION

Each sacrifice to Venus is, for the old man, a spadeful of earth on his head.

(Legrand, 1911).

The question of sexuality of patients is one that cannot easily be discussed because sex is a subject that often gives rise to ribaldry, probably because of insecurity about the topic. In a specialist area like genito-urinary surgery, mental handicap, gynaecology or psychiatry, the topic can be covered from a specific point of view relating to a particular problem. Older patients can have problems that relate to other specialist areas, but because of society's attitude to old people these problems are likely to be overlooked, or avoided by the nurses looking after the old people in hospital and the community. For the young nurse it may be difficult to imagine that the old patient under her care is an unmarried mother, homosexual, promiscuous, someone's lover, 'in love'.

From the point of view of the young these things would appear to stop well before 65. Nurses are quite happy to discuss sex roles from a sociological point of view, or the aspects of sexuality in terms of altered body image after surgery, but less happy with the practical aspects of sexual intercourse with an indwelling urinary catheter, alternative positions to adopt to prevent dyspnoea during intercourse, the nursing care of the elderly rape victim or the fears of the elderly Aids sufferer.

The first problem which has to be overcome by nurses talking about sexuality is their own prejudice. While sex appears to be an acceptable topic for discussion in these liberated days in fact all that has happened is that new taboos have been established. Extramarital sex, promiscuity, homosexuality, pornography and sexually transmitted diseases can all be discussed freely, but there is still embarrassment when discussing the sexuality of the disabled and the old. In our culture, where it seems that only the young, fit and beautiful have the right to a complete sexual life, the old and disabled and disfigured are assumed to find alternative expression for sexual feelings. When problems arise they may have a quasi-medical manifestation, for example in psychosomatic symptoms such as pain or fatigue. The average nurse student who may be quite young and already struggling with her own changing sexual role needs to know something about it. Nurses, especially students, need further training to become counsellors in this area. Nevertheless the close observation by the nurse and her intimate relationship with the patient means that she is in a position to discover or be asked about problems of sexuality, and she must be sensitive to her patient but frank and informative at the same time. She must know what an old person can expect to achieve in the way of sexual satisfaction, what can go wrong and what things can arise spontaneously as a topic of conversation. It is not, however, within the scope of this chapter to discuss ways of persuading people to talk about secret or private feelings.

WHAT OLD LOVERS CAN EXPECT

> In general care one can divide the life of women into three periods: in the first they dream of love; in the second, they make it; in the third, they regret its passing.
>
> (Reveille, 1853)

The sexual activity of an old person, rather like that of a young person, depends on opportunity, health and desire. The older woman who has lost her husband may, after a life-time of serving his needs and those of their children, have lost the social skills required to find another sex partner. The pain of the bereavement may take away the desire. If she herself is also ill, she may not feel desire for sexual contact, but rather loneliness. She may sublimate her feelings by devoting herself to her children and grandchildren, continuing to keep her house in order and attending clubs and meetings for women. A woman of the same age, married and fit, may have sexual intercourse as frequently and with as much pleasure as someone ten or twenty years younger, depending on how she regards her sexual life. Some people regard it as a tiresome conjugal duty, and would be relieved if it was no longer necessary or possible. To this end any physical change requiring a change in habit, such as an operation or heart disease, would be seized on as an excuse to terminate the sexual relationship. Even if the couple wanted to restart sexual activity after a period of illness, they may find it difficult to take the problem to a health care professional because they are afraid they will be seen as unrealistic in their desires. What the old lover can expect from sexual activity varies enormously, but is probably more than most young people would believe.

The change in a women's body at the menopause may either mark a negative change in her attitude towards sex, or mark a time of liberation from the anxiety about pregnancy. The response of her body during intercourse continues to change from adolescence to old age, and the confident mature woman and her partner will accept gradual change.

There is not much information available about the sexual activity of women over the age of 60. Plenty of advice is available through the popular women's press about the physical changes a women may expect, and how she can deal with the discomforts of the menopause and after, like 'hot flushes' and increasing body hair. There is an abundance of physical restoratives like plastic surgery, expensive diets, clothes and cosmetics. Susan Sontag (1978) describes the women who takes care of her appearance obsessively as a 'moral idiot', underlining from the radical feminist point of view the unfair advantage men seem to have in being able to incorporate signs of age, and the trick that women allow society to play on them waste so much time on trying to look younger than they are.

The older patient may have had a hard life, having brought up children during a war, having worked in industry, having been widowed perhaps more than once. Now that she has become a patient she will not look her best, and being ill she will be less able to make the little efforts that self-respect usually demands. The lack of interest in herself as a person may be a result of the poisoning effect of the medication she is on (most people over 65 are taking on average three different prescribed medications, apart from non-prescribed remedies); she may have psychological obstacles to taking care of herself, because of depression or confusion.

Old women enjoy love, affection and bodily contact, but may be slow to respond because of less frequent exposure to physical contact. During sexual intercourse women experience changes in their nipples and clitoris at all ages, but the reactions are slower in old age and the muscle tension built up in intercourse is less. Basically the older woman has fewer secretions from Bartholin's glands, and the changes in the wall of the vagina make her drier and more susceptible to injury in intercourse. During intercourse the older woman has vaginal contractions that are shorter than those of a younger woman.

Older men may not have erection of the penis so easily with purely psychological stimulation, and full engorgement may take longer. Production of secretions may be less urgent, and slower, with seepage of semen rather than the forceful ejaculation of youth. But the older man may be able to continue intercourse for longer without orgasm, to the satisfaction of his partner. He may not be able to repeat the process as quickly as in his youth. Masters and Johnson (1966) say, 'If elevated levels of sexual activity are maintained from earlier years and neither acute nor chronic physical incapacity intervenes, aging males usually are able to continue some form of active sexual expression into the 70- and even 80-year age groups.'

So what old people can expect depends on what they have been used to. Everything takes on a gentler pace and women are more likely to have problems of lubrication, which may lead to feelings of urinary urgency and burning afterwards.

But old people, in every sphere of their existence have come to expect little for themselves and are content with less. As has been said by Comfort (1974), 'old folks stop having sex for the same reasons they stop riding a bicycle – general infirmity, thinking it looks ridiculous, no bicycle – and of these reasons the greatest is the social image of the dirty old man and the asexual undesirable old woman'.

Frequency of intercourse does diminish over time on average, but barring death, infirmity or negative attitudes from society, the continuation of intimate relationships and sexuality can go on beyond the 70s and 80s.

WHAT CAN GO WRONG FOR THE OLDER LOVER

But there is an irony in the culture toward ageing as expressed in the manuals and general magazine articles. After World War Two it did a

> somersault. The basic message now is that age can be conquered. ... Sex, once disdained with horror, is now strongly encouraged as normal and healthy.
>
> (Stearns, 1977)

According to Masters and Johnson (1966), a number of factors can lead to loss of sexual functioning in old men.

- Monotony of a repetitious sexual relationship.
- Preoccupation with career or economic pursuits.
- Mental or physical fatigue.
- Overindulgence in food or drink.
- Physical or mental infirmities in either partner.
- Fear of performance associated with or resulting from any of the above.

Monotony

> In her first romance woman loves her lover.
> In all the others, all she loves is love.
>
> (Byron)

There is no reason why an old person, at a time when if anything the personality becomes more rigid, should alter radically in sexual behaviour. If a single partner has been the sole comfort of one person then promiscuity as a sudden behaviour change would be remarkable. If the old person has been promiscuous, then the availability of partners may become less as the attraction of the person in stereotypical physical ways seems less. If someone has been in the habit of visiting prostitutes then the shortage of available partners may make them rely on this even more in old age, with the concurrent problem of sexually transmitted diseases.

A new partner is a source of irritation to your family, if you are old, and it is even worse if you choose someone much younger as they may fear for a legacy, questioning your sanity and the motives of your young lover. Day centre nurses and home wardens may be horrified when old people fall romantically and sexually in love with one another.

The problem of monotony within a relationship may be set against the advantage to an old person of a safe permanent partner in the face of all of these obstacles to change. Heterosexual people may learn from homosexuals in this respect. Lesbians value old women in a way that the rest of society does not, perhaps as a measure of their greater valuation of women in general.

Preoccupation

Your father was a good man. He didn't bother me much.

Most old people no longer have to go to work, but they have the problem of surviving economically on a fixed income, which is probably much lower than that to which they were accustomed when they did work. These worries, real or imagined, will prevent the old person from relaxing enough to enjoy anything. Set against this is the advantage for the early retired couple who for the first time in years are able to spend time alone together. This time is one when old people can get to know each other's bodies again, in the relaxed atmosphere of retirement. That is if they can stand each other, after years of surviving without each other. Retirement can make the former worker feel worn out and useless, and the loss of self-esteem that goes with the loss of a role in life can cause problems.

Mental or Physical Fatigue

Not tonight, Josephine.

(Napoleon Bonaparte)

Old lovers may tire easily, but they may have more time to make love when they feel like it if they have adequate privacy and can relax. The amount of energy used in sexual intercourse is often exaggerated. Nevertheless, the mere business of survival can be complicated for old people and the fatigue involved could contribute to the cessation of their accustomed sex life.

Overindulgence in Food and Drink

From the practical point of view it is important that old people (and the not so old) should be aware of this problem. For old people the failure to have satisfactory sexual intercourse, which may have a simple physiological cause like overindulgence, may combine with the common misconceptions about sexuality to make the old couple think that their bodies are no longer capable of giving them pleasure and thus give up altogether.

Physical and Mental Infirmities

These will be dealt with in some detail as the nurse is most likely to come in contact with the patient because of other problems associated with the disease process, and will be in a position to advise the patient if there is a problem with sexuality.

Dementia

The first sign of dementia that is noted by close relatives is the change in the personality of patients. If they become moody or irritable then their spouses are less likely to want to make love. The patient may become more demanding sexually, and the satisfaction to the partner may be diminished, as if making love to a rude stranger instead of the well-known and loved partner of many years. With memory loss the husband or wife may deny knowledge of their partner, call them by the wrong name or demand angrily why they are in the same bed, or touching them. Caring staff may be repelled by the idea that a man finds his demented wife sexually attractive, as they regard her as a child to be protected, not treated like an adult.

As part of the dementing process the patient may become disinhibited in behaviour, exposing genital organs in public (often to urinate in an inappropriate place) or making inappropriate advances to people of the opposite sex. There is nothing worse than an indignant nurse complaining loudly about the dirty old man who touched her when she was helping him, unless it is the shrieks of laughter in his face. The appropriate professional response involves setting limits on his behaviour, ensuring his privacy and maintaining his dignity in the face of his confusion.

Cardiovascular Disease

Men have been described as having a morbid fear of dying during sexual intercourse (Comfort, 1974). The physical changes in orgasm are so profound and exciting that they may even be frightening in their intensity. The symptoms of heart disease include breathlessness, chest pain and fatigue. The angina sufferer may take glyceryl trinitrate prophylactically as with any other exercise. The problem of breathlessness may be helped by taking different positions, the breathless partner, for example, avoiding lying down flat, being propped up well with pillows. It is extremely rare for people to die during intercourse. From the common-sense point of view, nurses could advise their patients that if they really are at 'death's door' then they probably would not feel well enough to contemplate intercourse. The anecdotal accounts of death 'in flagrante delicto' usually involve the horror of being discovered dead in bed with a mistress, and tell more about the guilt and shame involved in sex rather than the physical danger.

The usual advice about health given to sufferers of heart disease with reference to smoking, weight loss and gentle exercise and the resultant improvement in general physical condition makes all functions easier, including sexual intercourse. Careless advice after myocardial infarction can lead to patients becoming excessively worried about their condition, and heart attack patients should be able to discuss with the nurses or doctor looking after them about the best time to resume normal activity.

From the woman's point of view it is likely that if she found her 'conjugal duties' tiresome she will look to the excuse of heart disease to excuse herself from them. On the other hand a considerate partner may avoid troubling her with what he sees as his need, and she may assume that her increasing age and ill-health have made her unattractive to him. It is most important that lovers of all ages should be able to talk to one another to avoid this kind of problem, but in the old it may be that sexual problems have never been discussed and they are unlikely to change radically in later years.

Stroke

The extent to which stroke affects the sex life of the sufferer depends on the extent of the stroke. The problems of communication, if the patient has become dysphasic, make it difficult for needs to be expressed and for the caring partner to relate to them.

> As a ward sister I remember one old man sitting for hours holding his wife, touching her and speaking to her, feeding and washing her, even though

> her only response was the look in her eyes that followed his every movement. In the privacy of his own home he might have been able to express his affection openly, but attempts to create a private environment in the ward led to staff briskly entering the space to find out if something was wrong, and strict injunctions not to enter led to curious speculation about what the couple were up to.

Patients who have suffered a stroke may have difficulty in looking attractive in their own terms, either because of the change in the face caused by paralysis of facial muscles, or because general debility prevents them from making sure for themselves that they are well groomed, and wearing well-fitting dentures and clothes. Food stains from eating problems and the problems of poorly controlled incontinence make the stroke patient feel unattractive and may repel the partner.

The practical problems of intercourse may be helped by adopting different positions, for example with the fit partner on top, which the couple may never have tried before, in many years together.

Fear of Performance Failure

> Nothing succeeds like success.

The performance failure is specifically a problem of the male partner. Even if he has a supportive partner who is interested in maintaining an active sex life, and is encouraged by her to go to the doctor with his problem, he may fear lack of sympathy and the response, 'What do you expect at your age?' Nurses should be aware of the treatable conditions which can lead to impotence and other sexual problems at any age.

PROBLEMS WITH SEX

Impotence

This is the inability to achieve or maintain an erection to permit penetration in intercourse. The causes (which are most likely to be among the psychogenic ones mentioned above) may include diabetes, various endocrine disorders, multiple sclerosis and the after-effects of perineal surgery. The nurse should be certain that her patient has had the chance to discuss with someone before surgery the effect that it may have on his sex life. Some common misconceptions exist among men, for example, that prostate operations lead to impotence. Drugs and depression are the most common real cause of erectile impotence.

Infertility

While this may be regarded as a liberation by many if not all post-menopausal women, there are men with younger partners who would like to conceive a child. Although fertility decreases throughout life, an old man may have children, and his infertility may be secondary to a treatable condition such as hypothyroidism, or may be helped by the kind of advice given to younger men regarding frequency and timing of intercourse.

Dyspareunia

Pain on sexual intercourse may be felt when penetration is attempted, or may occur after penetration has occurred. In either case the cause may be treatable. The mechanical problems caused by dry, thinned skin in the vagina can be helped by simple lubricants like water soluble gels, or by administration of hormone replacements. Deep pain may be a sign of pathological change, such as pelvic infection or malignancy.

Pruritis Vulvae

The inflamed and itching pudenda can be a source of great embarrassment and discomfort to the elderly woman, and in confused and disinhibited women it can lead to problems of scratching excessively, infection (which then can be transferred by the patient's hand to her eyes, for example) and socially inappropriate behaviour as she tries to relieve her discomfort. The cause may be a fungal infection, to which the elderly diabetic is particularly susceptible.

Cystitis

The problem of cystitis and its connection with sexual intercourse is illustrated by its association with the honeymoon. Like the young bride returning home sore and uncomfortable, the elderly woman can experience pain and frequency of micturition. The kind of advice that a nurse can offer includes strict personal hygiene, especially before and after intercourse for both partners, and a recommendation to maintain a high fluid intake and urinate as soon as possible after intercourse.

Recurrent urinary tract infections are more common in the elderly because of the residual urine in the bladder caused by outflow obstruction, as in enlarged prostate or in the distortion caused in women by prolapse of the anterior vaginal wall.

Other Practical Problems

The continence adviser and stoma nurse may be able to advise their clients about ways of overcoming problems with sexual intercourse. Patients should be aware of the fact that a man with an indwelling catheter can have an erection and that the catheter does not prevent intercourse for either men or women. The male partner should detach his catheter from the collecting bag and it can fit alongside his penis during penetration. While this may seem at first complicated and rather peculiar, it is probably no more so than some of the contraceptive devices the couple have had to deal with, and the benefit to their sex life of maintaining continence of urine in their bed is great. The woman with a catheter presents less of a practical problem, but the nurse should be aware of the fact that the patient may have doubts and fears, and she should be prepared to talk about them. The problems of the stomatist can be overcome in a number of ways including different positions, but the presence of a stoma bag, and the associations of smell and disfigurement need to be taken into account in the preparation of the old patient, as well as the young one, before surgery, and in the counselling made available after. Both partners should be involved if possible, as the self-esteem of the stomatist depends often on the reaction of the partner, and the partner may assume that the stomatist is no longer well enough to enjoy sex.

It is worth remembering that there are ways of expressing sexual feelings and achieving satisfaction other than sexual intercourse with penetration of a woman by her male partner. Old people who live alone, like young people, masturbate and this may be part of the range of sexual behaviour of a couple, as may contact with other parts of the body such as the mouth. These alternatives may become more attractive as the older body gets less supple and pain or other infirmity get in the way. Kissing and holding, eating and being alone together, helping each other with physical and mental tasks and resting together are all part of the range of activities that allow expression of sexuality between people of any age. As frequency of intercourse lessens, the other things may become more important. This presents a challenge for those who provide institutional care for the old. Why do more geriatric units not have rooms for couples? We admit parents with children but what about the life companion who is left alone at home at a time of crisis?

WHAT THE NURSE CAN DO

If nurses are aware of the fact that sex can continue to give pleasure to old people until well into their eighties then the first problem is over. As with her younger patients the nurse can be alert to signs of treatable conditions. She can treat the old patient like an adult with a right to privacy and dignity. She can respond like an adult when, because of the institutional setting, she witnesses the private sexual acts of old people, such as masturbation, and she can gently limit the extent to which the confused and disinhibited patient behaves inappropriately, without humiliation or mockery. The nurse can share in the joy of the old couple who find love for each other at a time when they had lost most other good things in life. She can help the old patient stay smart and attractive, with well-groomed hair, decent clothes and hearing aids that work, so that messages of caring do not get missed. Alternative opportuntities for affection and love can be encouraged. The nurse should touch and hold her patients in the course of her dealings with them, and be aware of the effect that her own sexuality has on them.

Case history

Jock MacLennon had been admitted because of the worsening of his chronic chest problem, but it became clear within a few hours of admission that he had other equally pressing issues on his mind. He asked to have the screen kept around his bed so that others would not see him.

Admitted from home, he had been discharged recently from a specialist cancer unit. The treatment there had involved the removal of the greater part of his nose. A suppurating and unsightly cavity was exposed, and Jock was still waiting for suitable prosthesis to be ready. He had not been out of his house for more than a week, he felt ugly and repugnant to others, said he did not feel 'like a man' any more and was withdrawn, wishing to spend most of his time in bed.

Within a day, this situation had reversed. He was laughing and joking with other patients and was, according to his family, 'back to his old self'. His nurse had achieved this through a plan of care which included:

- Ensuring Jock's privacy, with the offer of the use of a single-bed cubicle.
- Spending time with him, showing that he was accepted through an occasional cuddle and holding his hand, and giving no indication that his appearance was offensive.
- Applying a light dressing over his nasal area - which consisted of two small pieces of gauze, over which a further strip was lightly fastened. This gave the impression that Jock had a normal nose with a dressing over it. (It became a source of ribald humour with other patients as a result. 'Did the nurse biff you because you got too friendly, Jock?')
- Teaching him the simple techniques for applying the dressing himself until his prosthesis could be fitted.

We must remember that the old people in our care had to deal with practical and moral decisions about sex long before we were born, and we must also remember that they may have serious worries about it even now. Sex is good for you. It can help you relax and make you feel warm, well and comfortable, and with the right knowledge, and a bit of luck with health, it will do so until the day you die.

REFERENCES

Comfort, A. (1974) Sexuality in old age, *Journal of American Geriatrics Society*, Vol. 22, no. 10, pp. 440–2.

Legrand, (1911) *La longevité a travers les ages*, Paris (referred to in Stearns [1977] op. cit.).

Masters, W. H. and Johnson, V. E. (1966) *Human Sexual Response*, Little Brown, Boston.

Reveille, P. M. (1853) *Traité de la vieillesse hygiénique, medicale et philosophique*, Paris (referred to in Stearns [1977] op. cit.).

Sontag, Susan (1978) The double standard of ageing, in V. Carver and P. Liddiard (eds) (1978) *An Ageing Population*, Hodder & Stoughton/Open University, Sevenoaks, Kent.

Stearns, P. N. (1977) *Old Age in European Society*, Croom Helm, Beckenham, p. 37.

16. Worshipping

Lesley Surman

INTRODUCTION

In today's society religion appears to play a less dominant and important part in life than formerly but it still has many implications for the carer. Cox (1983) suggests that

> It has been argued that the rise in science may undermine religious faith. This is because the great success of science and technology may encourage man to feel that he can achieve mastery over the physical world whereas in previous eras he could only try to influence it by magical and religious rituals. Also a scientific way of thinking may encourage a 'rationalist' world view which has no room for the transcendental and the metaphysical.

The scientific achievements, as well as being easier to rationalize, are easier to comprehend because they provide answers to questions that can be seen, measured and evaluated. The transcendental and metaphysical associated with theological explanations demand a complexity of thought and a different approach to thinking and comprehension. Nurses are trained today to rationalize their thoughts and actions – everything must be explainable. Suddenly, in at least this area of concern, the carer is asked to conceptualize in a completely different manner, one that is little discussed or taught in schools of nursing. Hardly surprising then that carers find this conflict of approach very difficult. Mostly carers are aware of their shortcomings in catering for religious needs and honouring various beliefs and ideals of individuals, and most are striving to attain the broadness of mind that will allow them to be effective. Unfortunately there is no blueprint for achieving this. It is hoped that this chapter will shed some light on to a difficult area of care, and sow the seeds of other ways of thinking. We need to learn to accept that whatever the patient holds sacred is not necessarily wrong or right. If they are happy with their beliefs and ideals we are in no position to dispute them, but we are in a position to promote the well-being of the individual by allowing them the facilities to practise them in complete freedom.

Many sociologists have devoted much time to studying the significance of religion. Marx, Weber and Durkheim, viewed as the founding fathers of sociology have provided us with some foundations. However, Cox (1983) suggests that

> one point needs to be made at the onset. Sociology can describe religious behaviour and institutions, but it can never prove or disprove the ultimate truth or falsity of religious beliefs or the authenticity of religious experience. We as mere mortals travelling the road of life with our own beliefs, values and experiences are in no position to decry the same of others, even if it is done through ignorance or lack of experience or faith.

Differences have been identified between that which an individual believes and that which he practises; these are not always consistent with one another and are subject to change with circumstances and experience.

Religiousness may increase when a person is in distress. They may find much support and help in religion for overcoming the fear and torment caused by their illness and suffering. The support may come not just from the deepening or awakening of their own faith but from the strength and positive reinforcement generated by the social interaction intrinsic within these religious groups.

SUSTAINING THE PATIENT'S FAITH

If the nurse shares the same faith as the patient communication may be much easier, but even if she does not she can still try to discuss with the patient's situation in the light of their faith. It is our duty to respect all aspects of the patient's well-being and it should be viewed as an honour to be in this position to help them. Some see death and suffering as manifestations of 'God's Will' (Neuberger, 1987). What nurses cannot afford to do is to try and impose alternatives on the patient, which, while being more comfortable for the nurse, may have a detrimental effect.

Patients may or may not choose to share their beliefs with the nurse. If not the nurse must ensure they have access to the person they want to share with. If beliefs are shared with the nurse the experience can be beneficial to both parties.

Hospital chaplains have a difficult task in trying to integrate their work with that of the healers and carers. It takes time to build up a relationship and in areas where the turnover of patients is fast the difficulty is exacerbated. In caring for the elderly they are usually in a better position (except on the acute wards) to develop a relationship with a patient as they would with member of their own parish, the 'turnover' being slower in many instances and therefore availing the clergy more time.

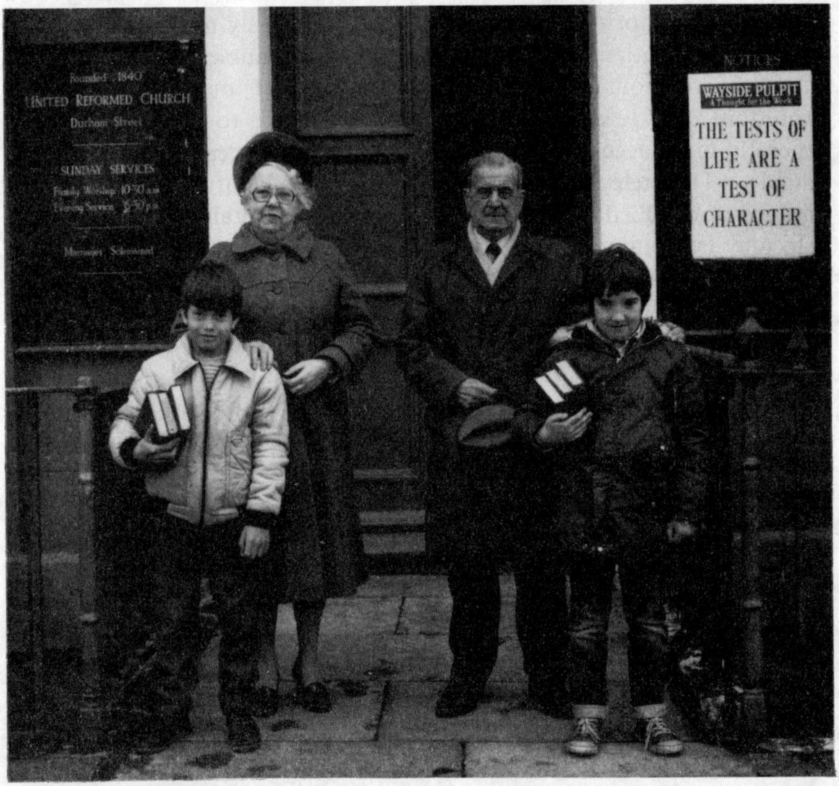

Religion is part of a 'social dimension' of life and it is therefore very important that patients be allowed and assisted, where it is physically, mentally and socially achievable, to continue with a liaison with their own church. For the elderly during the acute stages and exacerbations of illness this is obviously unrealistic, and in these instances the facility for worship should be brought to patients, either by their own or hospital clergy. However, as part of resocialization in preparation for discharge, or when patients are long stay in hospital or residential care, it is often feasable for them to attend a local church. As yet this is not widely practised and it does take some organization. It is, however, an opportunity for families to get involved. In many areas societies such as Age Concern have facilities to provide transport and personnel to help. Members of congregations also are known to offer their services in this respect.

Fortunately, there is no obvious religious discrimination that affects the elderly, although we do hear of situations that affect other age groups and minorities. It is necessary however for the nurse caring for a patient of a minority religious group to consciously make the effort to facilitate the patient's needs. The majority of nurses know sufficient about the religions they come into contact with most, the Catholic, Protestant and Jewish faiths, and the assistance to facilitate these is generally more accessible. Other faiths may require calling in help from outside. The telephone directory may be helpful in identifying organizations allied to specific faiths, and in hospitals information and help may be obtained from the administration or general offices.

Religious ceremonies frequently mark many of the memorable milestones in life, such as marriage, christenings, burials, confirmations, bar mitzvah. The elderly can find strength and peace in these memories and will often enjoy the contentment of relating the events to an interested nurse. Encouraging such discussion can assist the nurse to piece together a picture of her patient that will help her to empathize with the patient's perspectives on life, and appreciate the values and beliefs held by the patient.

Communal religious services help to provide social as well as spiritual support. Tucket (1976) discusses a 'lay-referral' system described by Friedson (1961) and he suggests that 'the perceived value of action to deal with symptoms is also something individuals learn from membership of a social group', the idea being that by being able to articulate anxieties with others, the anxiety is reduced. Others can share, if not the total experience, the thoughts and emotions and can advise on action to take.

FACILITATING RELIGIOUS PRACTICE

It is broadly advised that provision should be made in all homes and hospitals and other institutions for a quiet room that may be used for interviews and services or where grieving relatives or the patient themselves may have time alone.

Unfortunately most of the original buildings still in existence do not provide for this specific purpose, but it is heart-warming to observe that the majority of new buildings do include such facilities. Otherwise providing privacy taxes the nurse's ingenuity – a quiet part of the day room or an empty office perhaps.

Religious needs are often difficult for the nurse to appreciate, especially when her own are not in accordance with those of the patient. The admission assessment does give a good opportunity for exploratory discussion of this area. Generally there is an 'admission sheet' that is required to be completed as soon as possible. There is no real reason why the patients should not complete this themselves, abilities allowing, and make the initial assessment that much easier for the nurse.

There is a risk that whilst in hospital the patient may find his/her normal amount of time, or routine of religious practice, being limited. By good assessment and patient participation many potential problems can easily be avoided. Patient care can be modified according to specific needs. For example, if a patient requires a particular diet, this can be done through the hospital, but will probably be more appetizing and varied if provided by the family. Involving the family in satisfying the patient's needs, and hence enhancing well-being of their loved ones is very therapeutic. It gives the relatives a purpose and a function at a time when they can feel most helpless and frustrated.

Some specific religious needs may require forward activities to be planned around the patient's needs. If thought about and planned, they need present little or no problem to the overall running of a ward. Granted, there are some rituals which are more difficult to respect, willing as the staff may be.

Case history

A memo arrived on the ward from the administration advising all nursing staff that on the death of a person of the Muslim faith they should be laid out with the feet facing the south-east. Unsure of exactly where the south-east was in relation to the ward, the nursing staff requisitioned a compass. The following afternoon there was a telephone call from general office to say that it was not possible to grant the order, and could someone go out and buy one.

This possibly seems a somewhat extreme situation, but it actually did happen!

THE CLERGY

The ward minister means one who brings aid, who gives a service. Ministers of different faiths hold different titles and it is courteous for them to be addressed appropriately, at least by the staff. They are a member of the caring team and as such can be helped much by the nurses to be involved. Patients are not always so subtle.

Case history

Mary, an 80-year-old lady, selectively deaf, and maintaining all her mental faculties, was one day offered communion. The priest was visiting whilst the hospital clergy was on holiday. He was offered the facilities of a side ward where he could conduct a service for those who wished, but he declined saying that he was happy to give communion to those who wanted it on a one-to-one basis wherever they were.

Mary, one of the main characters of the ward, was sitting in the centre of the day-room, her favourite spot. She did not actually say that she wanted the communion but the priest proceeded to administer it anyway. He had just put the bread into Mary's mouth when, in her inimitable fashion, she looked past him to another patient and said, 'Is he a vicar or something?'

In this instance it was Mary's sheer devilry that prompted such a statement, but the nurse can help avoid embarrassment for the patient and minister by introducing them correctly, and ensuring the minister has any relevant information about the patient.

Dr Alex Comfort (1976) suggests that nobody actually needs to be told that they are dying because they instinctively know, and they are frequently trying to find ways and opportunities to tell you.

At this time the nurse's own fears and aversions or unwillingness to face the truth is often the greatest barrier for the patient. Frequently the religious needs are left to the priest, rabbi or minister, but in fact nurses are in a position to give religious as well as emotional support. By getting to know the patients and their families the nurse's understanding of their ways of coping, attitudes, life-styles and their religious and philosophic convictions will increase and planning their care will be more meaningful and effective.

To die with dignity is little to ask for as the final stages of life approach, and for many patients the meeting of their religious needs when conscious or not is a vital concern. Often patients will have their own minister, priest or rabbi, if they do not or they are unavailable to attend, most institutions have their own, or a liaison with clergy to meet the needs of those whose faith is Catholic, Jewish or Protestant. It is possible to obtain the services of clergy from other faiths if required.

The nurse may suggest that if patients so wish she could contact their own clergy or suggest one employed by the institutions. If the patients deny either, it does not automatically mean they do not wish any religious support. It may be inappropriate at that particular time or they may gain comfort from a member of the family or a nurse reading them passages from the Bible or prayer book.

If the patient does wish the clergy to visit, the nurse can facilitate and enhance the success of the meeting by ensuring there is time and uninterrupted privacy. Most dying patients, even if not actively religious in previous years, can gain tremendous consolation from active interaction during this time.

However, it may be suggested by family or friends that such a visit will be too upsetting for the patient. 'They will know something is wrong if the priest goes to him.' The fears of the relatives can be eased by the nurse explaining that the clergy are members of the team, and that it is not unusual to see them around. Patients rarely get suspicious or upset when visited by a minister. The patients do of course retain their rights to refuse the minister if they wish.

The visiting priest may require some help in administering his services. The sacrament and prayers offer hope and life, and since hope should never be taken away at any time it would seem reasonable to assist the minister in providing the support and comfort from which the patient can benefit.

Doctors and nurses are not generally trained to manage the religious and theological needs of the patients, but they can however participate in effective management and facilitate their satisfaction. By means of good liaison between the doctors and nurses and the clergy, the clergy will be better able to determine the state of mind, perception and awareness of patients towards their illness and adopt the appropriate approach. It should not be forgotten that the clergy are members of the caring team and can be of tremendous help to all when they are informed and involved.

Case history

Patrick was a 62-year-old Irish gypsy who had been a regular visitor to the hospital with pulmonary disease over the past year. The staff and priest had got to know the family well. The priest was especially helpful when Patrick was seriously ill and the family's concern exacerbated into tremendous emotional outbursts. The crying and hysteria could be heard throughout the unit. The nurse had little success in comforting the family and the priest was always willing to help and always had much more success.

Patrick's final admission caused more trauma than could ever have been imagined. He was settled into a large side ward, and as expected the family wanted to stay with him.

The family informed the nurses that his relatives in Ireland had been notified and were coming to England. What they had not told us was that there were at least forty of them. They descended *en masse* with the relatives and camp-mates from England just after seven o'clock one evening.

Patrick died. The relatives flooded around him, out into the corridor, down the stairs and out into the quad in front of the hospital. Chaos abounded.

The nurses had no idea what to do with this mass of relatives and the emotional upsurge of grief.

The priest arrived within minutes of being called. He took control of the whole situation with an authority any manager would have been proud of. Where he took the relatives we were not sure but at last the nurses could comfort and care for the other patients who were quite affected by the whole traumatic episode, as indeed were the nurses. But for the help and support of the priest, decorum could have been a long time in returning to that unit.

THE DIFFERENT RELIGIONS

Christian Denominations

The various Christian denominations have in common a faith in Jesus Christ and that there is a life after death. There are however some variations in the way in which they care for their ill and dying (McGilloway and Myco, 1985).

Church of England

This church follows an order from the book of common prayer where the priest aims to produce in the patient a successful path towards achieving individual peace of mind and soul. The basic pastoral aims are to pass through these stages:

(1) Penitence, where the person may express their sorrow and repeat for sins or offences made.
(2) Charity, to realize and restore a good will towards others, to intensify their love of humanity and to set affairs in order, such as ensuring all debts are paid and their will is made out.
(3) To increase, or reawaken and then increase the patient's faith and give support.

Roman Catholicism

This faith has a number of rites and sacraments to enhance the spiritual comforts of the dying patient and the family.

(1) Confession, or the sacrament of penance and reconciliation. Any patient wishing to make a confession should be provided with the privacy to do so. The priest gives 'absolution' on behalf of the church and assures complete forgiveness by a loving saviour. It is usually assumed that the patient needs to be able to speak to make a confession and attain absolution. This is not necessarily true. If the priest knows the patient has been informed of developments by the nursing staff he will probably be able to assess the temperament of the patient.
(2) When the illness progresses to a stage where it gives rise to concern the 'sacrament of the sick' is offered. Nurses frequently do not understand the difference between 'sacrament of the sick' and 'last rites'. which is probably because there is none nowadays. This sacrament was known in former years as the 'last rites' and recently it has been changed to 'sacrament for the sick'. The main purpose of this is to emphasize to the patient that it is a form of strength and consolation. The term 'last rites' seemed so final and hopeless and did not indicate the affirmative intention offered. The prayers of the sacrament are frequently a shared experience. Others may be present as it is not necessarily a private thing between priest and the patient.
(3) Holy Communion may be given. During this sacrament also special passages may be read from the scriptures. If it is obviously the last time the patient will receive Holy Communion then special prayers may be said to assist on this final journey. But frequently when death is near the priest is called upon and requested to visit. This may not be possible and if the sacrament for the sick has been administered it is not vital for the priest to be present to administer

the prayers for the dying person. Anyone present may read these, and again it may be shared with family and friends.

Free Church

The title *Free Church* encompasses all those whose belief follows that of the Christian faith. There are no special procedures or rites involved but readings from scriptures and visits from ministers and members of the congregation can give great spiritual comfort.

It is worth emphasizing that the free Churches have a close-knit congregation and highly regard scripture reading and communal prayer. They are very supportive to members of their congregation and frequently demonstrate a very caring attitude.

Non-Christian Denominations

Where you practise nursing will determine how much contact you have with non-Christian religions. In some areas there will be almost none, and in others a great deal, when it is accepted as the norm rather than the unusual. It can present as quite cultural shock for nurses initially but adapting to the needs of patients soon becomes a way life for the nurses.

Different religions adopt different rituals in association with dying and death. These frequently have implications other than spiritual and can reflect on the manner of physical care, presentation and diet.

Judaism

This is the most commonly encountered non-Christian religion, of which there are two groups, the Liberal Jews and the Orthodox Jews. It is important for the nurse to find out to which group the patient belongs as there are strict rules in both. The Liberal Jews have fewer special requirements, and those they have usually are concerned with diet. Many will eat only kosher food (which means that all pig meat and extracts are forbidden and all animals must be slaughtered in a specific way). Some may be vegetarian. They follow no special last rites but prayers for the dying are usually said, if not by a rabbi, then by family or friends.

Strict rules affecting the manner of daily living are followed by the Orthodox Jews. Again a strict diet is followed. Kosher food only is permitted and no food or extracts from the pig should be given. This includes extracts used to make drugs (such as porcine insulin).

The Orthodox Jew will wish for the presence of a rabbi. The patient will want (if able) to announce his sins and say special prayers.

In the absence of family or rabbi the nurses, after the death of a Jewish patient, are permitted only to close the eyes, straighten the limbs and tie up the jaw. Not all policies now include tying the jaw, but many problems have been overcome since nurses have been permitted to straighten the limbs after death! If the family or rabbi is present it is courteous to ask if they would perform these tasks. Once the body is in the mortuary a member of the family or synagogue will supervise proceedings and a specially trained official from the local burial society will wash the body. If the patient has no family or affiliation to any specific synagogue that can be traced, the Jewish Society do have a central headquarters in London. If the deceased has fully paid his dues they will appoint a person to oversee arrangements. If the patient lapsed completely and was not fully paid up in his dues the arrangements fall to the state.

There are three other religions that nurses are likely to come into contact with and these are the Buddhists, Hindus and Muslims.

Buddhism

Buddists are brought up to believe in Buddha and they believe in reincarnation, brotherhood and non-violence. Frequently they have a statue of Buddha with them, and it is important for them to practise meditation during the day. There are no specific requirements to care except the diet, as they may be vegetarian. Although there are no specific or special rituals and rites for the dying they may appreciate a visit by a Buddhist monk.

Islam

Muslims follow the Islamic religion. There are rituals the Muslims will wish to adhere to. Their faith demands that they pray to their God, Allah, at least five times a day. Prior to their praying, certain ablutions must necessarily be carried out. The faith commands that no Muslim women should be seen undressed by any man other than their husband and women may, therefore, demonstrate an unwillingness to undress or be examined by a male doctor. The nurse should allow for the discomfort and reluctances, and facilitate a female doctor to attend to the patient.

The Islamic religion does not have clergy as such but they have religious teachers who may be called upon to visit the patient. Prayers are usually read in Arabic and it is required that the patient face Mecca while doing so. (The feet will be pointing to the south-east!)

Muslims also have dietary restraints in that they do not eat any meat which comes from the pig, and they honour the festival of Ramadan during which they fast. Ill Muslims are exempt from fasting if it is considered seriously dangerous to their health.

There are rituals to be observed after death. Members of the family wash the body and then wrap it in special pieces of cloth. Because coffins are not used they usually wish for the burial to take place as soon after death as possible.

Hinduism

Hindus practise the worship of many gods and goddesses (known as polytheism). They have no single identifiable theological following. There are many philosophical schools of thought.

The cow is considered a sacred animal and practising Hindus will not eat meat from this animal, thereby giving rise to dietary considerations for the nurse. The Hindu women, like the Muslim women, may refuse to be examined by a male doctor or looked after in some aspects of daily living by a male nurse.

A Hindu priest is known as the Pundit and may be welcomed by the patient to read passages from their holy books. After the death the relatives will wash the body and then dress it in new clothes.

It can be seen from these brief descriptions that the family ties and involvement is very close, and is continuous even when transported out of their country of origin. In most instances the closeness and willingness to be involved can be of great help and support to both patient and nurse. Their natural grief-sharing can present difficulties to other patients in the ward. By providing an area away from others where the relatives may be together to share their grief and give support, the nurse can help everyone.

CONCLUSION

Catering to the religious needs of patients can demand careful thought, consideration and planning on the part of the nurse. She/he should find help and pleasure in the assistance the clergy can give, and derive great satisfaction in watching patients achieve the sense of calmness, understanding and tranquillity their faith can give them.

REFERENCES

Comfort, A. (1976) *A Good Age*, Crown Publications, New York.
Cox, C. (1983) *Sociology: An Introduction for Nurses, Midwives and Health visitors,* Butterworths, London.
Friedson, E. (1961) *Patients' View of Medical Practice*, Russell Saye Foundation, New York.
McGilloway, O. and Myco, F. (1985) *Nursing and Spiritual Care*, Harper & Row, London.
Neuberger, J. (1987) *Caring for Dying People of Different Faiths*, Austen Cornish, London.
Tucket, D. (1976) *An Introduction to Medical Sociology*, Tavistock, London.

17. Care of the Dying

Lesley Surman

INTRODUCTION

Nurses experience many difficult aspects of life at a very early age, not least of which is how to look after dying patients, their families and friends, and importantly the nurse herself. All too frequently the care of the staff is overlooked.

Much has been written and researched in recent years on this subject and at last it is being discussed widely in schools of nursing, being recognized as an important aspect of the curricula and given proper attention. However, it remains difficult for nurses to comprehend the process involved in dying. This chapter should help the nurse to recognize the processes taking place and enable her to plan care individually and successfully.

Winston Churchill (1881–1973) once said 'When I look back on all those worries, I remember the story of the old man who said on his deathbed that he had had a lot of trouble in his life, most of which had never happened.' The competent, conscientious, knowledgeable nurse can help prevent or alleviate many of those troubles!

Death is the inevitable end of life. For many years it has been a taboo subject. After a death many euphemisms are used to describe it and avoid the use of the word 'dead' or 'died'. Euphemisms such as 'passed over', 'gone to heaven', 'no longer with us' are frequently used.

SOCIETY'S MANAGEMENT OF DEATH

The sociologist Gorer (1965) suggests in his arguments that there are major differences between the way in which pre-industrial and industrial societies manage death. In pre-industrial societies people were encouraged to express their grief and share with others. During this time less than one-third of the population died in an institution of some kind, be it a hospital, asylum or workhouse. In our industrial society people generally die away from their own familiar environment, performing this last act of life neatly concealed within a place that is acceptable. Nowadays more than half of all deaths occur in hospitals (Charles-Edwards, 1983). This has lead to the whole process of death and grief being kept away from public view. After a death those left with their grief may acceptably show their emotions for a day or two, and indeed most employers will frequently give compasionate leave of between one and seven days, but after this the bereaved is requested by society to return to normal functioning and confine grief responses and reactions to the privacy of their own home.

Gorer argues that the means by which society manages death and grief today is not conducive to emotional stability and equilibrium. Suppressing grief and encouraging a hasty return to 'normal' only leads to greater suffering and emotional distress which may manifest itself at any time in the future. This may not be a matter of months but of years.

Case history

Joe and Barbara were the children of 84-year-old Ethel, who was dying. She knew and accepted this fact. In her last week her only hope was she could see her son Joe, who lived in Ireland. The family had had their traumas. Barbara was divorced for six years and the traumas of raising her three children alone had manifested in multiple psychological problems. Nevertheless she managed fairly well. She discussed with Sister a problem causing her grave concern. She knew her mother wanted to see Joe because she had been continually asking for him. Barbara was also aware that her mother knew she was dying.

Fourteen years previously Joe's wife had died leaving him with two very young children. Joe had never expressed his grief. He had picked up and carried on life as though his wife had never existed. Joe found solace and escape from his grief in alcohol. During the course of time Joe had distanced himself from all his friends and family and although he raised his children the best he could, he managed to isolate himself; people saw Joe, but no one knew Joe.

After discussion Barbara decided that she must ring Joe and ask him to come to England to see his mother.

Barbara was sick with worry as to how he would react. She knew he could be violent and very difficult. He arrived as soon as he could, on Boxing Day.

There was no violence and he was not difficult or unpleasant with anyone, but the staff and Barbara had to watch him fighting to maintain control over his emotions behind the guard he had erected so firmly over the years.

Ethel died shortly after Joe arrived. Eventually he could no longer maintain the decorum he fought to achieve and cried uncontrollably for days. He asked Barbara to help him and for the first time in fourteen years he put his arms around his sister, shared his grief and admitted he had a problem.

Joe sought help, and the last we heard, twelve months later, Joe was still receiving treatment but was coming to terms with his losses and his life.

The younger we are the less we think about 'real death'. The media expose us to death and violence quite frequently, but rarely do we think about our own deaths.

THE ELDERLY AND DEATH

The elderly, especially when inflicted with disease and disability, frequently speak of their own death as though it were a welcoming friend. They are frequently more concerned about the manner in which they end their lives than the end itself (Kübler-Ross, 1969). But they accept the end with a certain equanimity that the young may find difficult to comprehend. Many a nurse has been faced with a relatively fit and healthy elderly person saying to them, 'I'm ready to die now, whenever He wants to take me,' or, 'I want to die, I've lived my life now.' Doctors and nurses both find difficulty in appreciating what is being said, especially as the young doctor or nurse has different values on life, so much to do and achieve still that they would fight tooth and nail for longevity, not imagining that the quality of life can decline and become far less than previously experienced.

The relative youth of nurses may influence their attitude towards death. The elderly often do not get given the credit they should for their resignation to the inevitability of death, but, after all, they have far more experience to draw on. They have seen their families, friends and contemporaries die and have come to accept that they too will die. They do, however, frequently want to talk about it, about how they feel and why they are no longer striving to live longer. Unfortunately this is the sort of conversation that is brushed over and dismissed by the carer (Bond, 1980) with comments such as, 'Don't be silly, you're not going to die,' and, 'Don't worry, you'll be all right.' Well, maybe not yet, but the probability is that they *are* much nearer to death than their carers. They should be allowed to talk about it while they are feeling well. It is recommended that wills should be written when people are well and fit. Why then should they not talk about their death while in a fit state? Mostly it is dismissed because of the lack of understanding and ability to conduct such a conversation by the carer. Always the carer feels that she/he must be seen to 'achieve', and while listening often means that the nurse is helping, this sort of help is much more difficult to measure and evaluate than practical skills. The importance of listening and listening actively will be mentioned again in this chapter for it is one of the most vital roles of the doctor, nurse or carer that is not always easy to learn. Listening, whilst not inflicting your values on to another individual is all that is required in most instances (see Chapter 5).

RELATIONSHIPS WITH THE DYING

Death is the last life event and is a mystery, but it causes fear and apprehension not only for the dying but also for those left behind. Many have an idealistic image of the way in which they would like to die. But after all it is not a life experience that one can practise to perfect. Being a once-only experience, much responsibility falls on the carer to 'get it right'. There is a great deal that nurses can do above and beyond tending to the obvious physical needs of the patient, essential as these are. Many experienced nurses are training staff and learner nurses in this field of care, and there are beginning to be changes for the better in the management of these difficult and emotional situations (Barber, 1986).

Nurses encountering the death of a patient, especially in their early career, tend to feel an overwhelming sense of helplessness, inadequacy and some degree of fear. The nurse determines these feelings as painful, and unless they are brought forward and discussed and it is emphasized that awareness of feelings and being able to discuss them is a strength and will be of benefit, long-lasting damage to the persona, nursing ability and skill of that individual may occur (Strauss and Glaser, 1968). Nurses have of course survived in the past, but this does not give justification for perpetuating old trends. The expectations of the public are changing and the demands and requirements made of the nurse are growing. There must be education of nurses to help them to explore their own feelings, to feel comfortable and confident to spend time with the dying and their relatives, without fearing recrimination for sympathizing and expressing feelings with a fellow human being.

First impressions are most important and serve as a foundation for the development of future relationship building. The first meeting engages both parties in a nurse–patient, patient–nurse assessment, summing up and 'sussing out' each other. The patient is desperately trying to look for someone who cares about him as an individual with the experiences and feelings that are unique to him. The nurse is in all probability looking to see if the patient will be an 'easy' one to nurse. Stockwell (1984) identifies characteristics of the unpopular patient quite clearly in her research. Nurses, being mere human beings, are prone to look for the comfortable, conforming soul. However, armed with the knowledge that Stockwell has provided, the nurse would do well to refrain from judgement prematurely, for she is otherwise in danger of expressing a negative attitude that will in turn cause anxiety in her patient. The nurse's and patient's feelings will reinforce one another in an unhappy spiral.

The patient needs to feel he can have confidence in the nurse, and that he can trust her. The nurse must be able to recognize when the patient is experiencing emotions like loneliness, fear or pain and take the appropriate action to alleviate them without the patient having verbally to express them (see Chapter 4).

Time spent early on in the development of the relationship is without question supremely advantageous and beneficial to both parties (Chapter 5) the relationship will then have an opportunity to develop in a positive caring atmosphere, without stress and with trust. During this time, and to achieve the positive tranquillity of a relationship, the single most important act of the nurse is to be an empathetic, sympathetic caring *listener*.

If the patient does not trust the nurse he will not allow her to attain the full, comprehensive picture that is needed to identify and meet his needs. It is important for the nurse to work *with* the patient, to let the patient lead, be in charge of the decision-making. The nurse should have the knowledge foundation needed to identify for the patient the choices he has; from this point the nurse can discuss options and help the patient to make his own choices, thereby retaining control over what happens to him, when, where and how. This approach will maintain the patient's independence and dignity. Should the patient then reach a stage in the illness where he is no longer able to communicate outwardly, he will have the faith and the trust in his carer that the carer knows sufficient about him not to act in a hurtful way. The patient should feel safe and confident, knowing that when the nurse says, 'I'm going to give you an injection to keep the pain away,' that is all that will be done.

Nurses must realize and accept that the morals and values held by them are not necessarily the same as those held by the patient. It is important to consider this in relation to the value one has of life.

DEFENCE MECHANISMS

Most nurses, when encountering new situations, such as coping with the dying, adopt defence mechanisms of some sort or another. Bailey (1985) suggests that 'defence mechanisms such as the employment of suppression, and detachment may make "space" for the health professional to mobilize more open forms of problem-solving when emotional expression as a means of coping with stress is "inappropriate" '. This he accepts as reasonable in the short term but continues to say that the long-term defensive coping can take its toll on 'mental, emotional and physical health'. He also suggests that long term defensive coping strategies store up the stress and can lead to 'increased risk of burn-out and becoming one of the casualties of caring'. Senior nurses have a responsibility to their junior staff to watch for signs of stress and produce remedies. It is difficult for nurses to develop their own self-awareness of increasing stress when they are continually trying to identify and do right to the needs of others.

As Schröck (1980) suggests 'there must be a minimal degree of trust in essential truthfulness of communications with one's fellow men'. It has already been suggested that the patient needs to trust the nurse, and it is certainly time that nurses care and show that they care about each other! Friendship, counselling, understanding, acceptance of another's feelings, are as important in the nurse–nurse relationship as they are to the nurse-patient relationship (Sundeen *et al.,* 1976).

Bok (1978) suggests that 'It is time for health professionals to look closely at the threat which incompetence poses, and at the conflicts between loyalty and responsibility.'

Case history

In a role-play situation in class trained staff were enacting an interview between a sister and a patient's wife to show how not to conduct an interview. They had not rehearsed at all but several of the 'in vogue' lines came into the conversation.

The wife was becoming quite enraged and frustrated at not being able to get any straight answers to her questions from the sister. She suddenly said, 'Is my husband going to die?' The sister said, 'Well, we are all going to die sometime. What makes you think your husband is going to die?' Fiery responses from the wife threw the sister into a state of fear, and she demonstrated many defence mechanisms and avoidance strategies to overcome her inability to deal with responses that she had prompted.

The relationship was not good to start with and the interview had many ingredients to make it difficult and traumatic, if not a disaster. The Sister did not really want this interview and she managed to get herself into very difficult water. In the extract described the Sister made the statement, 'Well, we are all going to die sometime.' True as this statement is it was inappropriately placed and needed some follow-up, and is a good example of the use of an inappropriate 'trite expression' (Hames and Joseph, 1980). Nurses are often being asked how long someone has to live. This is always a difficult question to answer, yet the truth, that it is very difficult to say and if a time was estimated it could well be wrong, will raise the nurse's credibility and esteem in the eyes of the relatives far more than if she/he tries to know everything, being profoundly sure and then is proved wrong.

The sister in the above example then followed her first statement by asking a question, the answers to which she was not prepared (in either sense of the word) to deal. The saying 'a little knowledge is a dangerous thing' would seem to hold true here. The sister should have had more knowledge, that is her professional responsibility. Instead she put the ball back in the court of the wife and removed responsibility from herself. Inappropriate use of trite remarks emphasized her incompetence and highlights the difference between non-therapeutic and therapeutic communication (see Chapter 10).

In the majority of instances, if the nurses were left to decide, patients would be told the truth at the appropriate time. There is much evidence to support the view that the majority of patients do wish to be told the truth. Schröck (1980) suggests that 'claims that truthfulness is impossible, that patients do not want bad news and that truthful information might harm them rests largely on the paternalistic assumption of professional superiority'. How often has the consultant been heard to say that the patient should not be told, that they could not 'take it', or even have scribed in the notes, 'Patient not to be told diagnosis.' This presents an ethical dilemma. Does the nurse follow her own professional judgement and act accordingly or follow the doctor's orders? There is no straightforward answer. Each nurse must assess her own level of knowledge, confidence and capability within each given situation and then act accordingly. To simply follow doctor's orders is not commission for omission as the UKCC Code of Conduct (1985) suggests.

As previously mentioned, much work exists describing the patient's and carers' perspective on death, dying and bereavement. With a good knowledge foundation and understanding nurses can reduce their own apprehension and stress levels, and confidently respond to the patient's needs and wishes.

UNDERSTANDING THE PROCESS OF DYING

Management of a death and the most appropriate action to take and when, can be determined by assimilation of assessment of the impending death, by the form or character that it takes and its duration.

Strauss and Glaser (1968) describe a course of dying that they call the 'dying trajectory', trajectory meaning the curve or the route that the process takes. They also describe states of awareness, that is the understanding of each interacting person's knowledge of the other's perception, understanding and comprehension of the situation.

Strauss and Glaser have included in their writings a description of what they consider 'critical junctions'. Awareness of these three areas, which will be described, can provide a good working foundation for the carer and help her/him in her/his management and understanding of the stages of dying, frequently displayed by the patients and widely described by Kübler-Ross (1969).

DYING TRAJECTORIES

The death of a patient has two notably essential components: duration and a shape or form that can in fact be graphed. Nurses know that a dying patient may be quite 'up' before the final 'down'. Strauss and Glaser (1968) recognize several variations: 'it plunges straight down; it moves slowly but steadily downwards; it vacillates slowly, moving slowly up and down, before diving downwards radically; it moves slowly down at first, then hits a long plateau, then plunges to death.'

To understand this is especially important in providing care for the family and friends. With every gleam of improvement their hopes rise, soon to be shattered by the fall. The hope can never be taken away, nor should anyone ever try to remove it. It is, however, physically and emotionally draining; the longer the rise and fall trajectory persists the more exhausting for everyone. The carers also enjoy the 'up' times. It is more comfortable, less awkward and unpleasant questions are not asked, the atmosphere lightens. Family and friends frequently ask how long someone will live. It is impossible to predict this accurately, but they will formulate a time-span in their own minds for the impending death. Changes in the patient's course mean the family and friends have to readjust or process again their psychological preparation. This can be quite traumatic.

The 'awareness context' is described by Strauss and Glaser (1968) in four levels of relationships.

(1) *Closed awareness.* All those around the patient – family, friends and carers – are aware that he is dying, but the patient does not recognize it himself. He may die in this state, especially if sudden unconsciousness overtakes him.
(2) *Suspected awarenes.* The patient begins to explore, to ask questions and find out what the prognosis is, feeling it is possible that he may be dying. These suspicions may be reinforced (a relative he has not seen for many years suddenly visits, the nurses whisper as they pass his bed).
(3) *Mutual pretence awareness.* No one admits anything, everyone around the patient knows he is dying; he suspects but does not know for sure or talk about it. A complex verbal and non-verbal situation is set up as each party to the play avoids mentioning the truth.
(4) *Open awareness.* All know the truth of the diagnosis and recognize and admit the inevitability of death. They hence speak and act in accordance with this knowledge.

These states of awareness vary greatly with individuals, frequently depending on the path of the trajectory. They cannot be forced through. Patients will reach or develop the 'open awareness context' when and if they are ready to accept that the condition is terminal. The way care is managed can enhance feeling of safety and security that encourages a willing acceptance in the patient. But if those around do not provide the atmosphere and comfort it is unrealistic to expect patients to expose themselves, to be open and vulnerable.

Kübler-Ross (1969) has described stages of dying through which patients may travel. They will not necessarily experience all of them or in the order described below, but certainly some of the stages will be recognizable. The length of time spent in each or any stage is also variable. All this may depend upon the patients' perceptions of life, death and their illness, on their life experiences and beliefs. These stages of dying may also be referred to as the process of bereavement. Patients will try to come to terms with their inevitable death before the event. For those left behind the process generally occurs after death. Some will start grieving immediately, others may take a long while, but the process of grieving is necessary.

(1) *Denial and isolation* –'It's not me, they must have the wrong one.' This is often accompanied by desperate feelings of isolation and disbelief. It is a period for a lot of thinking but not necessarily producing many results. Patients frequently 'turn to face the wall' during this stage and communication can be difficult.

(2) *Anger* – 'Why me?' There is frequently outward expression of aggression during this stage. It is usually verbal but it is difficult for staff, family and friends to bear, as the expression of rage, resentment and bitterness can be very painful. Everyone tries to do what they can, to be kind, understanding and sympathetic, only to be rebuffed by the patient. Relatives find it particularly hard and frequently dread visiting, Kübler-Ross suggests, 'They then either respond with grief and tears, guilt or shame, or avoid future visits, which only increases the patient's discomfort and anger.' The perceptive knowledgeable nurse will identify the relatives' distress and can help them cope and understand with careful explanation of the process taking place.

(3) *Bargaining* –'If I'm good...' This can range in extremes from, 'If I stop smoking today I'll be better in a few days' time,' to, 'If I take the drugs you give me, will I be able to see my grandson come from Australia?' Frequently they are bargaining for more time, to put right what they feel they have done wrong, or for more time to achieve what they should have done earlier. It is thought that there may be deep guilt associated with these psychological promises.

(4) *Depression* – 'Yes, it is me who is going to die.' No longer can this impending death be denied. It is during this stage that it is perhaps suggested that the patient is given some drug therapy to alleviate depression. Is this fair? He does after all have a good reason to be depressed. Kübler-Ross believes that:

the patient should not be encouraged to look at the sunny side of things, as this would mean he should not contemplate his impending death. It would be contraindicated to tell him not to be sad, since all of us are tremendously sad when we lose a beloved person. The patient is in the process of losing everything and everybody he loves. If he is allowed to express his sorrow he will find a final acceptance much easier, and he will be grateful to those who can sit with him, just being around and not necessarily speaking, during this stage of depression without constantly telling him not to be sad.

(5) *Acceptance* – 'I'm going to die and now I'm ready to die.' The emotional turbulence is over and a state of peace and tranquillity resides within the patient. Family, friends and staff relax, the feeling of frustration and helplessness gradually lessens.

Whilst the patient is going through some of these stages tremendous turbulence can arise in the most loving of relationships. Patients and relatives may not all pass through the same grieving stages at the same time. However, openness and honesty with support from nurses can, as Murray-Parkes (1972) suggests, find the period of terminal care one of a time for growth and shared preparation. It can be the fulfilment and completion of marriage or 'can mar the memory of good relationships and undermine the health of the survivors for years'.

The nurse needs to assess the patient's awareness how much is known and how much knowledge is wanted. Patients should never have information thrust upon them. Many would argue that if patients do not want to know the truth they do not internalize it even when told. But by assessing their state of awareness and stage of dying, the management and care of a terminally ill person can be far more appropriately planned. The support the nurses will be able to give to relatives and friends will also be more effective.

The elderly settle and accept the inevitability of death with calm and dignity in most instances. They have the same fears of the journey as any other person of a lesser age, but generally they feel they have lived their lives having what the ancients called '*satietas vitae*', the fullness of life. (Kastenbaum, 1979).

THE PATIENT'S RIGHTS

The expression 'the nurse as the patient's advocate' (Wright, 1986) is quite widely used today, but the understanding of it and the enaction of it is not so simple to comprehend or execute. Although patients in the age group known as elderly may now be less submissive, more sure of what they want and their rights. It is though, still often through their children or another person that they speak of what they really want.

Case history

Mary was 95 years old and had been admitted due to progressive weakening over the last month. Amongst her other problems she had an inguinal hernia. The only real treatment was an operation and Mary did not want this, and had told the houseman, the nurses and her family so. The consultant did his ward round, examined Mary and decided the hernia was larger and firmer and needed operating on to find out what it was. He said to Mary, 'I'm going to arrange for you to have an operation for the lump at the top of your leg, all right?' Mary said, 'Yes.'

On asking Mary afterwards what made her change her mind she said that nothing had but he was the consultant and she must do what he said or she would be in trouble.

The difficulty in a situation like this is convincing Mary that she does not have to do anything she does not want, and certainly not without explanation, and then trying to convince the consultant that the patient was fearful of what would happen to her if she argued against him, and has, therefore, agreed to something she does not want. This is made doubly complicated when the doctor (in this case a consultant, but it could be anyone) does not recognize the power they have and perceive themselves as friendly and approachable (Wright, 1985).

It is not, however, all doom and gloom. Many doctors do appreciate the difficulties and do work with the nurses.

Case history

Betty was 73 years old. Her main medical problem was that of respiratory disease, but on admision she was found to have a lump in her breast. Betty was referred to the surgeons for a second opinion, not necessarily with a view to operation, but to identify what forms of treatment were available.

The surgeon came to see her, asked a few questions, examined Betty and then said, 'I'll operate and remove your breast next week. I'll arrange for you to be transferred to my ward.'

Betty was devastated by the cold calculated manner in which she was told this news. Sister went back to Betty after the consultant had left. Betty was frightened and did not want the operation. Betty's husband was contacted and asked to come in.

Betty and her husband were given time to discuss the situation after discussion with sister and the houseman. The doctor had explained clearly and carefully what the problem was and the choices of treatment. He stressed that the choice was hers, and that she did not have to undergo any treatment that she did not want. There was no rush to make up her mind and although Betty was sure she did not want an operation, the sister and doctor suggested that she thought it over for a while. The doctor would be back in the afternoon but she could take longer if she wished.

The sister and doctor returned as promised. Betty had some more questions, which were answered honestly. Betty chose the treatment she felt most comfortable with, that of simple drug therapy to slow down the progress of growth.

Everyone concerned had the feeling of achievement and 'feeling good' at the end of the day. The sister and doctor had worked well together to enable the patient to make her own choice. They had been honest but very supportive and the patient had visibly calmed and grown in strength as she realized her carers were working with her.

Again, this case really demonstrates the attitude and manner of the carers. In this instance it was demonstrated that neither the doctor nor the nurse had a need or wish to be all-powerful, and knew that by involving the patient, whatever the decision that was made, the patient would benefit far more than if any decision was made over her head and possibly against her will. Garrett (1983) supports the view that there are no second chances to amend care in the clinical situation. When there is support, and both sides are involved, the key to a meaningful and successful partnership between carer and patient has been found.

The psychological emotional and behavioural changes that a patient may demonstrate have already been discussed. Qvarmstron (1978) further identified some fears dying people frequently experience. These include the following:

- Fear of pain and suffering that may come from the illness and the situation.
- Fear of loneliness and of dying alone.
- Fear for the relatives and how they will cope with the situation.
- Fear of what will happen after death.

With the knowledge that they are not going to 'get better' the dying person suffers a massive complex of fears and anxieties. They no longer fit into the 'programme for recovery' and both patient and relatives fear that they will be neglected. These fears can manifest themselves in changes in behaviour. The patient becomes demanding, the relatives are always complaining and the care never satisfies them. These are usually subconscious reactions to their desperate need for attention, to be given time to talk, ask questions, and feel part of the social scene.

Charles-Edwards (1983) suggests three guiding principles that nurses should follow:

(1) To listen well. By doing this the nurse will realize that the patients are telling us what they know, what they want to know and at the pace at which they can work. They will also tell of what they want and fear.
(2) Never lie to patients. Nurses are frequently trying to assess patients' abilities to cope, but patients have a right to the truth, and if the nurse has listened well she will know the right time and how much information to give at any particular time.
(3) Never remove all hope. While there is breath there is hope and to remove this is brutal and as cruel as withholding analgesia.

THE PLACE OF DYING

The dying person's Bill of Rights states, 'I have the right to be cared for by those who can maintain a sense of hopefulness, however changing this might be ' (AJN, 1975). Hope is a small word with great depth and meaning. As George Bernard Shaw once said,'The worst sin towards our fellow creatures is not to hate them, but to be indifferent to them; that's the essence of inhumanity.' The majority of people would rather die at home amongst their own. This is not always feasible for many reasons. More and more people are dying in institutions. The increasing establishment of hospices has served not only to provide the dying with an alternative surrounding but to share knowledge and explore with those nurses working in other areas. There are many practices and philosophies used in hospices that can and have been taken into the hospital setting.

Patients dying at home need much support and the health care team need to consider the carer as much as the patient. There are special considerations such as ensuring that there is adequate availability of drugs and equipment, and that access to a hospital bed is possible should one be required. There should be sufficient appropriately trained staff to provide the 24-hour support needed, with the time to enable patients and their families to discuss their fears and anxieties and problems. The communication links are much broader and need to be maintained at a superior level to maintain effective continuation of care.

Hospices are places that have been established specifically to care for the terminally ill person. They have been in existence for many centuries but it is only recently that they have increased in number in the UK. The word hospice means 'traveller's house of rest', which was their original function. They gradually became to be used for the sick. Although originally designed as separate institutions many of their philosophies are now being integrated into the work in hospital. Mainly care in them is planned and executed for the individual and the whole caring team is involved to tend to the needs of the individual, be they physical, social, psychological or spiritual.

Hospices provide a much more open environment, with more awareness of what is going on, and the family is as involved as possible. The atmosphere of a hospice is something to treasure, and it would be too difficult to explain all one can experience in this type of establishment. Anyone involved in caring for the dying would benefit greatly from the experience of visiting a hospice. Most are very welcoming to visitors, so arrange a visit. It will be time well spent.

There are difficulties nursing the dying in hospital, but how many of these are of a practical nature and how many are a matter of attitudes? This is a question that should be given much consideration.

There have been some very sobering studies undertaken by Sudnew (1967) who has suggested that the 'social' and 'biological' death of a person does not necessarily occur at the same time. Staff nursing patients who have been considered 'as good as dead' have in fact treated them as such.

Medical personnel still have a tendency to regard death as 'failure'. Bond (1980) describes Western culture as 'death-denying', and heroic activities and traumatic treatments being given to patients in an attempt to keep them alive all costs can still be seen. The emphasis on the 'acute' patient who is getting well may lead to the dying patient, who represents failure and yet who needs help that the nurses feel unable to give, being avoided.

Hospital staff always seem to be concerned with where the patient dies, where the bed is in the ward and that the patient should die neatly and tidily in his bed. Their position in the ward matters in so far as it actually affects the patient and the family, and other patients. Some may like to be in a side ward and so long as the patient is not neglected in there, this would seem quite reasonable. In some areas the dying elderly are put at the end of the ward, tucked away neat and tidy, while in others they make a steady, progressive journey around the ward to finish in a bed nearest sister's office or the nurses' station. The need for this is questionable, and even more questionable is the practice of drawing curtains around the bed of a patient who is dying. It may be pertinent in some instances but the positioning and curtaining should be assessed in view of the patient's requirements and not because it makes the onlookers feel happier.

CONCLUSION

Death is a unique event in our lives. Individuals trust and honour nurses by allowing them to participate in helping them to a dignified end to their lives. Nurses then have a responsibility not to violate this trust. There are no second chances to 'get it right' and therefore, any nurse involved in caring for the dying is under an obligation to ensure that she has the knowledge foundation and the skills with which to assist the patient and their family and friends. As nurses we can ease or erase many of their fears and anxieties. We may never be able to completely fulfil this, but if we ensure that we are available and willing to help by sharing the remaining worries, the support we give may be sufficient to enable patients to overcome them themselves.

REFERENCES

American Journal of Nursing (1975) The Dying Person's Bill of Rights, *AJN,* Vol. 75, no. 1.

Bailey, R. (1985) Stress and coping with demands of caring seminar at School of Nursing and School of Medicine, University of California, San Francisco.

Barber, I. (1986) Bereavement, *Nursing Practice,* Vol. 1, no. 2, pp.159 - 66.

Bok, S. (1978) *Dying: Moral Choice in Public and Private Life,* Harvester Press, Hassocks, Surrey.

Bond, S. (1980) A taboo of our times, *Nursing Mirror,* 13 March.

Charles-Edwards, A. (1983) *The Nursing Care of the Dying Patient,* Beaconsfield Publishers, Beaconsfield.

Garrett, G. (ed.) (1983) *Health Needs of the Elderly,* Macmillan Press, London.

Gorer, G. (1965) *Death, Grief and Mourning in Contemporary Britain,* Cresset Press, London.

Hames. E. C. and Joseph, D. H. (1980) *Basic Concepts of Helping: A Holistic Approach,* Appleton-Century-Crofts, New York.
Kastenbaum, R. (1979) *Growing Old: The Years of Fulfilment,* Harper & Row, London.
Kübler-Ross, E. (1969) *On Death and Dying,* Macmillan, New York.
Murray-Parkes, C. (1972) *Bereavement Studies of Grief in Adult Life,* Tavistock, London.
Qvarmstron, N, (1978) Patients' reactions to impending death. Unpublished PhD thesis, University of Stockholm.
Schröck, R. A. (1980) A question of honesty, *Journal of Advanced Nursing,* Vol. 5, pp.135–48.
Stockwell, F. (1984) *The Unpopular Patient,* RCN, London
Strauss, A. and Glaser, B. (1968) Patterns of dying, in Cox, C. and Mead, A. (eds) (1968) *A Sociology of Medical Practice,* Macmillan Press, London.
Sudnew, D. (1967) *Passing On: The Social Organisation of Dying,* Prentice-Hall, Englewood Cliffs, New Jersey.
Sundeen, S., Stuart, E. D., Ranklin, E. D., and Cohen, S. P. (1976) *Nurse-Client Interaction,* Mosby, St Louis.
Surman, L. (1986) Death with dignity, *Nursing Practice,* Vol. 1, no. 2, pp. 152–8.
United Kingdom Central Council for Nursing, Midwifery and Health Visiting (1985) *Code of Professional Conduct,* London.
Wright, S. G. (1985) Conflict or co-operation – new nurses, new boundaries, *Nursing Practice,* Vol. 1, no. 1, pp.37–48.
Wright, S. G. (1986) *Building and Using a Model of Nursing,* Arnold, London.

18. Conclusion

Linda Thomas

THE ROLE OF NURSES IN CARING FOR ELDERLY PEOPLE

This role has never been more clearly defined than in the preceding chapters; clichés and jargon are noticeable for their absence as the concept of the nurse as an independent practitioner is explored to the full. Indeed, the tone of the book is set by an Ancient Briton's 'flavour of defiance' in the first chapter.

Independence through good health remains the keynote to a fulfilled life throughout old age. As society persists in viewing elderly people as a nameless, faceless group, the frustration of looking old whilst feeling young is graphically described. This introduction is refreshingly straightforward in setting out some basic ground rules for good nursing, all of which hinge on accepting each elderly patient as an individual with unique needs.

This is just one of many themes underpinning the whole text, and the problems inherent in regarding 'the elderly' as a homogeneous group are discussed again in the context of ageism in Chapter 2. Most nurses are familiar with the story of the old man whose painful knee is dismissed by the doctor with the words, 'What can you expect at your age?' 'But the other knee's the same age and it's not painful,' retorts the old man. The need for nurses to understand the normal process of ageing in order to identify the abnormal is recognized if they are to make a significant contribution to health education and promotion for elderly people. The ways in which specialist nursing care for elderly people has been influenced by medical developments is also examined, posing the question as to whether this has, in the end, served the best interests of either patients or nurses.

The low status afforded to older people and those who nurse them is mentioned again in Chapter 3. In organizing nursing care, the danger of 'creeping institutionalization' for both patients and nurses is recognized as very real, some nurses still viewing patients as a collection of tasks to be completed. If nurses are to become effective agents of change in establishing nursing philosophies and models and agreeing common goals, the need for them to understand the theories of change management is paramount. This chapter discusses in some detail the gradual evolution of nursing, identifying those major themes which promote quality of care for elderly people. Until nurses are clearly able to identify their role and what nursing is, they continue to be treated with scant respect by other members of the health care team.

The title of Chapter 4, 'Promoting safety and comfort', has a somewhat cosy ring to it; in fact, this is one of the most challenging chapters of the book, highlighting as it does the potential hostility of the so-called 'caring' environment. The right to privacy and personal space is often forfeited in institutions and nurses need to know how to make space sympathetic. Norman (1980) has identified the fact that the whole ethos of nursing care is directed towards protecting the patient from harm and this chapter shows how nurses can become over-protective. However, they do have a major role to play in ensuring patients' safety and comfort in other respects, for example in effective assessment and monitoring of pain control. The uniqueness of each elderly patient's experience of pain is stressed.

The fact that some nurses hide behind a shield of tasks in an attempt to avoid communicating with patients as individuals is brought out in Chapter 5. As well as discussing the more practical aspects of communications - speech and hearing problems, for instance - this chapter also looks at less well-recognized barriers to communication. Patients' lack of trust and nurses who fall into the jargon trap are examples quoted which mitigate against therapeutic communication. The difficulties which very young nurses may experience in empathizing with elderly patients is also mentioned.

The nurse's role in achieving comfort and relief for patients with breathing problems is outlined in Chapter 6. In order to appreciate the significance of both acute and chronic breathing problems in elderly people, nurses need to understand the normal effects of ageing on the cardiopulmonary system and these are outlined in some detail, together with the profound psychosocial effects breathing problems may have on an elderly person's life-style, producing the isolated 'respiratory cripple'.

Winter brings along not only an exacerbation of respiratory problems for elderly people, but also an increase in the incidence of hypothermia. The crucial role of the nurse in prevention, by giving information and advice, is discussed in Chapter 7. Nurses also have a vital role to play in recognizing hypothermia (which may occur in institutions as well as at home) and in restoring normal temperature. Although the maintenance of normal body temperature is invariably associated with hypothermia, the dangers of hyperthermia and pyrexia are also identified. Most nurses caring for elderly people will be familiar with the misery a heatwave may bring, particularly into non-air-conditioned hospital environments.

The task-oriented approach to care is mentioned again in Chapter 8 in relation to maintaining patients' hygiene. Level of dependency is not always a factor in determining how a patient is bathed, for example, and what should be a private and therapeutic experience becomes a public nightmare.

The complex issues related to mobility are addressed in Chapter 9, the laudable old man who continues to participate in fun runs perhaps serving to illustrate that only a minority of elderly people is affected by multiple pathologies resulting in loss of functional ability. Nevertheless, the environmental issues which affect elderly people's mobility are discussed - lack of accessible transport can have as fundamental an effect on an old person's mobility as the most profound physical handicap (Norman, 1981).

The need for effective multidisciplinary teamwork and creative planning are stressed in this chapter. In examining the common problems experienced by patients who are not independent, the needs of nurses are not ignored. Regrettably, nurses caring for elderly people suffer a high incidence of back pain and back injury and are sometimes lost to the profession. The practical advice on lifting and handling skills is very helpful in preventing discomfort to both patients and nurses.

In Chapter 10 the myth that 'you can't teach an old dog new tricks' is dismissed in examining the role of the nurse as a health educator in the care of elderly people. Patients (and carers, if appropriate) should play their part in planning their own care, a world away from the task-oriented, maternalistic view of nursing. This may be as difficult a concept for the patient to grasp as for the nurse - after all, nurses are surely meant to do things for patients. Once again, the need for therapeutic communication becomes obvious if patient education is to be taken seriously.

Maintaining a balanced diet is a vital ingredient of good health at any age. In Chapter 11, the inability to maintain a normal diet due to the psychosocial and physical changes of ageing is examined. Admission to an institution is no guarantee against malnutrition for elderly people, as limited choice of food together with rigid meal patterns may mitigate against them receiving proper nourishment. This chapter explores the ways in which nurses can employ both imagination and common sense in helping elderly patients with nutritional problems.

Nurses often regard themselves as experts in managing incontinence. However, as Chapter 12 points out, incontinence has a variety of causes and presents in many different ways, all of which require different approaches. Similarly, in promoting continence, the introduction of the same toileting regime for every patient is doomed to failure. The need for individualized assessment, the commitment of every member of the nursing team and the value of positive thinking are all essential in tackling a problem which may be demoralizing not only for the patient but also for those involved in the patient's care.

Chapter 13 moves away from the somewhat jaded view that recreational activities for elderly patients should revolve around enforced communal bingo sessions. Everyone needs something interesting or exciting to look forward to, and recreation in institutional care should have a purposeful outcome to make it worthwhile. Staff may sometimes need convincing of the value of, say, reminiscence or horticultural or pet therapy but eventually nursing time will be saved as patients are roused from apathetic inertia and begin to regain a degree of independence as their interest in life is reawakened.

The infamous words 'slept well' of a million nursing care plans take on a whole new meaning when viewed in the context of the complexities of rest and sleep explored in Chapter 14. Nurses tend to know little of the nature of sleep and often fail to take account of the effects of institutionalization on patients' sleeping patterns – alteration in routine, the hustle and bustle, lack of stimulation or downright exhaustion. A host of remedies is suggested through nursing intervention before drug therapy needs to be considered.

The extent to which stereotypical images affect elderly people's behaviour, resulting in the self-fulfilling prophecy of uselessness in old age is never more profoundly exhibited than in relation to sexuality in old age. In Chapter 15 the prejudice of nurses and their reluctance to discuss this subject through embarrassment is examined. If nurses are to be of any help in advising on sexual problems in old age, they must do so from a sound basis of knowledge.

On the other hand, the fact that nurses are aware of their shortcomings in catering for religious needs is accepted in Chapter 16. Religious needs may be difficult for nurses to appreciate, especially if the patient's religion is an unfamiliar one. Nevertheless, certain aspects of some religions may affect nursing care and the brief résumés of different religious beliefs should prove very helpful to nurses.

While death may be welcomed as a friend by some elderly people, others may experience great fear, sometimes of the manner of dying rather than death itself. The need to develop a trusting relationship between patient and nurse is very important in allowing the patient to talk about dying and death, however difficult this may be for the nurse. To a certain extent, it is true, it may be easier for nurses to accept the death of an elderly patient than a young one, but it is a rare nurse who remains unmoved when a patient she/he has cared for dies.

> I have often seen really good nurses distressed, because they could not impress the doctor with the real danger of their patient; and quite provoked because the patient 'would look' either 'so much better' or 'so much worse' than he really is 'when the doctor was there'. The distress is very legitimate, but it generally arises from the nurse not having the power of laying clearly and shortly before the doctor the facts from which she derives her opinion, or from the doctor being hasty and inexperienced, and not capable of eliciting them.
>
> (Florence Nightingale, 1969)

It is remarkable that these thoughts of Florence Nightingale, written more than a century ago, should still have such a ring of truth about them today. Indeed, many of the topics included in her *Notes on Nursing* can be found within this text. Miss Nightingale would surely have approved of the aim of this book to work on a nursing, rather than a medical model.

NURSING ELDERLY PEOPLE: CURRENT TRENDS

There can be little doubt that the nursing care of elderly people has progressed a long way in a relatively short space of time. The brutality and appalling conditions exposed in *Sans Everything* (Robb, 1967) may not have vanished completely, as occasional 'shock-horror' stories in the newspapers remind us; nevertheless, there are nurses with vision who have escaped from the 'sick nursing' medical model of care and adopted the more appropriate supportive model described by Wade (1983), characterized by consultation and involvement of elderly people in the care regime and maximizing their physical and mental independence.

Despite progress and innovation, nurse researchers continue to identify the same problem areas. Wade (1983) refers to the fact that 'the delegation of nursing care for the very old and very frail to untrained auxiliaries betrays strong allegiance to the medical model of care. It also betrays an underlying assumption that training in social skills is unnecessary or unimportant.' This echoes the view of Wells (1980) that 'auxiliary nurses, the most numerous caregivers for the hospitalized elderly, had little or no idea of the cause and care of common problems in the elderly'.

These findings are very relevant in terms of nursing as a whole. Realistically, despite the attraction to the specialty of an increasing number of well-qualified and articulate, trained nurses, it is unlikely that there will be any significant change in the high numbers of unqualified staff. The burden of responsibility on trained staff will continue to be very great, emphasizing Kitson's (1984) research findings on the therapeutic function of the ward sister/charge nurse.

As Fielding (1986) points out, one of the greatest nursing problems in the care of old people, whatever the setting, is one of attitudes. Attitudes have a profound impact on the quality of care delivered, significantly affecting standards of care. Fielding highlights the implications for nursing research in general and attitude research in particular as a result of her study. The implications for nursing education and nursing practice which she identifies are summarized very briefly below:

- *Nursing education.* A more structured component on the specialized care of elderly people is required in general nursing education. Nurse tutors must become more conversant with recent advances in the specialty and must develop ways of incorporating these advances into the content of the courses they teach. There is a need for teaching communication skills to nurses.

- *Nursing practice.* In order to implement an individualized approach to nursing elderly patients, nurses need to listen to what old people want out of life and goals should be set from that perspective. Early nursing assessment of elderly patients in medical wards should take place. There should be a recognition of the limitations of rehabilitative care given in such wards so that resources can be redirected appropriately.

In examining attitudes to elderly people in institutional care, it is worth bearing in mind Phillipson's (1982) comment that simply because they live longer, women are much more likely than men to spend their last years in some form of institutional care. He goes on to suggest that this fact may in itself partly explain low standards of care, reflecting in institutions the attitudes of society at large towards women in general and elderly women in particular.

This combination of discrimination - ageism and sexism - is an interesting, if controversial, area of speculation. As Ford and Sinclair (1987) state,

> Because women form the largest proportion of the very old, where the most severe problems of care are concentrated, the notion of elderly women as problematic becomes even more pronounced and generalized. What is necessary is a counter-balance to the problem-centred stance, an approach that draws out a more holistic picture of their lives by focusing on the routine daily round, the everyday taken-for-granted, and which charts the fears, achievement, problems and pleasures of being an older woman.

NURSING ELDERLY PEOPLE: FUTURE TRENDS

Several factors are likely to influence the nursing care of elderly people in the future.

- Demographic changes, leading to a growth in the number of very elderly people at the end of the century, could affect the manner in which 'specialist' hospital units for elderly people are designated.

- Elderly people will continue to be the major occupiers of all hospital beds and the major consumers of health and social services.
- The trend away from hospital long-term care towards community-centred continuing care is likely to accelerate.
- The emphasis on swift 'through-put' of elderly patients recovering from acute illnesses will continue to place a considerable strain on community nursing services.
- Radical reform of the nurse education system is inevitable, and long overdue.
- There is likely to be much greater emphasis in the future on the role of nurses as health educators for all age groups.

It cannot be too strongly emphasized that all nurses need expertise in the care of elderly people because virtually every nurse will be involved in the care of this client group at some stage in his or her career. If nurses are to be properly educated to meet the needs of the most numerous of their clients, then this fact must be taken into account in the basic learning curriculum. For those who wish to specialize following qualification, a range of opportunities already exists. Recognizing the need for a more radical approach, for example, the Welsh National Board has approved a multidisciplinary post-basic course comprising a core or foundation course of twenty days, together with five modules also of twenty days each, of which two must be completed to gain a certificate. The National Nursing Boards offer a variety of courses specializing in the care of the elderly for nurses to advance their knowledge and skill.

A number of suggestions have been made in the previous section about current developments in the care of the elderly. Keeping abreast of new knowledge and the accelerating nature of change can be a daunting task for nurses. Many of the chapters in this book have suggested further sources of help, and it is true to say that there is no dearth of organizations and individuals offering help and information.

The addresses at the end of this book contain many such useful sources of assistance. Each of the national nursing boards for example (England, Scotland, Wales and Northern Ireland) will supply details on their current courses and policies, as will the offices of the Departments of Health and Social Security. The numerous professional organizations such as the Royal College of Nursing or the Health Visitors Association, also have special groups offering support to those caring for the elderly.

Other organizations are at the forefront of advancing the needs and rights of elderly people, and nurses are actively involved in many of these. Age Concern has achieved national prominence for its effort, as has the Centre for Policy on Ageing. Organizations such as Extend, Cosmic Nursing, Age Exchange and the University of the Third Age are at the forefront in promoting innovation in meeting the needs of older persons. Others, meanwhile, offer support to groups with specific needs such as the Alzheimer's or Parkinson's Disease Societies. The reader is urged to advance her or his own knowledge and skill by contacting appropriate addresses listed at the end of the book where help and advice are readily available.

COMMUNITY CARE

The idea of managing certain groups of people, generally regarded as 'the priority care groups', in huge Victorian institutions has gradually been replaced over a number of years by a more humane philosophy of community care. Few people have argued with this philosophy, although defining 'community' is sometimes difficult.

Certainly, the increased discharge rate of elderly people from hospital imposes very substantial demands on nursing services in the community. It does seem illogical that nurse training concentrates so heavily on hospital services, perpetuating the rigid dividing line between hospital and community and creating the need for a role which should, in an ideal world, be superfluous – that of the community liaison nurse who acts as a go-between for hospital and community nurses.

The emphasis on community care from a succession of government documents is also beginning to highlight the needs of informal carers. Their initial commitment to caring for an elderly dependant is often a totally open-ended one, with no thought of the possibility of increasing frailty and dependency as the years go by. Support may not be readily available from statutory services as research has indicated (e.g. Family Policy Studies Centre, 1984). It may be that potentially nurses are the most appropriate professionals to provide the necessary advice, recognition and information for the carer before a crisis occurs and breaking point is reached.

Community care is a complex issue particularly if it is interpreted as covering residential care and nursing homes in the independent, voluntary and local authority sectors. While legislation covering independent and voluntary nursing homes is relatively straightforward, the situation is more complicated within residential care settings.

The Royal College of Nursing experienced little difficulty in producing guidelines for nurses working in registered nursing homes (Royal College of Nursing, 1987). However, controversy continues to rage over the role of nurses in residential care homes, supposedly only meant to offer 'personal' rather than 'nursing' care to their residents.

As to local authority homes (Part III), the stresses placed on unqualified and often poorly prepared care assistants by an increasingly frail population of elderly residents, both physically and mentally, will continue to grow. Nursing must have a role to play in this area, as the appointment of community nurses to act in an advisory capacity to these homes is beginning to demonstrate. It is likely that more and more nurses will be employed as officers within residential care homes; recognition must be given to their nursing qualifications.

Improved collaboration and co-ordination between all agencies is vital if there is to be any progress in caring for elderly people in the community. Where collaborative schemes have been introduced effectively, the results are often impressive as elderly 'customers' are offered a package of care tailored to meet their own unique individual needs.

Like some young people, there are some old people who want nothing more than a sheltered existence in which all their basic needs are met. But like most young people, most old people would prefer to live a life of opportunity and risk.

The exciting potential of realistic collaboration between different organizations and disciplines involved in the care of elderly people is only just beginning to make an impact. Nursing is one small but important piece in the overall jigsaw of care.

REFERENCES

Family Policy Studies Centre (1984) *The Forgotten Army: Family Care and Elderly People*, London.

Fielding, P. (1986) *Attitudes Revisited: An Examination of Student Nurses' Attitudes towards Old People in Hospital,* Royal College of Nursing, London.

Ford, J. and Sinclair, R. (1987) *Sixty Years on: Women Talk about Old Age,* Women's Press, London.

Kitson, A. (1984) A study of geriatric wards, their patients and nursing staff in Northern Ireland. Unpublished report, New University of Ulster Nursing Studies Department.

Florence Nightingale (1969) *Notes on Nursing: What it is and What it is Not,* Dover Publications, New York.

Norman, A. (1980) *Rights and Risk: A Discussion Document on Civil Liberty in Old Age*, Centre for Policy on Ageing, London.

Norman, A. (1981) Barriers to mobility, in D. Hobman (ed.) *The Impact of Ageing: Strategies for Care*, Croom Helm, Beckenham.

Phillipson, C. (1982) *Capitalism and the Construction of Old Age*, Macmillan Press, London.

Robb, B. (1967) *Sans Everything: A Case to Answer*, Nelson, London.

Royal College of Nursing Forum for Independent Nurse Managers (1987) *Caring for the Elderly in Registered Nursing Homes*, Royal College of Nursing, London.

Wade, B. E. (1983) *Different Models of Care for the Elderly*, Nursing Times Occasional Paper No. 79, p. 12.

Wells, T. J. (1980) *Problems in Geriatric Nursing Care: A Study of Nurses' Problems in Hospital*, Churchill Livingstone, Edinburgh.

Appendix: Useful Addresses

The Abbeyfeld Society
35A High Street
Potters Bar
Herts

Action on Smoking and Health (ASH)
5–11 Mortimer Street
London W1N 7RH

Age Concern England
Bernard Sunley House
60 Pitcairn Road
Mitcham
Surrey CR4 3LL

Age Exchange
15 Camden Row
Blackheath
London SE3 0QA

The Albany Trust
32 Shaftesbury Avenue
London WIV 8EP

Alcohol Concern
305 Grays Inn Road
London WC1X 8QF

Alcoholics Anonymous
PO Box 514
11 Redcliffe Gardens
London SW10 4BQ

Alzheimers's Disease Society
3rd Floor
Bank Buildings
Fulham Broadway
London SW6 1EP

The Arthritis and Rheumatism Council for Research
41 Eagle Street
London WC1R 4AR

Association of Hospital and Residential Care Officers
Redwalls Community House
Weaverham Road
Sandiway
Cheshire CW8 2ND

Association of Nurses in Substance Abuse
c/o Alcohol Problem Advisory Services
National Temperance Hospital
Hampstead Road
London NW1 2LT

British Association for the Hard of Hearing
6 St James Street
London WC1N 3DA

British Association for Services to the Elderly
119 Hassell Street
Newcastle
Staffs ST5 1AX

British Association of Retired Persons
14 Frederick Street
Edinburgh EH2 2HB

British Dental Foundation
2B Ravensdale Avenue
London N12 9HS

British Diabetic Association
10 Queen Anne Street
London W1M 0BD

British Diabetic Association
Daimler House
Paradise Circus
Queensway
Birmingham B1 2BJ

British Epilepsy Association
92 Tooley Street
London SE1

British Heart Foundation
102 Gloucester Place
London W1M 4DH

British Holistic Medical Association
179 Gloucester Place
London NW1

British Homeopathic Association
27A Devonshire Street
London W1N 1RJ

The British Library of Tape Recordings for Hospital Patients
12 Lant Street
London SE1 1QH

British Medical Association
BMA House
Tavistock Square
London WC1M 7JF

British Migraine Association
178A High Road
Byfleet
Weybridge
Surrey

British Red Cross Society
Aids for the Disabled
9 Grosvenor Crescent
London SW1X 7EJ

British Society for Music Therapy
69 Avolea Avenue
East Barnet
Herts EN4 8NB

Cancer Aftercare
Lodge Cottage
Church Lane
Timsbury
Bath BA3 1LF

Cancer Help Centre
Grove House
Cornwallis Grove
Clifton
Bristol BS8 4PG

Centre for Policy on Ageing
25-31 Ironmonger Row
London EC1V 3QP

Chest, Heart and Stroke Association
Tavistock House North
Tavistock Square
London WC1M 7JE

The Colostomy Welfare Group
38-39 Eccleston Square
London SW1V 1RB

Company Pensions Information Centre
7 Old Park Lane
London W1Y 3LJ

Confederation of Health Service Employees (COHSE)
Glen House
High Street
Banstead
Surrey SM7 2LM

Consumers Association
4 Buckingham Street
London WC2

Cosmic Nursing
93 Chorley Road
Bispham Green
Parbold
Lancs

Counsel and Care for the Elderly
131 Middlesex Street
London E1 7JF

Council for Music in Hospitals
340 Lower Road
Little Bookham
Surrey

Council for Professions Supplementary to Medicine
Park House
184 Kennington Park Road
London SE11 4BU

Crossroads Care Attendant Scheme
11 Whitehall Road
Rugby
Warwickshire

CRUSE
126 Sheen Road
Richmond
TW9 1UR

Department of the Environment
2 Marsham Street
London SW1

Department of Health and Social Security
Alexander Fleming House,
Elephant and Castle
London SE1 6BY

Department of Health and Social Services (Northern Ireland)
Dundonald House
Upper New Fownards Road
Belfast BT4 3SF

Depressives Associated
19 Merley Way
Wimbourne Minster
Dorset BH21 1QN

Disability Alliance
21 Star Street
London W2 1QB

Disabled Living Foundation
346 Kensington High Street
London W14 8NS

Disablement Income Group Charitable Trust
Attlee House
28 Commercial Street
London EC1

Distressed Gentlefolks Aid Association
Vicarage Gate House
Kensington
London W8

District Nursing Association
57 Lower Belgrave Street
London SW1W 0LR

English National Board for Nursing, Midwifery and Health Visiting
Victory House
170 Tottenham Court Road
London W1A 0HA

Equal Opportunities Commission
1 Bedford Street
London WC2A 8PS

'Extend'
3 The Boulevard
Sheringham
Norfolk NR26 8LJ

Forty-plus Career Development Centre
High Holborn House
49–51 Bedford Row
London WC1V 6RL

The Friends of the Elderly and Gentlefolks Help
42 Ebury Street
London SW1

The General Dental Council
37 Wimpole Street
London W1M 8DQ

General Medical Council
44 Hallam Street
London W1N 6AE

Geriatric Nursing and Home Care
Scutari Projects Ltd
Viking House
17–19 Peterborough Road
Harrow HA1 2AX

Health and Safety Commission
Regina House
259 Old Marylebone Road
London NW1 5RR

Health Education Council
78 New Oxford Street
London WC1A 1AH

Health Service Commissioner
Church House
Great Smith Street
London SW1P 3BW

Health Visitors Association
50 Southwark Street
London SE1

Hearing Aid Council
40A Ludgate Hill
London EC4

Help the Aged
Research and Education Division
16–18 St James's Walk
London EC1R 0BE

Help the Hospices
BMA House
Tavistock Square
London WC1H 9JP

Holiday Care Service
2 Old Bank Chambers
Station Road
Horley
Surrey

Holidays for the Disabled
12 Ryle Road
Farnham
Surrey GU9 8RW

Ileostomy Association
Amblehurst House
Chobham
Woking
Surrey GU24 8PZ

King's Fund Centre
126 Albert Street
London NW1 7NF

The Leonard Cheshire Foundation
26–29 Maunsel Street
London SW1P 2QN

Lion Clubs International
4 The Drive
Hove
Sussex

Marie Curie Memorial Foundation (for the Welfare of those with Cancer)
28 Belgrave Square
London SW1

Marriage Guidance Council
76A New Cavendish Street
London W1M 7LP

Mastectomy Association
25 Brighton Road
South Croydon CR2 6EA

Motability
Boundary House
91–93 Charterhouse Street
London EC1M 6BT

Multiple Sclerosis Society
71 Grays Inn Road
London WC1X 8TR

National Association of Citizens Advice Bureaux
110 Drury Lane
London WC2 5SW

National Association of Health Authorities
Garth House
47 Edgbaston Park Road
Birmingham B15 2RS

National Association for Mental Health (MIND)
22 Harley Street
London W1N 2EO

National Association of Laryngectomies Clubs
4th Floor
Michael Sobell House
30 Dorset Square
London NW1 6QL

National Council for Carers and Elderly Dependants
29 Chilworth Mews
London W2

National Council for Voluntary Organizations
26 Bedford Square
London WC1B 3HM

National Federation of Housing Associations
32 Southampton Street
The Strand
London WC1

National Listening Library
49 Great Cumberland Place
London W1

National Society for Cancer Relief
Michael Sobell House
30 Dorset Square
London NW1 6QL

National Union of Public Employees (NUPE)
Civic House
20 Grand Depot Road
Woolwich
London SE18 6SF

Northern Ireland National Board for Nursing Midwifery and Health Visiting
RAC House
79 Chichester Street
Belfast BT1 4JE

Nuffield Foundation
Nuffield Lodge
Regents Park
London NW1 4RS

Office of Population, Censuses and Surveys
St Catherine's House
10 Kingsway
London WC2 6JP

Open University
The Admissions Office
Walton Hall
Milton Keynes MK7 6AA

Orthopaedic Bedding Advisory Service
Britannia House
Dace Road
London E3

Parkinson's Disease Society
36 Portland Place
London W1N 3DG

The Patients Association
Room 33,
18 Charing Cross Road
London WC2H 0HR

Pharmaceutical Society of Great Britain
1 Lambeth High Street
London SE1

Pre-retirement Association of Great Britain and Northern Ireland
19 Undine Street
London SE17 8PP

Registered Nursing Homes Association
Catthorpe House
Hagley Road
Edgbaston
Birmingham B16 8Q7

Royal Association in Aid of the Deaf and Dumb
27 Old Oak Road
Acton
London W3 7AN

Royal Association for Disability and Rehabilitation
25 Mortimer Street
London W1N 8AB

Royal College of Nursing Society of Geriatric Nursing
20 Cavendish Square
London W1M 0AB

Royal National Institute for the Blind
224 Great Portland Street
London W1N 6AA

Royal National Institute for the Deaf
105 Gower Street
London WC1E 6AM

Royal Society for Mentally Handicapped Children and Adults
National Centre
123 Golden Lane
London EC1Y 0RT

Royal Society for the Prevention of Accidents (ROSPA)
Cannon House
The Priory
Queensway
Birmingham B4 6BS

SAGA (Senior Citizens) Holidays Ltd
119 Sandgate Road
Folkestone
Kent CT20 2BN

St Andrews Ambulance Association
Milton Street
Glasgow G4

Scottish Association for the Deaf
Moray House
Edinburgh EH8 8AQ

Scottish Association for Mental Health
67 York Place
Edinburgh EH1 3JD

Scottish Committee for Disability
5 Shandwick Place
Edinburgh EH3

Scottish Health Education Group
Woodburn House
Canaan Lane
Edinburgh EH10 4SG

Scottish Home and Health Department
St Andrew's House
Edinburgh EH1 3DE

Scottish National Board for Nursing, Midwifery and Health Visiting
22 Queen Street
Edinburgh EH2 1JX

Scottish Retirement Council
212 Bath Street
Glasgow G2

Sexual and Personal Relationships of the Disabled
The Diorama
14 Peto Place
London NW1 4DT

Shape
1 Thorpe Close
London W10 5XL

Talking Newspapers Association of the United Kingdom
48 Leigh Road
Eastleigh
Hants

United Kingdom Central Council for Nursing, Midwifery and Health Visiting
23 Portland Place
London W1N 3AF

The University of the Third Age
6 Parkside Gardens
London SW19 5EY

Urinary Conduit Association
36 York Road
Denton
Manchester

Index